Quantitative Trait Loci Analysis in Animals

For Hayim, Shelly, Sarit, Asher and Malka

Quantitative Trait Loci Analysis in Animals

Joel Ira Weller
Institute of Animal Sciences
ARO, The Volcani Center
Bet Dagan 50250
Israel

CABI *Publishing*

CABI *Publishing* is a division of CAB *International*

CABI Publishing
CAB International
Wallingford
Oxon OX10 8DE
UK

CABI Publishing
10 E 40th Street
Suite 3203
New York, NY 10016
USA

Tel: +44 (0)1491 832111
Fax: +44 (0)1491 833508
Email: cabi@cabi.org
Web site: http://www.cabi.org

Tel: +1 212 481 7018
Fax: +1 212 686 7993
Email: cabi-nao@cabi.org

©CAB *International* 2001. All rights reserved. No part of this publication may be reproduced in any form or by any means, electronically, mechanically, by photocopying, recording or otherwise, without the prior permission of the copyright owners.

A catalogue record for this book is available from the British Library, London, UK.

Library of Congress Cataloging-in-Publication Data

Weller, Joel Ira.
 Quantitative trait loci analysis in animals / Joel Ira Weller.
  p. cm.
 Includes bibliographical references (p.).
 ISBN 0-85199-402-4 (pbk. : alk. paper)
 1. Livestock--Breeding. 2. Livestock--Genetics. 3. Quantitative Genetics. I. Title

SF105.W36 2001
636.08'21--dc21   2001025568

ISBN 0 85199 328 1

Printed and bound in the UK by Cromwell Press, Trowbridge, from copy supplied by the author.

Contents

	Page
Preface, theory vs. results	1
Chapter one: Historical overview	3
1.1 Introduction	3
1.2 From Mendel to Sax	3
1.3 Quantitative genetics 1920-1980, or who needs Mendel?	5
1.4 QTL detection 1930-1980, theory and experiments	6
1.5 From biochemistry to biotechnology, or more markers than we will ever need	7
1.6 Genetic mapping functions	9
1.7 Physical and genetic mapping, questions of scale	12
1.8 Summary	14
Chapter two: Principles of Parameter Estimation	15
2.1 Introduction	15
2.2 Desired properties of QTL parameter estimates	16
2.3 Moments method of estimation	17
2.4 Least-squares parameter estimation	17
2.5 Least-squares solutions for a single parameter	18
2.6 Least-squares solutions for the general linear model	19
2.7 Maximum likelihood estimation for a single parameter	20
2.8 Maximum likelihood multi-parameter estimation	22
2.9 Confidence intervals and hypothesis testing for MLE	23
2.10 Methods to maximize likelihood functions	24
2.11 Derivative-free methods	25
2.12 Second derivative-based methods	26
2.13 First derivative-based methods (EM)	26
2.14 Bayesian estimation	27
2.15 Minimum difference estimation	28
2.16 Summary	29
Chapter three: Random and Fixed Effects, the Mixed Model	30
3.1 Introduction	30
3.2 The mixed linear model	30
3.3 The mixed model equations	32
3.4 Solving the mixed model equations	33

3.5 Some important properties of mixed model solutions	34
3.6 Equation absorption	34
3.7 Multivariate mixed model analysis	35
3.8 The repeatability model	37
3.9 The individual animal model	38
3.10 Grouping individuals with unknown ancestors	39
3.11 The reduced animal model	40
3.12 Maximum likelihood estimation with mixed models	41
3.13 Estimation of variance components, analysis of variance type methods	41
3.14 Maximum likelihood estimation of variance components	42
3.15 Restricted maximum likelihood estimation of variance components	45
3.16 The problem of variance components outside the parameter space	46
3.17 Summary	47

Chapter four: Experimental Designs to Detect QTL, Generation of Linkage Disequilibrium — 48

4.1 Introduction	48
4.2 Assumptions, problems and types of effects postulated	48
4.3 Experimental designs for detection of QTL in crosses between inbred lines	52
4.4 Linear model analysis of crosses between inbred lines	53
4.5 Experimental designs for detection of QTL in segregating populations - general considerations	57
4.6 Experimental designs for detection of QTL in segregating populations - large families	60
4.7 Experimental designs for detection of QTL in segregating populations - small families	63
4.8 Experimental designs based on additional generations	67
4.9 Comparison of the expected contrasts for different experimental designs	70
4.10 Gametic effect models for complete population analyses	71
4.11 Summary	73

Chapter five: QTL Parameter Estimation for Crosses between Inbred Lines — 75

5.1 Introduction	75
5.2 Moments method of estimation	76
5.3 Least-squares estimation of QTL parameters	77

5.4 Least-squares estimation of QTL location for sib-pair analysis with flanking markers	81
5.5 Linear regression mapping of QTL with flanking markers	83
5.6 Marker information content for interval mapping, uninformative and missing marker genotypes	85
5.7 Maximum likelihood QTL parameter estimation for crosses between inbred lines and a single marker	87
5.8 Maximum likelihood tests of significance for a segregating QTL	88
5.9 Maximum likelihood QTL parameter estimation for crosses between inbred lines and two flanking markers	89
5.10 Estimation of QTL parameters by the expectation-maximization algorithm	90
5.11 Biases in estimation of QTL parameters with interval mapping	92
5.12 The likelihood ratio test with interval mapping	93
5.13 Summary	94
Chapter six: Advanced statistical methods for QTL detection and parameter estimation	**96**
6.1 Introduction	96
6.2 Higher order QTL effects	97
6.3 QTL interaction effects	97
6.4 Simultaneous analysis of multiple marker brackets	99
6.5 Principles of composite interval mapping	101
6.6 Properties of composite interval mapping	101
6.7 Derivation of maximum likelihood parameter estimates by composite interval mapping	102
6.8 Hypothesis testing with composite interval mapping	103
6.9 Multi-marker and QTL analysis by regression of phenotype on marker genotypes	104
6.10 Estimation of QTL parameters in outbred propulations	105
6.11 Solutions for analysis of field data from segregating populations	107
6.12 Maximum likelihood analysis of QTL parameters for the daughter design with linkage to a single marker	109
6.13 Maximum likelihood estimation of QTL parameters from other complex pedigrees	111
6.14 Non-linear regression estimation for complex pedigrees	112
6.15 Maximum likelihood estimation with random effects included in the model	114

6.16 Maximum likelihood estimation of QTL effects on categorical traits ... 115
6.17 Estimation of QTL effects with the threshold model ... 117
6.18 Estimation of QTL effects on disease traits by the allele-sharing method ... 118
6.19 Summary ... 119

Chapter seven: Analysis of QTL as Random Effects ... 120

7.1 Introduction ... 120
7.2 ML estimation of variance components for the Haseman-Elston sib-pair model ... 121
7.3 The random gametic model of Fernando and Grossman, computing G_v ... 123
7.4 Computing the inverse of G_v ... 125
7.5 Analysis of the random gametic model by a reduced animal model (RAM) ... 126
7.6 Analysis of the random gametic QTL model with multiple QTL and marker brackets. ... 128
7.7 Computation of the gametic effects variance matrix ... 129
7.8 The gametic effect model for crosses between inbred lines ... 131
7.9 REML estimation of the QTL variance and recombination for the model of Fernando and Grossman ... 132
7.10 REML estimation of the QTL variance and location with marker brackets ... 133
7.11 Bayesian estimation of QTL effects, determining the prior distribution ... 134
7.12 Formula for Bayesian estimation and tests of significance of a segregating QTL in a simulated grand-daughter design ... 138
7.13 Comparison of ML and Bayesian analyses of a simulated grand-daughter design ... 139
7.14 Markov Chain Monte Carlo algorithms, Gibbs' sampling ... 140
7.15 Summary ... 141

Chapter eight: Statistical Power to Detect QTL, and Parameter Confidence Intervals ... 142

8.1 Introduction ... 142
8.2 Estimation of power in crosses between inbred lines ... 143
8.3 Replicate progeny in crosses between inbred lines ... 144
8.4 Estimation of power for segregating populations ... 146
8.5 Power estimates for likelihood ratio tests - general considerations ... 150

8.6 The effect of statistical methodology on the power of QTL detection	150
8.7 Estimation of power with random QTL models	151
8.8 Confidence intervals for QTL parameters - analytical methods	152
8.9 Simulation studies of confidence intervals	153
8.10 Empirical methods to estimate CI, parametric and non-parametric bootstrap and jackknife methods	154
8.11 Summary	156

Chapter nine: Optimization of Experimental Designs — 157

9.1 Introduction	157
9.2 Economic optimization of marker spacing when the number of individuals genotyped is non-limiting	157
9.3 Economic optimization with replicate progeny	158
9.4 Selective genotyping	160
9.5 Sample pooling - general considerations	163
9.6 Estimation of power with sample pooling	163
9.7 Comparison of power and sample sizes with random genotyping, selective genotyping, and sample pooling	166
9.8 Sequential sampling	167
9.9 Summary	168

Chapter ten: Fine Mapping of QTL — 169

10.1 Introduction	169
10.2 Determination of the genetic map critical interval for a marker locus with a saturated genetic marker map	169
10.3 Confidence interval for QTL location with a saturated genetic marker map	171
10.4 Fine mapping of QTL via advanced intercross lines	172
10.5 Selective phenotyping	173
10.6 Recombinant progeny testing	174
10.7 Interval specific congenic strains	174
10.8 Recombinant inbred segregation test	176
10.9 Fine mapping of QTL in outcrossing populations by identity by descent	176
10.10 Summary	177

Chapter eleven: Complete Genome QTL Scans - the Problem of Multiple Comparisons — 178

11.1 Introduction	178
11.2 Multiple markers and whole genome scans	179

11.3 QTL detection by permutation tests	181
11.4 QTL detection based on the false discovery rate	181
11.5 *A priori* determination of the proportion of false positives	185
11.6 Analysis of multiple pedigrees	186
11.7 Biases with estimation of multiple QTL	188
11.8 Summary	189
Chapter twelve: Multiple Trait QTL analysis	**190**
12.1 Introduction	190
12.2 Problems and solutions for multiple trait QTL analyses	190
12.3 Multivariate estimation of QTL parameters for correlated traits	191
12.4 Comparison of power for single and multitrait QTL analyses	193
12.5 Pleiotropy vs. linkage	196
12.6 Estimation of QTL parameters for correlated traits by canonical transformation	197
12.7 Determination of statistical significance for multitrait analyses	199
12.8 Selective genotyping with multiple traits	200
12.9 Summary	203
Chapter thirteen: Principles of Selection Index and Traditional Breeding Programmes	**205**
13.1 Introduction	205
13.2 Selection index for a single trait	205
13.3 Changes in QTL allelic frequencies due to selection	207
13.4 Multitrait selection index	208
13.5 The value of genetic gain	209
13.6 Dairy cattle breeding programmes, half-sib and progeny tests	211
13.7 Nucleus breeding schemes	214
13.8 Summary	215
Chapter fourteen: Marker-assisted Selection - Theory	**217**
14.1 Introduction	217
14.2 Situations in which selection index is inefficient	217
14.3 Potential contribution of MAS for selection within a breed - general considerations	218
14.4 Phenotypic selection vs. MAS for individual selection	219
14.5 MAS for sex-limited traits	220

14.6 Two-stage selection: MAS on juveniles, and phenotypic selection of adults — 221
14.7 MAS including marker and phenotypic information on relatives — 222
14.8 Maximum selection efficiency of MAS with all QTL known, relative to trait-based selection, and the reduction in RSE due to sampling variance — 223
14.9 Marker information in segregating populations — 224
14.10 Inclusion of marker information in "animal model" genetic evaluations — 225
14.11 Velogenetics - the synergistic use of MAS and germ-line manipulation — 225
14.12 Summary — 226

Chapter fifteen: Marker-assisted Selection - Results of Simulation Studies — 227

15.1 Introduction — 227
15.2. Modeling the polygenic variance — 227
15.3 The effective number of QTL — 229
15.4 Proposed dairy cattle breeding schemes with MAS – overview — 230
15.5 Inclusion of marker information into standard progeny test and MOET nucleus breeding schemes — 230
15.6 Progeny test schemes, in which information on genetic markers is used to preselect young sires — 232
15.7 Selection of sires based on marker information without a progeny test — 234
15.8 Long-term considerations, MAS vs. selection index — 235
15.9 MAS for a multitrait breeding objective with a single identified QTL — 238
15.10 MAS for a multitrait breeding objective with multiple identified QTL — 241
15.11 Summary — 241

Chapter sixteen: Marker-assisted Introgression — 243

16.1 Introduction — 243
16.2 Marker-assisted introgression - general considerations — 245
16.3 Marker-assisted introgression of a major gene into an inbred line — 246
16.4 Marker-assisted introgression of a QTL into a donor population under selection — 247
16.5 Marker-assisted introgression for multiple genes — 248

16.6 Summary   249

Glossary of commonly used symbols   250

    Latin symbols   250
    Greek symbols   258
    Other symbols   260

References   261
Author index   274
Subject index   277

Preface, theory vs. results

Joseph stored up huge quantities of grain, like the sand of the sea; it was so much that he stopped keeping records because it was beyond measure.

Genesis 41:49

Although detection of quantitative trait loci (QTL) has become a "hot" topic since the late 1980s, the basic principles and methodology have been around since the 1920s, almost immediately after the demonstration of the chromosomal theory of inheritance, and Fisher's polygenic theory of quantitative variance. One of the first actual experiments was performed by Sax in 1923, and positive results were obtained. This then begs the question, "Why was this methodology more or less ignored for over 60 years?" Of course we must first answer that a number of very fine papers on QTL detection and estimation were written during this period, but nowhere near the explosion of literature during the past two decades. Until 1980 QTL detection was definitely a scientific backwater. Most standard genetic texts written prior to 1980 do not even mention the topic.

The obvious answer is the lack of segregating genetic markers in species of interest. Until 1980, the genetic markers available were morphological, blood groups, and biochemical polymorphisms. These were insufficient to provide complete genome coverage. In addition, most markers were biallelic with one allele predominating in the population, and many displayed complete dominance. These markers were not optimal for QTL detection. With the advent of DNA level genetic markers, in the early 1980s, and especially DNA microsatellites from 1990, the problem of finding suitable genetic markers can be considered solved. It is now clear that a genetic map saturated with polymorphic codominant Mendelian markers can be generated for almost any species. Nearly saturated genetic maps have already been produced for most species of economic or scientific interest.

Because of the paucity of actual results until 1980, the theory of QTL detection was ahead of experimental results. A number of theoretical papers were written under the premise: "Assuming we had segregating genetic markers in the species of interest, how should we use them?" Most of these studies, based on the current state of knowledge, assumed that genetic markers would remain few and far between. However, the recent explosion in DNA technology has put the horse back in front of the cart. During the 1990s experimental opportunities pulled ahead of the theory and methodology necessary for analysis. The almost unlimited availability of genetic markers created new problems not considered by the early theoretical studies.

Although one of the main objectives in QTL detection in agricultural species is to incorporate this new source of information in breeding programs, much less has been written on marker-assisted selection (MAS) than on QTL detection or estimation. Furthermore, much of what has been written is quite pessimistic. Clearly in certain situations and breeding, gains from MAS will be minimal. However, most studies have investigated the contribution of marker information into existing breeding programmes. As with most new technologies, it will probably be necessary to modify breeding programmes to fully exploit MAS. Now that we are finding the genes, we must have methodology that gives reasonable answers for application of this information to improve actual breeding programs for plants and animals.

The objectives of this book are to summarize the scientific literature on methods for QTL detection and analysis, and marker-assisted selection, especially that pertaining to agricultural animal species. Although a large portion of the information covered is also applicable to QTL analysis in plant and human populations, this book emphasizes the special problems associated with animal breeding. Information related to marker technology will be given only as it relates to the methodologies considered. Likewise, this book does not cover the literature related to detection of genes affecting quantitative traits without relying on genetic markers, although some of the same methodologies may apply.

The reader is assumed to have a basic understanding of the principles of quantitative genetics and statistics. Several sections require a familiarity with matrix algebra and mixed model methodology. Readers unfamiliar with these topics can skip these sections without loss of continuity.

Shevat, 5761

Chapter one:

Historical Overview

1.1 Introduction

Detection of quantitative trait loci (QTL) and parameter estimation required developments in statistics, "classical genetics" or breeding, and biochemistry. The basic theory and tools for QTL detection were all in place by 1923 when Sax completed his landmark experiment with beans (*Phaseolus vulgaris*). In Section 1.2 we will discuss the basic discoveries prior to 1923 that made Sax's experiment feasible. Section 1.3 is a cursory review of the major statistical advances that have had direct bearing on genetics and practical breeding, especially with respect to QTL detection. Section 1.4 considers the major theoretical advances with respect to QTL detection and parameter estimation prior to 1980. Section 1.5 considers the important advances first in biochemistry, and more recently in biotechnology, that have resulted in the possibility of saturated genetic marker maps for any species. Section 1.6 considers functions to translate recombination frequencies into genetic map units, and Section 1.7 compares briefly the scope of the major techniques currently available for QTL localization, including genetic and physical mapping. The major advances of this century pertaining to QTL detection and analysis are summarized in Figure 1.1.

1.2 From Mendel to Sax

Modern genetics is usually considered to have started with the rediscovery of Mendel's paper in 1900. However, there were major advances in both statistics and cytogenetics prior to this watershed date, the importance of which became apparent only later. In the realm of statistics, Pearson in 1890 defined the correlation coefficient, and showed that it could be used to describe the relationship between two variables. During the last decades of the nineteenth century, important advances were also made in cytology: chromosomes were discovered, and the stages of both meiosis and mitosis were observed and described.

The rediscovery of Mendel's laws lead to a rapid first synthesis of genetics, statistics, and cytology. Sutton (1903) and Boveri, in the following year, first proposed the "chromosomal theory of inheritance", that the Mendelian factors were associated with the chromosomes. Using *Drosophila*, Morgan (1910) demonstrated that Mendelian genes were linked, and could be mapped into linear

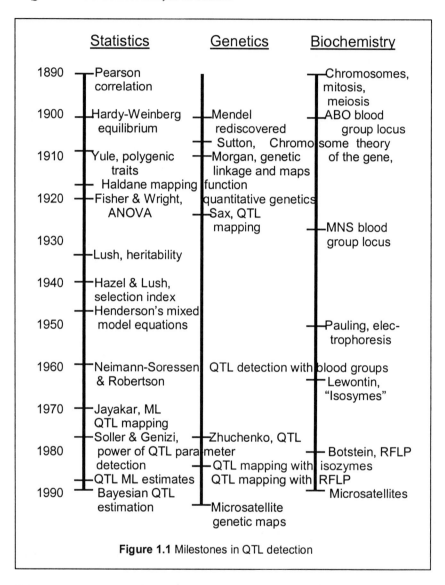

Figure 1.1 Milestones in QTL detection

linkage groups of a number equal to the haploid number of chromosomes. Hardy and Weinberg in 1908 derived their famous equation to describe the distribution of genotypes in a segregating population at equilibrium. In 1919 Haldane derived a formula to convert recombination frequencies into additive "map units" denoted "Morgans" or "centi-Morgans", assuming a random distribution of events of recombination along the chromosome. This formula will be considered in detail in Section 1.6.

Most traits of interest display continuous variation, rather than the discrete distribution associated with Mendelian genes. Despite the early synthesis between Mendelian genetics and cytogenetics, there seemed to be no apparent connection between Mendelian genetics on the one hand, and quantitative variation and natural selection on other.

Experiments by Johansen (1903) with beans demonstrated that environmental factors are a major source of variation in quantitative traits, leading to the conclusion that the phenotype for these traits is not a reliable indicator for the genotype. Yule in 1906 first suggested that continuous variation could be explained by the cumulative action of many Mendelian genes, each with a small effect on the trait. Fisher in 1918 demonstrated that segregation of quantitative genes in an outcrossing population would generate correlations between relatives. Payne (1918) demonstrated that the X chromosome from selected lines of *Drosophila* contains multiple factors, which influenced scutellar bristle number. Thus, by 1920, the basic theory necessary for detection of individual genes affecting quantitative traits was in place.

In Sax's 1923 experiment with beans he demonstrated that the effect of an individual locus on a quantitative trait could be isolated though a series of crosses resulting in randomization of the genetic background with respect to all genes not linked to the genetic markers under observation. Even though all of his markers were morphological seed markers with complete dominance, he was able to show a significant effect on seed weight associated with some of his markers. The rationale behind this experiment will be discussed in more detail in Chapter four.

1.3 Quantitative genetics 1920-1980, or who needs Mendel?

Since the beginning of history, plant and animal breeding was based on selecting individuals with the desired phenotype as parents for the next generation. Comparison between domestic populations and their wild progenitors demonstrates that artificial selection has been quite successful in altering phenotypes without any formal knowledge of genetics. Wright, Haldane, and Fisher completed the synthesis between Darwinism and Mendelism in a series of papers from 1924 though 1931 that demonstrated how natural selection could work on Mendelian factors controlling quantitative traits under selection. Fisher also demonstrated that Mendelian factors could explain the phenotypic similarity between relatives. These principles became the basis for scientific breeding of animals and plants from the 1930s onwards.

Using the genetic and statistical knowledge accumulated up to 1940, Lush and Hazel developed the principles of selection index to optimize artificial selection based on known relationships among individuals and phenotypic trait information. Selection index proved to be a remarkably efficient and flexible methodology for practical breeding of plants and animals. Not only could selection be economically optimized, the expected gains from selection could also be predicted.

Selection index theory had very little connection to Mendelian genetics. The "Infinitesimal model" advanced by Fisher (1918) assumed that each quantitative trait was controlled by very many independently segregating Mendelian genes all acting in an additive manner, and each individual locus had an infinitesimal contribution to the total genetic variance. However, nearly identical results would be obtained if the trait was controlled by only a few loci. Only "additive" genetic variation was considered in the basic model. Dominance (interactions among alleles within a gene), and interactions among genes (epistasis) were beyond the scope of selection index.

This biometrical methodologyced during the 1950s, 1960s, and 1970s chiefly by C. M. Henderson and his colleagues. Using matrix notation Henderson developed the "Mixed Model" equations combining least-squares estimation with selection index in order to derive unbiased estimates of genetic values of individuals sampled in different environments, such as herds or blocks. He also devised methods to derive unbiased estimates of the genetic and environmental variance components required for solving these equations. Finally he developed a simple algorithm for inverting the "numerator relationship" matrix. This made possible the incorporation of information from all known relatives in the derivation of genetic evaluations. Mixed model methodology will be described in detail in Chapter three. None of this methodology, however, required any information on the specific genetic architecture of the traits under selection.

1.4 QTL detection 1930-1980, theory and experiments

During these 50 years, there were relatively few successful experiments that found marker-QTL linkage in plant and animal populations, and of these even fewer were independently repeated. A major problem that continues to today is the relatively small size of most experiments. In most cases in which QTL effects were not found, power was too low to find segregating QTL of a reasonable magnitude (Soller et al., 1976). During the period 1960-1980 there were important methodological advances in QTL detection and parameter estimation, even though the lack of segregating markers was, beyond doubt, the main limiting factor for this technology.

In 1961 Neimann-Soressen and Robertson proposed a half-sib design for QTL detection in commercial dairy cattle populations. Their model will be described in detail in Chapter four. Although the actual results were disappointing, this was the first attempt to detect QTL in an existing segregating population. All previous studies were based on experimental populations produced specifically for QTL detection. This study was also ground breaking in other aspects. It was the first study to use blood groups rather than morphological markers, and the proposed statistical analyses, a χ^2 (chi-squared) test, based on a squared sum of normal distributions, and ANOVA were also unique. This was the first study that attempted to estimate the power to detect QTL, and to consider the problem of multiple comparisons. Law (1965) completed the first successful QTL mapping experiment (as opposed to mere detection) in an agricultural species. He localized a QTL in wheat using substitution lines.

Jayakar (1970) proposed that maximum likelihood could be used to map QTL. Two years later, Haseman and Elston (1972) proposed a sib-pair analysis method for QTL detection in human populations. They also presented a likelihood function to estimate recombination frequency and QTL parameters. Soller *et al.* (1976) and Soller and Genizi (1978) developed formula to estimate statistical power of QTL for crosses between inbred lines and segregating populations. For segregating populations they considered large half-sib and full-sib families. Their studies clearly showed that very large samples, generally more than 1000 individuals, were required to obtain reasonable power to detect a QTL explaining 1% of the phenotypic variance.

1.5 From biochemistry to biotechnology, or more markers than we will ever need.

Marker-QTL linkage studies require polymorphic genes with classical Mendelian inheritance. In *Drosophila*, strains carrying multiple mutants served this purpose very effectively. However, this is not the case for humans or agricultural species. In plants the only markers initially available were genes that resulted in morphological differences. Clearly, these were insufficient to cover the genome. In addition, most morphological markers display complete dominance. Finally, the direct effect on the phenotype of most of these markers was quite dramatic. Thus, even if an effect was found on the trait of interest associated with the marker, it was very likely that this effect was a pleiotropic effect of the marker. In farm animals, marker-QTL linkage studies are generally carried out within populations, and require as markers loci that are polymorphic within the population of interest. Prior to 1980, the only suitable Mendelian loci were blood groups, which were naturally prevalent in all populations, often multiallelic, and had no visible affect on the phenotype for any traits of interest. However, it eventually became clear that the total number of polymorphic blood loci was quite limited. Thus, blood groups were not a solution for QTL detection in animal populations.

The first biochemical polymorphism was detected for sickle cell anemia by Pauling in 1949. Lewontin and Hubby showed in 1966 that electrophoresis could be used to disclose large quantities of naturally occurring enzyme polymorphisms in *Drosophila*. Almost all enzymes analysed showed some polymorphism that could be detected by the speed of migration in an electric field. This large quantity of naturally occurring polymorphism created quite a shock for the scientific community. There seemed to be no adequate explanation as to why this variation was maintained. Later studies with domestic plant and animal species found that electrophoretic polymorphisms were much less common in agricultural populations. During the 1980s there was a number of QTL detection studies in agricultural plants based on isozymes using crosses between different strains or even species in order to generate sufficient electrophoretic polymorphism (Edwards *et al.*, 1987; Kahler and Wherhahn, 1986; Tanksley *et al.*, 1982; Weller *et al.*, 1988). It was clear though, that naturally occurring biochemical polymorphisms were insufficient for complete genome analyses in populations of interest.

The first detected DNA-level polymorphisms were restriction fragment length polymorphisms (RFLP). Grodzicker *et al.* (1974) first showed that restriction fragment band patterns could be used to detect genetic differences in viruses. Kan and Dozy (1978) used methods developed by Southern (1975) to detect polymorphism near the human hemoglobin gene. In the following year Solomon and Bodmer (1979) and Botstein *et al.* (1980) proposed RFLP as a general source of polymorphism that could be used for genetic mapping. Although RFLPs are diallelic, initial theoretical studies demonstrated that they might be present throughout the genome. Beckmann and Soller (1982) proposed using RFLP for detection and mapping of QTL. The first genome-wide scan for QTL using RFLP was performed on tomatoes by Paterson *et al.* (1988). Since then, many additional QTL mapping studies based on RFLP have been carried out successfully in plant species. In animal species, however, RFLP markers, because of their diallelic nature, were homozygous in most individuals, and therefore have not been as useful for QTL mapping as was initially anticipated.

A major breakthrough came at the end of the decade with the discovery of DNA microsatellites. Mullis *et al.* (1986) proposed the "Polymerase Chain Reaction" (PCR) to specifically amplify any particular short DNA sequence. Using the PCR, large enough quantities of DNA could be generated so that standard analytical methods could be applied to detect polymorphisms consisting of only a single nucleotide. Since the 1960s it has been known that the DNA of higher organisms contains extensive repetitive sequences. In 1989 three laboratories independently found that short sequences of repetitive DNA were highly polymorphic with respect to the number of repeats of the repeat unit (Litt and Luty, 1989; Tautz, 1989; Weber and May, 1989). The most common of these repeat sequences were poly(TG), which was found to be very prevalent in all higher species. These sequences were denoted "simple sequence repeats" (SSR) or "DNA microsatellites".

Finally the ultimate genetic marker was at hand. Microsatellites were prevalent throughout all genomes of interest. Nearly all poly(TG) sites were polymorphic, even within commercial animal populations. These markers were by definition "codominant", that is the heterozygote genotype could be distinguished from either homozygote. Furthermore, microsatellites were nearly always polyallelic. Thus, most individuals were heterozygous. In short, "Just what the doctor ordered"! Relatively dense genetic maps based on microsatellites are being generated for most agricultural species and are available on the Internet (e.g. http://sol.marc.usda.gov/genome), although these maps still contain gaps spanning more than 10 centi-Morgans.

Recently new classes of markers have also come into use. Chief among them are "single nucleotide polymorphisms" (SNP) (reviewed by Brookes, 1999). A SNP is generally defined as a base pair location at which the frequency of the most common base pair is lower than 99%. Unlike microsatellites, which usually have multiple alleles, SNPs are generally diallelic, but are much more prevalent throughout the genome, with an estimated frequency of one SNP per 300 to 500 base pairs. In human populations differences in the base pair sequence of any two randomly chosen individuals occur at a frequency of approximately once per 1000 kb (Brookes, 1999). Thus, SNPs can be found in genomic regions that are microsatellite poor. SNPs are apparently more stable than microsatellites, with lower frequencies of mutation, and methods are being developed for automated scoring of large numbers of individuals.

1.6 Genetic mapping functions

Distances between loci on genetic maps are measured in units called Morgans (M), the expected number of events of recombination, or centi-Morgans (cM). One cM distance between two chromosomic sites is equivalent to a 1% probability of recombination between them. However, if two loci are not very closely linked, not all events of recombination will be detected. If two events of recombination occur, the original linkage phase is observed. Various functions have been proposed to convert recombination frequencies between markers into genetic maps. Morgan (1910, 1928) proposed the first "mapping function". He assumed equivalence between recombination frequency and map distance. That is $R = M$, where R is the probability of recombination between two loci. This relationship is approximately correct for closely linked loci. Over greater chromosomal distances recombination frequencies are not strictly additive.
Numerous mapping functions have been proposed. In addition to Morgan's function we will consider in this chapter only the Haldane and Kosambi mapping functions. For a more extensive discussion of mapping functions see Lui (1998).

Assume that markers a, b, and c are located in that order on the same chromosome. Further assume that the recombination frequencies between markers a and b is 10%, while the recombination frequency between markers b and c is 5%. In general the recombination frequency between markers a and c will be less than 15%, because of double recombinations. That is if recombination occurs both between a and b, and b and c, then no recombination is observed between a and c. In general the frequency of recombination between a and c will be the probability of recombination between a and b, plus the probability of recombination between b and c, minus twice the probability of simultaneous recombination in both segments. The reason that the probability of simultaneous recombination is deducted twice is that this probability must be deducted from the probability of recombination both between a and b, and between b and c.

Many studies have shown that recombination at a specific point of the chromosome can affect recombination rates in adjacent regions. This is termed "crossover interference" or "recombination interference". "Zero interference" is defined as the situation in which recombination frequencies between adjacent regions are statistically independent. Thus the probability of recombination in the example given above of two adjacent chromosomal segments will be the probability of recombination between a and b, multiplied by the probability of recombination between b and c. The probability of recombination between a and c can then be computed as follows:

$$R_{ac} = R_{ab} + R_{bc} - 2R_{ab}R_{bc} \qquad \{1.1\}$$

where R_{ac}, R_{ab}, and R_{bc} are the corresponding probabilities of recombination for the three chromosomal segments.

The Haldane mapping function (Haldane, 1919) is based on the assumption of zero interference throughout the genome. In this case the number of event of recombination in any given chromosomal segment follows a Poisson distribution. That is the probability of having x events of recombination in a given chromosomal segment (P_x) is:

$$P_x = e^{-M}M^x/x! \qquad \{1.2\}$$

where M is the mean expected number of events of recombination within the segment. As noted above, the units of M are denoted Morgans. Recombination between two points on the chromosome will be observed only if there is an odd number of events of recombination between them. The Haldane mapping function is derived by summing P_x over all odd values of x from 1 through infinity. This summation reduces to the following simple relationship:

$$R = \tfrac{1}{2}(1 - e^{-2M}) \qquad \{1.3\}$$

Thus the map distance between to genes in Morgans as a function of the frequency of observed recombination between them is derived as follows:

$$M = -\tfrac{1}{2}\ln(1 - 2R) \qquad \{1.4\}$$

The Haldane mapping function is the most widely used, and will be considered the standard throughout this text. The Morgan mapping function assumes complete interference, that is, zero frequency of double recombinants. In this case, $R_{ac} = R_{ab} + R_{bc}$, and $R = M$.

The Kosambi mapping function (Kosambi, 1944) assumes a moderate amount of positive interference. That is, the frequency of double recombinants is less than expected assuming a random distribution of recombination events. This requires rewriting equation {1.1} as follows:

$$R_{ac} = R_{ab} + R_{bc} - 2C_r R_{ab} R_{bc} \qquad \{1.5\}$$

where C_r is the coefficient of coincidence and $1 - C_r$ is the recombination interference. In the Haldane mapping function $C_r = 1$, and interference $= 0$. In the Morgan mapping function, $C_r = 0$, and there is complete interference. Therefore in the Morgan function $R = M$. In the Kosambi function $C_r = 2R$. That is positive interference of $1 - 2R$ is assumed. Thus, interference increases as R decreases, which seems to correspond to the biological reality. In the Kosambi mapping function the relationships between R and M are as follows:

$$R = \frac{1 - e^{-4M}}{2[1 + e^{-4M}]} \qquad \{1.6\}$$

$$M = 0.25 \ln[(1+2R)/(1-2R)] \qquad \{1.7\}$$

M as a function of R is plotted in Figure 1.2 for all three mapping functions. As can be seen, the Kosambi function lies between the Morgan and Haldane functions. For the Haldane function differences between R and M can be quite large for relatively large values of R. For example, for $R = 0.4$, $M = 0.8$ for the Haldane function.

A disadvantage of the Kosambi mapping function, as compared to either the Morgan or Haldane functions, is that map distances are not additive. That is, the map distances in Morgans for the segments ab and ac should sum to the map distance for ac in the Haldane mapping function, but not the Kosambi function.

With multiple markers, computation of map distances can get quite complicated. In the example given previously, of three linked markers, recombination frequencies will generally not correspond exactly to any mathematical mapping function. Furthermore, if markers are close together it is often not possible to unequivocally determine marker order. In addition, with multiple markers some of the markers genotypes will be missing or "uninformative" for some of the individuals analysed. Algorithms and computer programs have been developed based on maximum likelihood to determine the most likely marker order and map distances from a sample of genotypes of related individuals (see Ott, 1985 and http://linkage.rockefeller.edu/soft/crimap). A discussion of multimarker

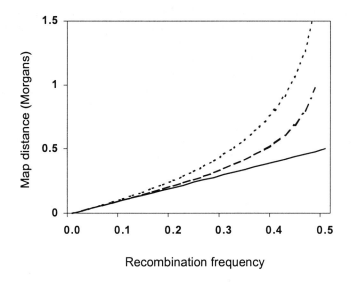

Figure 1.2 The relationship between recombination frequency and genetic map distances for three mapping functions. —, Morgan's function; - - -, Haldane's function, — —, Kosambi's function

mapping algorithms is outside the scope of this text. Maximum likelihood estimation will be explained in detail in Chapter two, and "informativity" of marker genotypes will be considered in Chapter four.

1.7 Physical and genetic mapping, questions of scale

The genome can be considered on various levels, and various techniques have been developed for gross and fine mapping of specific sites. The basic units used to measure the genome are DNA base pairs (bp), genes, recombination frequencies, genetic map units (M or cM), and chromosomes. The relationships among these units are more than a simple question of scale, such as converting meters to inches. Although on the average 1 cM is approximately equal to one million bp, it has been shown that on the level of the physical map, certain regions have a high frequency of recombination, while other regions have a low frequency of recombination. Furthermore, recombination frequency is affected by other factors, such as sex.

The number of chromosomes is known without error, while genome lengths in base pairs and cM can now be determined quite accurately. However, the total number of genes is still just an educated guess. For example, the bovine genome consists of 29 autosomes, about 3000 cM, and 3.75×10^9 bp. The total number of genes has been estimated as 60,000. Thus, the average bovine autosome has about 100 cM. Likewise, on average, a 10 cM chromosomal segment will have about 200 genes, and 1.25×10^7 bp. However, there is significant variation in the correspondence between the physical and genetic maps.

The physical genome in bp and the genetic map in cM are compared in Figure 1.3 on a log scale. Using *in situ* hybridization it is only possible to determine the general chromosomal region of a target DNA sequence. The effective ranges for genetic mapping and the various techniques that can be used for physical gene mapping are also indicated. Genetic mapping, which is the focus of this book, occupies the middle ground of the log scale, from about 0.1 to 20 cM, or from 10^5 to 10^7 bp.

Genetic mapping cannot be used to identify individual loci, but other techniques, such as pulse-field electrophoresis, yeast artificial chromosomes, chromosome walking and jumping, and radiation hybrid mapping are available to accomplish this objective. These techniques are outside the scope of this text.

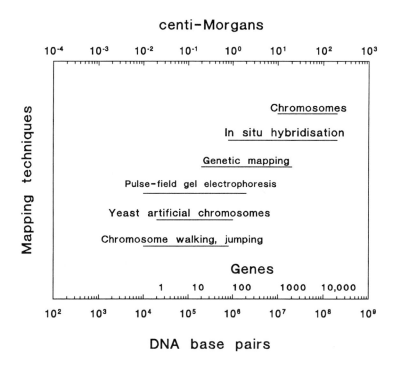

Figure 1.3 Comparison of the physical genome in bp and the genetic map in cM on log scales. Horizontal lines indicate the effective ranges for various mapping techniques. (Adapted from Smith and Smith, 1993)

1.8 Summary

In this chapter we reviewed the history of QTL detection from the three aspects of statistics, formal genetics, and biochemistry. By 1923 genetics understood that individual Mendelian genes controlled traits with continuous distributions, and that the effects of these genes could be detected with the aid of genetic markers using an appropriately designed experiment. Statistical methods to accurately estimate QTL parameters were only developed 50 years later. Even though the basic theory was in place by 1980, QTL detection only became a major field of scientific research towards the end of the 1980s with the discovery of prevalent DNA-level polymorphism. The objective of this book is to describe the statistical methods useful for QTL detection and analysis, thus we will not consider genotyping techniques, mapping of Mendelian genes, or modern methods of physical mapping in detail.

Chapter two:

Principles of Parameter Estimation

2.1 Introduction

Variables are generally divided into two groups, fixed and random. Random variables are assumed to be sampled from a distribution with known parameters, while no such assumptions are made about fixed variables. "Parameters" are defined as fixed variables that describe the statistical distribution of a population. For example, a population with a normal distribution is described by two parameters: the mean and the variance. Generally parameters are estimated based on a sample derived from the population. Parameter estimates derived from sample data are denoted "statistics".

In the next chapter we will briefly describe analysis of mixed models, models that include both fixed and random variables. In Chapter four we will consider experimental designs that can be used to detect segregating QTL and to estimate the main parameters of interest: means and variances of QTL genotypes, and recombination frequencies between the genetic markers and the QTL. Methods of estimating QTL parameters will be discussed in detail in Chapters five to seven. It will be demonstrated that in nearly all cases, estimation of QTL parameters is not trivial.

The basic concepts of parameter estimation are usually covered in only a very cursory way in introductory statistic courses. Since these principles are central to the methods that will be considered in the following chapters, an overview of the principles of parameter estimation is now presented. In the following section we will explain the desirable properties of parameter estimates. In this chapter we will consider only the basic methods that have been used for QTL parameter estimation. Some of the material covered requires matrix algebra. Readers not familiar with the principles of matrix algebra can either skip this material, or read a short introduction to matrix algebra given in either *Economic Aspects of Animal Breeding* (Weller, 1994), or *Genetics and Analysis of Quantitative Traits* (Lynch and Walsh, 1998). A more extensive treatment of all relevant aspects of matrix algebra is given in *Matrix Algebra Useful for Statistics* (Searle, 1982).

Throughout the remainder of this text we will try to maintain the conventions that parameters are denoted by Greek symbols, while statistics are denoted with Latin symbols. In sections that use matrix algebra, vectors will be denoted in **lower case bold** and matrices will be denoted in **UPPER CASE BOLD**. The transpose of a matrix will be denoted by an apostrophe. The inverse of a matrix will be denoted by the −1 superscript.

Least-squares and maximum likelihood (ML) estimation will be described in detail in Sections 2.4 to 2.13. The "moments" method of estimation, Bayesian estimation, and minimum difference estimation will be described in a more cursory form. Bayesian estimation of QTL effects will be considered in more detail in Chapter seven.

2.2 Desired properties of QTL parameter estimates

For the general question of parameter estimation, there are four main desired properties of estimators: unbiasedness, minimum estimation error variance, estimates within the parameter space, and consistency. For simple situations, it is possible to derive estimators with all of these properties, but for more complicated cases, it will not be possible to obtain estimates with all the desired properties, and there will be a question of trade-offs. We will now describe these properties in detail.

Unbiasedness: assume that $\hat{\theta}$ is an estimator of a parameter θ. $\hat{\theta}$ is unbiased if: $E(\hat{\theta}) = \theta$, that is the expectation of the estimator is equal to the parameter value. As an example, in estimating the variance based on the sample mean we divide by the sum of squares by n−1, where n is the sample size. If instead we divide by n then the estimator will be a biased estimate of the variance.

Minimum estimation error variance: is defined as the value of $\hat{\theta}$ for which: $E[(\hat{\theta} - \theta)^2]$ is minimal. This property is the basis of least-squares estimation. The estimator with minimum estimation error variance is also called the "best" estimate.

Estimates within the parameter space: simple examples of estimators outside the parameter space are negative variance component estimates, correlation estimates > 1 or < −1, or estimates for recombination frequency < zero or > 0.5. Although the requirement of estimates within the parameter space may appear trivial, this is often not the case. In many situations it is not possible to obtain an estimate that is both unbiased and within the parameter space. The problem of parameter estimates outside the parameter space will be considered in more detail in the next chapter, within the context of estimation of variance and covariance components. Maximum likelihood estimates are always within the parameter space, because a parameter estimate outside the parameter space has a likelihood of zero by definition.

Consistency: an estimator, $\hat{\theta}$, is considered "consistent" if $\hat{\theta}$ tends to θ as the sample size tends toward infinity. An estimator can be consistent even if it is biased. Consider the example given above of estimating the variance of a sample. If we divide by n instead of n−1, the estimator is biased, but consistent, because as n tends to infinity, n tends to n−1. Although this property also appears trivial, it is especially important for QTL detection, because of incomplete linkage between QTL and genetic markers. In most cases, the effect on a quantitative trait associated with a genetic marker is an inconsistent estimate of the QTL effect.

An additional desirable property of estimators is **robustness**. This property measures how the estimator is affected by inaccuracies in the assumptions employed to derive the estimator. For example, most of the estimation methodologies that will be employed assume an underlying normal distribution of residuals. Of course no variable has a completely normal distribution. One potential problem is "outliers", observations that deviate further than expected from the mean, due to effects not included in the analysis model. These observations can potentially have a very significant effect on parameter estimates, especially if the estimator is based on minimizing the squared differences. Generally, robustness will decrease, as more specific assumptions are made with respect to the assumed distribution

2.3 Moments method of estimation

This method is not currently in general use, and its interest can be considered purely historical. The Moments method of estimation was used by Zhuchenko *et al.* (1979a, 1979b) to estimate QTL parameters in a backcross design. The mth central moments of a sample, T^m, is computed as follows:

$$T^m = (1/N)\sum_{}^{N}(y - \bar{y})^m \qquad \{2.1\}$$

where N is the sample size and $\bar{y}$ is the sample mean. The first central moment is equal to zero, and the second central moment of a sample is an estimate of the variance of the distribution. The statistics g_1 and g_2, which are used to estimate the skewness and kurtosis of a distribution, are derived from the third and fourth central moments, respectively.

The advantages of the Moments method are that it is easy to apply, the estimates are unbiased, and no assumptions are made about the properties of the underlying QTL distributions. The disadvantages are that parameter estimates outside the parameter space can be obtained, such as negative variance estimates, or recombination frequency outside the range of 0 to 0.5, and that not all information in the data is utilized. Many of the parameter estimates derived by Zhuchenko *et al.* (1979a, 1979b) were outside the parameter space.

2.4 Least-squares parameter estimation

We will use matrix notation to briefly describe least-squares estimation. Assume that there is a series of observations for some variable, y, which we wish to model in terms of other variables for which data is also available. We will denote y as the "dependent variable" and the other variables as the "independent variables". The objective is to "explain" the dependent variable in terms of a series of parameter estimates linking the dependent variables to the independent variable. That is, to derive a function of the independent variables that approximates the observations for y. Generally it will not be possible to completely explain y in terms of the dependent variables. The difference between the estimates of y, based on the independent variables and the parameter estimates is denoted the "error" or "residual" of the model.

Least-squares estimation is based on deriving the parameter estimates that minimize the expectation of the sum of squared errors. Thus, by definition this method has minimum estimation error variance. In matrix form a completely general model can be written as follows:

$$\mathbf{y} = f(\theta') + \mathbf{e} \qquad \{2.2\}$$

where $\mathbf{y}$ = vector of observations, θ = vector of parameters, $f(\theta')$ is some function of θ, and $\mathbf{e}$ = vector of residuals. The least-squares solution, $\hat{\theta}$, is the vector that minimizes $[\mathbf{y}-f(\hat{\theta})]^2 = \mathbf{e}^2$. For a linear model, Equation {2.2} can be written as follows:

$$\mathbf{y} = \mathbf{X}\theta + \mathbf{e} \qquad \{2.3\}$$

where $\mathbf{X}$ is a matrix of coefficients of θ. Effects in linear models can take one of two forms, class or continuous. Discrete effects such as a specific herd, block, or sex are denoted "class effects". Although the levels of these effects can be numbered, there is no relationship between the number of a specific herd and effect associated with it. For continuous effects a linear relationship is assumed between the value for the independent variable and the dependent variable. Each row of X corresponds to the coefficients of θ for a specific record in y. For class effects the elements in $\mathbf{X}$ will be either zero or one. For continuous effects, each element in $\mathbf{X}$ corresponds to the observed value for the independent variable.

2.5 Least-squares solutions for a single parameter

The least-square solutions are solved by finding the parameter estimates than minimize the sum of squares of the residuals. This will first be illustrated for the following simple linear regression model:

$$y_i = \mu + x_i b + e_i \qquad \{2.4\}$$

where y_i is the dependent variable for observation i, μ is a constant, x_i is the independent variable for observation i, b is the regression coefficient, and e_i is the random residual. The residual sum of squares are computed as follows:

$$\Sigma(y_i - \mu - x_ib)^2 = \Sigma e_i^2 \qquad \{2.5\}$$

$$\Sigma y_i^2 + \Sigma \mu^2 + \Sigma(x_ib)^2 - \Sigma(2y_i\mu) - \Sigma(y_ix_ib) + \Sigma 2(\mu x_ib) = \Sigma e_i^2 \qquad \{2.6\}$$

where Σ denoted summation over the sample. Equation {2.6} can be further simplified by noting that constants can be moved outside the summation signs, and that the sum of constant is equal to the constant times the sample size, N.

$$\Sigma y_i^2 + N\mu^2 + b^2 \Sigma x_i^2 - 2\mu\Sigma y_i - 2b\Sigma(y_ix_i) + 2\mu b\Sigma x_i = \Sigma e_i^2 \qquad \{2.7\}$$

The least-squares estimates for μ and b are derived by computing the partial derivatives of Equation {2.7} with respect to these two parameters, and setting these derivatives equal to zero. Differentiating with respect to μ, and setting the derivative equal to zero gives:

$$2N\mu - 2\Sigma y_i + 2b\Sigma x_i = 0 \qquad \{2.8\}$$

and the least-squares solution for μ is: $(\Sigma y_i - b\Sigma x_i)/N$. Differentiating with respect to b, and setting this partial derivative equal to zero gives:

$$2b\Sigma x_i^2 - 2\Sigma(y_ix_i) + 2\mu\Sigma x_i = 0 \qquad \{2.9\}$$

and the least-squares solution for b is: $[\Sigma(y_ix_i) - \mu\Sigma x_i]/\Sigma x_i^2$. Thus a system of two equations with two unknowns is obtained. Substituting the for μ into equation {2.9} and rearranging gives the following solution for b:

$$b = \frac{\Sigma(y_ix_i) - (\Sigma y_i \Sigma x_i)/N}{\Sigma x_i^2 - (\Sigma x_i)^2/N} \qquad \{2.10\}$$

Equation {2.10} is the sample covariance divided by the variance of x, which is the formula for the coefficient of regression.

2.6 Least-squares solutions for the general linear model

The least-squares solution for the general linear model given in equation {2.3} is derived in a similar manner. The residual sum of squares in matrix notation is computed as follows:

$$(y - X\theta)'(y - X\theta) = e'e \qquad \{2.11\}$$

$$y'y - 2(X\theta)'y + (X\theta)'X\theta = e'e \qquad \{2.12\}$$

Setting the differential with respect to θ equal to zero and solving gives:

$$\theta = (X'X)^{-1}X'y \qquad \{2.13\}$$

Equations {2.13} are termed the "Normal Equations," and are used extensively in modern statistics. If the observations are correlated, or do not have equal variances or both, then the normal equations can be modified as follows:

$$X'V^{-1}X\theta = X'V^{-1}y \qquad \{2.14\}$$

where **V** is the variance matrix among the observations. **V** is a diagonal matrix with rows and columns equal to the number of observations. The diagonal elements of **V** are the variance of each observation, and the off-diagonal elements are the covariances between the corresponding pair of observations. Solutions to equations {2.14} are called "generalized least-squares" solutions, and minimize **e'e**, subject to the restriction of the known variance matrix. These equations are difficult to apply as written, because they require the inverse of **V**, which is difficult to compute for large data sets.

For a linear model the parameter estimates will also be unbiased, consistent, and within the parameter space. If **y** is not a linear function of θ, then the least-squares solution can generally not be derived analytically, although various iterative methods have been developed. Only effects on the mean of **y** are included in the model, thus effects on the variance of **y** or higher order moments cannot be estimated by least-squares.

2.7 Maximum likelihood estimation for a single parameter

Maximum likelihood (ML) is much more flexible than least-squares estimation, but requires rather complex programming, except for models which can be analysed by available software, such as program LE of BMDP (Elkind *et al.*, 1994). There are three steps in ML parameter estimation:

1. Defining the assumptions on which the statistical model is based.
2. Constructing the likelihood function, which is the joint density of the observations conditional on the parameters.
3. Maximizing the likelihood function with respect to the parameters.

The basic methodology for ML estimation of a single parameter will be illustrated using an example from a binomial distribution. Assume that from a sample of 10 observations, three are "successes" and the other seven are "failures". We wish to derive the ML estimate (MLE) of p, the probability of success. The binomial probability for this result as a function of p is:

$$L = \frac{10!(p)^3(1-p)^7}{3!7!} \qquad \{2.15\}$$

where L is the probability of obtaining this result, conditional on p. L is denoted the "likelihood function". The MLE for p is that value of p which maximizes L. The MLE is computed by differentiating L with respect to p, and solving for p, with this derivative set equal to zero. In practice it is usually easier to compute and differentiate the log of L. With respect to maximum likelihood, this is equivalent to differentiating L, because a function of a variable and the log of the function will be maximal for the same value of the variable. The MLE of p is then derived as follows:

$$\text{Log } L = \log(10!) - \log(3!7!) + 3(\log p) + 7[\log(1-p)] \qquad \{2.16\}$$

$$d(\text{Log } L)/dp = 3/p - 7/(1-p) = 0 \qquad \{2.17\}$$

$$p = 3/10 \qquad \{2.18\}$$

This is, of course, the proportion of successes derived in the sample. Thus, for this simple case, the MLE is the intuitive estimate value. From the above discussion, it should be clear why MLE must lie within the parameter space. A parameter estimate outside the parameter space will, by definition, have a likelihood of zero, and can therefore not be the MLE.

For a continuous distribution, the likelihood is computed as the statistical density of the distribution, conditional on the sample. Statistical density, f(y), for a continuous variable, y, is defined as the ordinate of the distribution function for a given value of y. For example, assume that a sample was taken from a normal distribution. To obtain the MLE for the mean, it is necessary to compute the joint statistical density of the sample. For a single observation the likelihood will be:

$$L = \frac{e^{-(y-\mu)^2/2\sigma^2}}{\sqrt{2\pi\sigma^2}} \qquad \{2.19\}$$

where σ is the standard deviation, e is the base for natural logarithms and is approximately equal to 2.72, μ is the mean, π is the ratio of the circumference and the diameter of a circle and is approximately equal to 3.141, and y is the variable value. For a sample of N observations, the likelihood will be the product of the likelihoods for each individual observation. As in the previous case, the MLE for μ can be derived by computing the derivative of the log of the likelihood with respect to the mean, and setting this function equal to zero. The derivative of log L for a sample from a normal distribution is computed as follows:

$$L = \prod_{i}^{I} \left[\frac{e^{-(y_i-\mu)^2/2\sigma^2}}{\sqrt{2\pi\sigma^2}} \right] \quad \{2.19\}$$

$$\text{Log } L = \sum_{i}^{I} \log \left[\frac{e^{-(y_i-\mu)^2/2\sigma^2}}{\sqrt{2\pi\sigma^2}} \right] \quad \{2.20\}$$

$$d(\text{Log } L)/d\mu = \Sigma(y_i - \mu) \quad \{2.21\}$$

where $\prod$ signifies a multiplicative series, parallel to Σ, and y_i is element i of y. Setting $\Sigma(y_i - \mu)$ equal to zero, we find that the MLE of μ is $(\Sigma y_i)/n$, the sample mean, which is again the intuitively correct result.

The MLE for the variance could be derived in the same manner, and would again yield the intuitive result of the sample variance. This result will be considered again in the following chapter in relation to estimation of variance components. Although in the two examples given so far, ML has been used to derive estimates that could have been derived by other methods, it will be demonstrated in the following chapters that for more complicated problems, ML and Bayesian estimation are the only estimation methods that can utilize all the available data.

2.8 Maximum likelihood multi-parameter estimation

ML can also be used to estimate several parameters simultaneously, for example, to estimate both the mean and variance in a normal distribution. In that case it is necessary to maximize the likelihood with respect to both parameters. This can be done by computing the partial derivatives of the log likelihood with respect to each parameter, and setting each partial derivative equal to zero. It is then necessary to solve a system of equations equal to the number of parameters being estimated. In general the likelihood function for estimation of m parameters, (θ_1, θ_2,..., θ_m), from a sample of N observations (y_1, y_2,..., y_N) can be written as follows:

$$L = p(y_1, y_2,...y_n|\theta_1, \theta_2,...\theta_m) =$$

$$= p(y_1|\theta_1, \theta_2,...\theta_m)p(y_2|\theta_1, \theta_2,...\theta_m)...p(y_n|\theta_1, \theta_2,...\theta_m) \quad \{2.22\}$$

$$= \prod p(y_i|\theta_1, \theta_2,...\theta_m)$$

$$= \prod p(y_i|\theta)$$

where $p(y_i|\theta)$ represents the probability of obtaining y_i, conditional on the vector of parameters. If the distribution is continuous, then $p(y_i|\theta)$ will be replaced by $f(y_i|\theta)$, i. e. the density of y_i, conditional on θ. Thus, ML can be applied to solve any problem that can be phrased in terms of Equation {2.22}.

Although it is generally possible to write the likelihood function and differentiate log L with respect to the different parameters, for QTL detection models it will not be possible to solve analytically the resultant system of equations. Iterative methods to derive solutions will be described in Sections 2.10 to 2.13.

2.9 Confidence intervals and hypothesis testing for MLE

In addition to deriving parameter estimates, it is also important to determine the accuracy of the estimates. Generally the standard errors of the estimates are used for this purpose. The square of the standard error is denoted the "prediction error variance". The following equation can generally be used to derive the prediction error variance for MLE of a single parameter:

$$\text{Var}(\hat{\theta}) = \frac{-1}{E[d^2(\log L)/d\theta^2]} \quad \{2.23\}$$

where $\hat{\theta}$ is the MLE of θ, and $E[d^2(\log L)/d\theta^2]$ is the expectation of the second derivative of L with respect to θ. Equation {2.23} will be correct if the first derivative of θ is a multiple of the difference between the true parameter value and its estimate. Otherwise the prediction error variance will be slightly greater than the right-hand side of Equation {2.23}. Under a wide range of conditions, Equation {2.23} will be "asymptotically correct"; that is, as the sample size increases, the difference between the left-hand and right-hand sides of the equation tends towards zero. The square root of the prediction error variance, the standard error of the estimate, can be used to determine the confidence interval of the estimate.

The prediction error variances for the multi-parameter estimation problem can be derived in a manner parallel to that described in Equation {2.23}. The parameter estimates and the first derivatives will each consist of a vector with the number of elements equal to m, the number of parameters. The second derivatives and the prediction error variances will both be square m × m matrices. Using brackets to denote matrices and vectors, the matrix of prediction error variances can be computed with the following equations:

$$\text{Var}[\hat{\theta}] = -\left[\frac{\partial^2 \text{Log L}}{\partial [\theta]^2}\right]^{-1} \qquad \{2.24\}$$

where the right-hand side is the inverse of the matrix of second partial derivatives with respect to $[\theta]$. The diagonal elements will be the prediction error variances of the estimates, and the off-diagonal elements will be the prediction error covariances between the elements. These are needed to test hypotheses based on linear functions of the parameters.

Even if the prediction error variance is not computed, ML can still be used to test a hypothesis by a "likelihood ratio test". In a likelihood ratio test the maximum likelihoods obtained under two alternative hypotheses are compared. In the null hypothesis, one or more of the parameters that are maximized in the alternative hypothesis are assumed fixed. For example, the mean is set equal to zero. The alternative hypothesis is termed the "complete" model, because ML estimates are derived for all parameters, while the null hypothesis is termed the "reduced" model, because some of the parameter values are fixed. Under the assumption that the null hypothesis is correct, the natural log of the maximum likelihood ratio of the complete and reduced models will be asymptotically distributed as: $(1/2)\chi^2$, where χ^2 is the Chi-squared statistic. The number of degrees of freedom (df) will be equal to the number of parameters that are maximized in the alternative hypothesis, but fixed in the null hypothesis. This ratio will have a χ^2 distribution only if the null hypothesis is "nested" within the alternative hypothesis. Hypothesis are "nested" if some parameters that are fixed in the null hypothesis are set to their maximum likelihood values in the alternative hypothesis, but all parameters that are fixed in the alternative hypothesis are also fixed in the null hypothesis.

2.10 Methods to maximize likelihood functions

Numerous iterative methods have been proposed to maximize multi-parameter likelihood function. The initial solutions for all methods are selected arbitrarily. These methods will be compared based on ease of application, speed of convergence, and probability of convergence. Of all the methods that will be considered below, only expectation-maximization (EM) is guaranteed to converge to a maximum, provided a maximum exists within the parameter space. However, even for EM, the convergence point may be only a local maximum. It is possible that there may be other maxima with higher values. Generally the problem of multiple maxima is addressed by iterating from several different sets of initial values. If all runs converge to the same parameter estimates, then it is likely, but not certain, that this parameter set is a global maximum.

Iterative maximization methods can be divided into three categories: derivative free methods, methods based on computation of first derivatives, and methods based on computation of second derivatives. For all derivative-based methods, the parameter estimates of the ith iterate are computed by solving a system of equations equal in number to the number of parameters being estimated. These reduced equations are themselves functions of the parameter estimates from the previous iteration. Generally, iteration is continued until changes between rounds fall below a sufficiently small value. Although this is the generally accepted criterion for approximate convergence, this is not necessarily this case. If convergence is slow, it is possible that changes between consecutive rounds of iteration can be small, even if the estimates are not close to the actual solutions. Convergence is generally most rapid for second derivative methods, but convergence is not guaranteed, even if there is a maximum within the parameter space. We will consider first derivative-free methods, then methods based on computation of second derivatives, and finally methods based on computation of first derivatives.

2.11 Derivative-free methods

Several general-purpose algorithms that find the maximum of a function without computing derivatives have been devised. These methods are available in many software packages, and can be applied to virtually any continuous function. These methods are based on predicting the direction of the maxima based on the set of current solutions. For example, assume that the likelihood is a function of two parameters. Likelihood values are derived for three sets of initial solutions. These three points define a plane on the likelihood surface. The direction of highest increase in the likelihood can then be determined for these three points. A new set of solutions is then computed in the direction of steepest ascent of the likelihood function. This method can be extended to any number of parameters. At each step the number of points analysed is one more than the number of parameters.

Although derivative-free methods are relatively easy to compute for any function, they have serious drawbacks. The direction is only approximate, and there is no method to estimate how far to go in that direction. Thus, it is quite easy to "overshoot" the maximum, and the new solution set may have a lower likelihood than the previous solutions. In general, derivative-free methods tend to be inefficient for large samples or many parameters. Derivative-free methods

2.12 Second derivative-based methods

In Newton-Raphson (Dahlquist and Bjorck, 1974), both the first derivatives and the matrix of second derivatives are computed analytically. Solutions for the ith round of iteration are computed by solving the following system of equations:

$$[\hat{\theta}_i] = [\hat{\theta}_{i-1}] - \frac{\partial \text{Log L}}{\partial [\theta]} \left[\frac{\partial^2 \text{Log L}}{\partial [\theta]^2} \right]^{-1} \qquad \{2.25\}$$

where $[\hat{\theta}_i]$ is the estimate of q for the ith iterate, $[\hat{\theta}_{i-1}]$ is the previous estimate of $[\theta]$, and the other terms are as defined above, with derivatives computed for the i–1 estimate of $[\theta]$.

The main advantage of Newton-Raphson is that convergence is generally rapid. The disadvantages are that the algorithm may not converge, even if the likelihood does have a maximum within the parameter space, and computation of the matrix of second derivatives is often a non-trivial task. This problem is alleviated somewhat if numerical methods are used to estimate the differentials (Bailey, 1969; Jensen, 1989). Thus, the algebra is simplified somewhat, but there is some sacrifice in both efficiency, in terms of computing time, and the accuracy of the estimates and the prediction error variances. However, as shown above, this matrix can be used to derive estimates of the standard errors of the estimates, which is of itself an important objective.

2.13 First derivative-based methods (EM)

Expectation-maximization (EM) is based on computation of first derivatives. The principle behind EM is to consider two sampling densities, one based on the complete data specification (unknown), and the second based on the incomplete data specification (known). The EM algorithm consists of two steps: the estimation step, in which the sufficient statistics are estimated for the complete data density function; and the maximization step, in which this function is maximized with respect to the parameters. A "sufficient statistic" is a statistic derived from the sample which contains all the information in the sample relevant to the parameter being estimated. For example, the sample mean is a sufficient statistic to estimate the population mean. This method will be explained in more detail in Chapter five using an example based on detection of QTL parameters.

EM is generally considered the method of choice, because it is guaranteed to converge to a local maximum, provided that one exists within the parameter space. However, the rate of convergence may be very slow, and there is no guarantee that the maximum found is the global maximum. The only way to approximately address this problem is to begin iteration from several different sets of initial values. If all the runs converge to the same solutions, then it is likely that there is only a single maximum within the parameter space.

An additional advantage of EM is that it is possible to include "nuisance" parameters in the analysis, such as block or herd effect, even if these parameters have a very large number of levels. This will also be illustrated in Chapter five.

2.14 Bayesian estimation

Bayesian estimation differs from ML in that instead of maximizing the likelihood function, the "posterior probability" of θ, $p(\theta|y)$ is maximized as a function of the likelihood function multiplied by the "prior" distribution of θ. Bayes Theorem in general terms for multiple parameters and observations is computed as follows:

$$p(\theta_1, \theta_2,...\theta_m | y_1, y_2,...y_n) = p(\theta_1, \theta_2,...\theta_m) p(y_1, y_2,...y_N | \theta_1, \theta_2,...\theta_m) \quad \{2.26\}$$

where $p(\theta_1, \theta_2,...\theta_m | y_1, y_2,...y_N)$ is the "posterior" probability of the parameters, $p(\theta_1, \theta_2,...\theta_m)$ is the "prior probability" of the parameters, and $p(y_1, y_2,...y_N | \theta_1, \theta_2,...\theta_m)$ is the likelihood function. Similar to ML, it is possible to maximize the posterior probability or density function relative to the parameter values. Assuming that prior information of the parameters is available, Bayesian estimation, which makes use of this information, should be preferable to ML, which ignores any prior information on the parameters.

Instead of maximizing the posterior density, it is possible to define a "loss function" which determines the economic value "lost" by incorrect parameter estimation. Common examples are linear and quadratic loss functions. In the linear loss function, the value of the loss is a linear function of the difference between the parameter estimates and their true values. In the quadratic loss function, the loss increases quadratically as a function of the difference between the parameter estimate and its true value. Minimizing the linear loss function is equivalent to maximizing the posterior density. Minimizing the quadratic loss function is equivalent to maximizing the mean of the posterior distribution.

Similarly a Bayesian test of alternative hypothesis is based on minimizing the expectation of the loss function. If a decision must be made between two alternative hypotheses, the economic value of the "loss" is determined for each incorrect decision. The expectation of the loss will be the probability of each incorrect decision (the type I and type II errors) multiplied by its economic value. The decision is then based on minimizing the expected loss.

There are two major drawbacks to Bayesian estimation. First, prior information on the parameters is often vague, and it is not possible to mathematically represent this information in terms of a statistical distribution function without additional assumptions, which cannot be verified. Second, if many records are included in the analysis, then the likelihood function tends to "overwhelm" the prior distribution of θ. In this case, the Bayesian estimates tend to converge to the ML estimates. An example of Bayesian estimation of QTL parameters will be given in Chapter seven.

2.15 Minimum difference estimation

Although Bayesian estimation requires extensive assumptions *a priori* about the data, both least-squares and ML also make some assumptions about the underlying distribution of the data. With least-squares a normal distribution of residuals is nearly always assumed. Generally both least-squares and ML are robust to violations of the assumed distribution. However, this may not be the case in the presence of "outliers", observations that deviate greatly from the assumed distribution

Minimum difference (MD) estimators are the parameter values that minimize some function of the theoretical distribution, given the parameter estimates, and the empirical distribution of the data. The most common function used is the sum of squares deviation, called the Cramer-von Mises distance, which is computed as follows:

$$\delta = \sum_{i=1}^{n} [(\Phi(y_i|\theta_1, \theta_2,...\theta_m) - (i - 0.5)/N]^2 \qquad \{2.27\}$$

where δ is the distance to be minimized, $\Phi(y_i|\theta_1, \theta_2,...\theta_m)$ is the cumulative normal distribution function up to observation y_i, with the observation sorted in ascending order and given parameter estimates $\theta_1, \theta_2,...\theta_m$, and the other terms are as defined previously. The objective is then to find the parameter estimates than minimize δ. That is, the theoretical distribution that most closely approximates the empirical distribution of the data.

This method is only dependent on the rank of the observations, not their absolute values, and is therefore less affected by extreme values of y. In the presence of outliers, this method has been found to be more robust that ML for estimation of QTL parameters in a backcross design (Perez-Enciso and Toro, 1999).

Theoretically, δ can be derived by taking the partial derivatives of the left-hand side of Equation {2.27} with respect to the parameters, and setting this system of equations equal to zero. In practice, similar to ML, this system of equations cannot be solved analytically, and iterative methods are required. If the number of parameters is low, Equation {2.27} can be minimized by trial-and-error. Alternatively, similar to ML, approximate Newton-Raphson iteration can be applied. The first and second partial derivatives can be approximated by computing δ over a series of possible parameter values, and these derivatives can then be used in Equation {2.25} to derive parameter estimates for the next iteration.

2.16 Summary

In this chapter we considered first the desirable properties of estimators in general. We then considered various methods for parameter estimation of crosses between inbred lines, emphasizing least-squares and ML. ML is not trivial to apply, but can be applied to many models which are not amenable to solution by other methods. Unlike other estimation methods, ML estimates must be within the parameter space. General methods were presented to compute estimation error variances of MLE and to test hypotheses related to parameter values. Least-squares models give nearly identical results to ML, and can be applied using standard statistical packages, such as SAS® (SAS Institute Inc, Cary, NC), but are much more limited as to possibilities of model specification. For all models of interest likelihood functions cannot be maximized analytically. We also considered iterative methods to maximize likelihood functions. None of these methods guarantee that, even if a maximum is found, it will be the global maximum. In the final sections we considered Bayesian estimation and the method of minimal distance. Solutions by these methods, like ML, can only be computed iteratively. Application of these methods to estimation of QTL parameters will be considered in detail in Chapters five to seven.

Chapter three:

Random and Fixed Effects, the Mixed Model

3.1 Introduction

So far we have assumed that all effects included in the model, except for the residual, are fixed. For random effects, it is assumed that each effect is sampled from an infinite population of possible effects with a known distribution. In Chapter seven we will consider models in which QTL effects are considered random. The basis of selection index theory is that polygenic breeding values for quantitative traits should be considered random, because these effects are "sampled" from a normal distribution of effects with a known variance. In genetic evaluation based on field records, it will also be necessary to include fixed effects, such as herd or block, in the model. Therefore, analysis models will include both fixed and random effects in addition the residual. The models that include both fixed and random effects are termed "mixed models".

We will first consider the general strategy for solving mixed models, based on the "mixed model equations" (Henderson, 1973) in Sections 3.2 to 3.6. In Sections 3.8 to 3.11 we will consider a number of models used to derive genetic evaluations for quantitative traits, and note the advantages and disadvantages of each model. We will consider maximum likelihood parameter estimation from mixed models in Section 3.12.

In general it will be assumed that random effects are sampled from a normal distribution with a mean of zero and a known variance. Therefore, estimates for random effects can only be derived if their variances are known. In the final four sections we will consider methods for variance component estimation in mixed models, based on constant fitting and maximum likelihood, and restricted maximum likelihood (REML).

3.2 The mixed linear model

As an example we will first consider the following simple mixed model used to derived breeding values of bulls for milk production:

$$Y_{ijk} = H_i + S_j + e_{ijk} \qquad \{3.1\}$$

where Y_{ijk} is the milk production record of cow k in herd i, H_i is the effect of herd i, S_j is the effect of the cow's sire j on her production, and e_{ijk} is the random residual. The herd effect will be assumed to be a fixed effect, and the sire effect will be assumed to be random. In general terms the mixed model can be written in matrix notation as follows:

$$y = X\beta + Zu + e \qquad \{3.2\}$$

where β is a vector of fixed effects, u represents the vector of random effects, X and Z are incident matrices, and e is the vector of random residuals. The additive breeding values are considered random effects, with a known variance matrix. Both u and e are assumed to have a normal distribution. Thus y has a multivariate normal distribution with a mean of $X\beta$, and a variance V computed as follows:

$$V = ZGZ' + R \qquad \{3.3\}$$

where G is the variance matrix of u, and R is the variance matrix of the residuals. If sires are not related, then the variance matrix of the sire effect will be $I\sigma_s^2$, where I is an identity matrix, and $\sigma_s^2 = \frac{1}{4}$ of the additive genetic variance. The sire effect variance is equal to one-quarter of the additive genetic variance, because each sire passes half of his genes to each daughter. When squared to compute the variance, the one-half additive genetic effect becomes one-quarter of the additive genetic variance.

If the sires are related, then $G = A\sigma_s^2$, where A is the numerator relationship matrix among the sires. The diagonal elements of A will be equal to unity, and the off-diagonal elements will reflect the fraction of genes that the two individuals, corresponding to the appropriate row and column of A, have identical by descent, for example 0.5 for father and son, and 0.25 for half-sibs. Both A and G are always symmetrical matrices, that is $G = G'$ and $A = A'$.

As in the fixed model, the residuals will be generally be assumed to be uncorrelated and have equal variance. In this case $R = I\sigma_e^2$, where σ_e^2 is the residual variance. For the sire model given above in Equation $\{3.1\}$, if relationships among sires are ignored the distribution of a specific record can be written as follows:

$$Y_{ijk} = \left[\frac{e^{-(s_j)^2/2\sigma_s^2}}{\sqrt{2\pi\sigma_s^2}} \right] \left[\frac{e^{-(Y_{ijk} - H_i - S_j)^2/2\sigma_e^2}}{\sqrt{2\pi\sigma_e^2}} \right] \qquad \{3.4\}$$

where σ_s^2 is the variance of the sire effect.

3.3 The mixed model equations

Theoretically the least-squares solutions for the fixed effects can be derived from equations {2.14}. Defining the solutions for the fixed effects as $\hat{\beta}$, Henderson (1973) showed that solutions for the random effects can then be computed as: $GZ'V^{-1}(y - \hat{\beta})$. However, the variance matrix, $V = ZGZ' + R$, is not diagonal, and therefore cannot be inverted for large data sets. Solutions for β and u for large data sets can be derived by solving the following set of equations, denoted the "mixed model equations" (Henderson, 1973):

$$\begin{bmatrix} X'R^{-1}X & X'R^{-1}Z \\ Z'R^{-1}X & Z'R^{-1}Z + G^{-1} \end{bmatrix} \begin{bmatrix} \hat{\beta} \\ \hat{u} \end{bmatrix} = \begin{bmatrix} X'R^{-1}y \\ Z'R^{-1}y \end{bmatrix} \quad \{3.5\}$$

where R^{-1} is the inverse of the residual variance matrix, and G^{-1} is the variance matrix for u. The left-hand side of these equations consists of a square, symmetrical, matrix termed the "coefficient matrix", and $\hat{\beta}\,\hat{u}$ the vector of solutions. As noted previously, for analysis of a single trait it is generally assumed that the residual variances for each record are equal and uncorrelated. In this case, the residual variance matrix is equal to $I\sigma_e^2$, and $R^{-1} = I/\sigma_e^2$. Thus the mixed model equations can be simplified by multiplying both sides by σ_e^2 as follows:

$$\begin{bmatrix} X'X & X'Z \\ Z'X & Z'Z + G^{-1}\sigma_e^2 \end{bmatrix} \begin{bmatrix} \beta \\ u \end{bmatrix} = \begin{bmatrix} X'y \\ Z'y \end{bmatrix} \quad \{3.6\}$$

For the "sire model" given in Equation {3.1}, $X'X$ will be a diagonal matrix with rows and columns equal to the number of herds. The diagonal element of each row will be the number of records in the corresponding herd, and all off-diagonal elements will be zero. Similarly, $Z'Z$ will be diagonal with each diagonal element equal to the number of daughter records of each sire. $X'Z$ will have rows equal to the number of herds, and columns equal to the number of sires. Each element will be the number of records in the corresponding herd × sire combination. $X'y$ will be a vector of length equal to the number of herds, and each element will be the sum of the record values in the corresponding herd. The length of $Z'y$ will be the number of sires, and each element will be the sum of the records of all the daughters of the corresponding sire.

3.4 Solving the mixed model equations

Solutions to the mixed model equations can be obtained by multiplying the right-hand side vector by the inverse of the coefficient matrix. An exact solution requires inverting the coefficient matrix, but generally the coefficient matrix will be much smaller than **V**. The number of rows and columns of **V** is equal to the total number of records, while the number of columns and rows in the coefficient matrix is equal to the number of levels of effects included in the model, which is generally many fewer.

If many effects are included in the model, approximate solutions can be obtained by iteration. There are several iteration methods that can be applied to solve the mixed model equations. Gauss-Seidel iteration is generally the method of choice, because it is relatively rapid, and guaranteed to converge, provided the equations have a solution (Quaas and Pollak, 1980). In Gauss-Seidel iteration the solution for each equation in iteration i is computed as follows:

$$B_i = [Y_i - \sum_{j=1}^{i-1} B_j c_{ij} - \sum_{j=i+1}^{J} B_j c_{ij}] / c_{ii} \qquad \{3.7\}$$

where B_i is the solution for equation i at iteration k, Y_i is the right-hand side for equation i, B_j is the solution for equation j at iteration k–1, c_{ij} is the element of the coefficient matrix at column i and row j, and c_{ii} is the diagonal element of column i. The larger the diagonal elements of the coefficient matrix relative to the off-diagonal elements, the faster will be the convergence with Gauss-Seidel iteration. Thus, sire models may converge in less than 10 rounds of iteration, because the diagonal elements are generally very large compared to the off-diagonal elements. Animal models, described below, generally required hundreds of rounds of iteration to achieve approximate convergence.

Computing the coefficient matrix still requires inverting **G**. For a sire model $\mathbf{G}^{-1} = \mathbf{A}^{-1}/\sigma_s^2$, and $\mathbf{G}^{-1}\sigma_e^2 = \mathbf{A}^{-1}\sigma_e^2/\sigma_s^2$. σ_e^2/σ_s^2 is a constant, which is generally assumed known. As noted above, σ_s^2 is equal to one-fourth of the additive genetic variance. Thus σ_e^2 includes three-fourths of the genetic variance, plus all the remaining variance. Thus σ_e^2 is equal to $1-h^2/4$ of the total variance, where h^2 is the heritability, the ratio of the additive genetic variance to the phenotypic variance. Therefore, in terms of the heritability, σ_e^2/σ_s^2 is equal to $(4-h^2)/h^2$. Henderson developed a simple algorithm to invert **A** from a list of individuals and their sires and dams (Henderson, 1976). Thus, the only matrix that must be inverted is the coefficient matrix, which will be a square matrix of size equal to the number of effects included in the model.

3.5 Some important properties of mixed model solutions

Solutions to the Normal equations presented in the previous chapter are termed "best linear unbiased estimates" (BLUE). Unbiasedness was defined in the previous chapter. The meaning of "best" is that if $\hat{\beta}$ is an estimate of β, $E(\hat{\beta}-\beta)^2$ is minimal among the class of linear unbiased estimates. Henderson (1973) termed the solutions of random effects in the mixed model "best linear unbiased predictors" (BLUP). Under the assumed variance structure, the random solutions in the mixed model equations, $\hat{u}$, will be "best" in the sense that $E(\hat{u}-u)^2$ will be minimized, within the assumed constraints. Since the random effects are not parameters, their solutions were termed "predictors" rather than "estimates". BLUP solutions have several important properties that will be summarized here.

The prediction error variances of the fixed and random effects can be estimated by inverting the coefficient matrix of the mixed model equations. This inverse can be partitioned into four sub-matrices corresponding to the four sub-matrices in the mixed model equations. That is:

$$\begin{bmatrix} X'R^{-1}X & X'R^{-1}Z \\ Z'R^{-1}X & Z'R^{-1}Z + G^{-1} \end{bmatrix}^{-1} = \begin{bmatrix} C_{11} & C_{12} \\ C_{21} & C_{22} \end{bmatrix} \quad \{3.8\}$$

The diagonal elements of C_{11} will correspond to the prediction error variance for the fixed effect solutions, and the diagonal elements of C_{22} will correspond to the prediction error variance for the random effect solutions. Solutions for fixed effects will have greater variance than the actual effects, while prediction error variances of the random effect solutions, which are regressed towards the mean, will be less than the variance of the actual effects. In general:

$$\text{var}(u) = \text{var}(\hat{u}) + \text{pev}(\hat{u}) \quad \{3.9\}$$

where var (u) and var $(\hat{u})$ are the variances of u of $\hat{u}$, and pev$(\hat{u})$ is the prediction error variance of $\hat{u}$. Henderson (1973) also showed that the covariance of u and $\hat{u}$ is equal to var $(\hat{u})$. Thus, the regression of u on $\hat{u}$ is equal to unity. That is, if the actual difference between two random effects is equal to x, the expected difference between their solutions will also be equal to x. This is not the case for fixed effects.

3.6 Equation absorption

For many common models in genetic analysis, the number of equations can be further reduced by a technique called "absorption". This technique can be applied both to fixed and mixed models, and will be illustrated with the following set of equations:

$$\begin{bmatrix} X_1'X_1 & X_1'X_2 \\ X_2'X_1 & X_2'X_2 \end{bmatrix} \begin{bmatrix} \beta_1 \\ \beta_2 \end{bmatrix} = \begin{bmatrix} X_1'y \\ X_2'y \end{bmatrix} \qquad \{3.10\}$$

where the subscripts 1 and 2 refer to any division of the equations into two groups. These equations can be rewritten as follows:

$$X_1'X_1\beta_1 + X_1'X_2\beta_2 = X_1'y$$
$$X_2'X_1\beta_1 + X_2'X_2\beta_2 = X_2'y \qquad \{3.11\}$$

Solving for β_1 in the first set of equation gives:

$$\beta_1 = [X_1'y - X_1'X_2\beta_2][X_1'X_1]^{-1} \qquad \{3.12\}$$

β_1 in the second set of equation can then be replaced by the solution for β_1 in Equations {3.11}. The second set of equations is now only a function of β_2 and can be solved separately. Once solutions are derived for β_2, "back solutions" can be derived for β_1 by solving for β_1 in Equations {3.11}.

Of course, this procedure requires a solution for $[X_1'X_1]^{-1}$. In many cases, $X_1'X_1$ is diagonal, as noted above for the sire model given in Equation {3.1}, and can therefore be readily inverted. For this model, the $X'X$ matrix will be diagonal with the number of records in each herd as the diagonal element, and the inverse will be the reciprocal of each diagonal element. Random effects can also be absorbed, provided that the coefficient matrix has an appropriate diagonal, or block diagonal, structure.

3.7 Multivariate mixed model analysis

The mixed model equations can also be used to analyse several correlated traits, for example milk and butterfat production of cows. A multitrait sire model can be described as follows:

$$Y_{ijkl} = H_{il} + S_{jl} + e_{ijkl} \qquad \{3.13\}$$

where Y_{ijkl} is the production record of cow k in herd i for trait l, H_{il} is the effect of herd i on trait l, S_{jl} is the effect of the cow's sire j on trait l, and e_{ijkl} is the random residual associated with trait l. In this case it will generally be assumed that both the additive genetic effects and the residuals have a multivariate normal distribution. As in the univariate case, the distribution of each record will be given by the distribution of the random genetic effect times the residual effect distribution. For two correlated traits, x and y, the distribution of the residuals for each individual will be as follows:

$$[2\pi\sigma_x^2\sigma_y^2(1-\rho^2)]^{-1/2} e^\phi \qquad \{3.14\}$$

where σ_x^2 and σ_y^2 are the residual variances for traits x and y, $\rho = \sigma_{xy}/\sigma_x\sigma_y$ is the residual correlation, and ϕ is computed as follows:

$$\phi = -\frac{1}{2(1-\rho^2)}\left[\frac{(x-\mu_x)^2}{\sigma_x^2} - 2\rho\frac{(x-\mu_x)^2(y-\mu_y)^2}{\sigma_x^2\sigma_y^2} + \frac{(y-\mu_y)^2}{\sigma_y^2}\right] \qquad \{3.15\}$$

where μ_x and μ_y are the means for traits x, and y, and are equal to $H_{il} + S_{jl}$ for each trait. The distributions for the genetic effects are computed in a similar manner.

Now consider the general mixed model equations given in Equations {3.5}. The residual variance matrix will no longer by diagonal, but will be "block diagonal". For two traits, the residual matrix will have the structure $I \otimes R_i$, where I is an identity matrix, and R_i is a 2 × 2 matrix with elements as follows:

$$R_i = \begin{bmatrix} \sigma_x^2 & \sigma_{xy} \\ \sigma_{xy} & \sigma_y^2 \end{bmatrix} \qquad \{3.16\}$$

$\otimes$ denotes the "Kronecker product", which means that each element of I is multiplied by R_i. Similarly the variance matrix of the sire effect will be $A \otimes S$, where S is a 2 × 2 matrix as follows:

$$S = \begin{bmatrix} \sigma_{sx}^2 & \sigma_{sxy} \\ \sigma_{sxy} & \sigma_{sy}^2 \end{bmatrix} \qquad \{3.17\}$$

where σ_{sx}^2 and σ_{sx}^2 are the sire effect variances for traits x and y, and σ_{sxy} is the covariance between them. Although both the residual and sire effect matrices can be easily inverted, the simplification obtained in Equations {3.6} by multiplying by the residual variance is no longer possible. The total number of equations will be the number of level of effects times the number of traits.

3.8 The repeatability model

The model given in Equation {3.1} is appropriate if each cow has only a single record. If cows have multiple records, there will generally be an effect common to all records of the same animal. One way to handle this situation is to consider the multiple records of animals as correlated traits. Multiple records of the same individual will then have non-zero residual and genetic covariances. The number of equations will then be equal to the number of levels of herds and sires, times the maximum number of records per individual. This model also requires that the residual and genetic variances among records of the same animal be known.

A somewhat simpler solution is the "repeatability model". This model assumes that the same sire effect is common to all individuals, and that the residual covariances among all records of the same individual are the same. In this case, the model of Equation {3.1} can be modified as follows:

$$Y_{ijkl} = H_i + S_j + C_{jk} + e_{ijkl} \qquad \{3.18\}$$

where: H_i now refers to a herd-year-season, and C_{jk} is the effect common to all records of cow k. C_{jk} will also be a random effect with a variance matrix of $I\sigma_c^2$, where σ_c^2 is the variance due to the common cow effect. This model assumes that the common cow effects are not correlated, which is only an approximation, because related individuals will have a positive covariance. As noted above the sire effect includes one-fourth of the additive genetic effect, while the cow effect will include the remaining three-fourths of the additive genetic effect, plus an additional effect termed the "permanent environmental" effect. This effect will include non-additive genetic effects, and environmental effects common to all records of the individual. In matrix notation this model can be written as follows:

$$y = X\beta + Z_1 s + Z_2 c + e \qquad \{3.19\}$$

where Z_1 is the coefficient matrix for the sire genetic effects, Z_2 is the coefficient matrix for the common individual effects, s and c are the vectors of sire genetic and common individual effects, respectively. The mixed model equations for this model will be:

$$\begin{bmatrix} X'X & X'Z_1 & X'Z_2 \\ Z_1'X & Z_1'Z_1 + G^{-1}\sigma_e^2 & Z_1'Z_2 \\ Z_2'X & Z_2'Z_1 & Z_2'Z_2 + I\gamma \end{bmatrix} \begin{bmatrix} \beta \\ s \\ c \end{bmatrix} = \begin{bmatrix} X'y \\ Z_1'y \\ Z_2'y \end{bmatrix} \qquad \{3.20\}$$

where $\gamma = \sigma_e^2/\sigma_c^2$. The number of equations will be equal to the total number of levels. However, since $Z_2'Z_2 + I\gamma$ is a diagonal matrix, these equations can be readily absorbed (Ufford et al., 1979).

3.9 The individual animal model

The repeatability model ignores all relationships among females. Henderson (1973) first proposed that the mixed model equations could be used to estimate polygenic breeding values for all animals in a population accounting for all known relationships, via the "individual animal model" (IAM). A simple IAM is given below:

$$Y_{ijk} = H_i + a_j + p_j + e_{ijk} \qquad \{3.21\}$$

where Y_{ijk} is record k of individual j in "herd" or "block" i, H_i is the fixed effect of herd i, a_j is the random additive genetic effect of individual j, p_j is the random permanent environmental effect for individual j, and e_{ijk} is the random residual associated with each record. As with the repeatability model, a permanent environmental effect is required if individuals can have multiple records, because there will generally be an effect common to all records of each individual. In matrix notation this model can be written as follows:

$$y = X\beta + Z_1 a + Z_2 p + e \qquad \{3.22\}$$

where Z_1 is the coefficient matrix for the additive genetic effects, Z_2 is the coefficient matrix for the permanent environmental effects, a and p are the vectors of additive genetic and permanent environmental effects, respectively.

In a completely fixed model, the additive genetic and permanent environmental effects would be completely confounded, because each level of these two effects are related to the same, single, individual. In the IAM these effects can be estimated separately, because both are random, but their variance structures are different. The variance matrix for the permanent environmental effect will be $I\sigma_p^2$, where σ_p^2 is the variance component of the permanent environmental effect. The variance matrix for the additive genetic effect will be $A\sigma_A^2$, where σ_A^2 is additive genetic variance. After multiplying by the residual variance, the mixed model equations for this model are:

$$\begin{bmatrix} X'X & X'Z_1 & X'Z_2 \\ Z_1'X & Z_1'Z_1 + G^{-1}\sigma_e^2 & Z_1'Z_2 \\ Z_2'X & Z_2'Z_1 & Z_2'Z_2 + I\gamma \end{bmatrix} \begin{bmatrix} \beta \\ a \\ p \end{bmatrix} = \begin{bmatrix} X'y \\ Z_1'y \\ Z_2'y \end{bmatrix} \qquad \{3.23\}$$

where $\gamma = \sigma_e^2 / \sigma_p^2$.

In most cases not all individuals included in the population will have records. For example, if the trait analysed is milk production, only females will have production records. Individuals without records, such as sires of cows, can be included in the analysis via the relationship matrix. Additional equations can be added for these individuals in the mixed model equations as follows:

$$\begin{bmatrix} X'X & X'Z_1 & 0 & X'Z_2 \\ Z_1'X & Z_1'Z_1+G^{11}\sigma_e^2 & G^{12}\sigma_e^2 & Z_1'Z_2 \\ 0 & G^{21}\sigma_e^2 & G^{22}\sigma_e^2 & 0 \\ Z_2'X & Z_2'Z_1 & 0 & Z_2'Z_2+I\gamma \end{bmatrix} \begin{bmatrix} \beta \\ a_1 \\ a_2 \\ P \end{bmatrix} = \begin{bmatrix} X'y \\ Z_1'y \\ 0 \\ Z_2'y \end{bmatrix} \quad \{3.24\}$$

where G^{11} and G^{22} are the blocks of the inverse of the genetic variance matrix pertaining to individuals with and without records, respectively, G^{12} and G^{21} are the off-diagonal blocks, and a_1 and a_2 are the solutions for individuals with and without records, respectively. All other elements of the equations for animals without records will be zero. The total number of equations will be equal to the number of herds, plus the number of individuals with records, plus the total number of individuals included in the relationship matrix.

Even though this system of equations will generally be very large, it will also be quite "sparse", that is most elements will be equal to zero. These equations can also be solved by Gauss-Seidel iteration, as described in Section 3.4. As noted above, the number of iterations required for convergence is a function of the size of the diagonal elements in the coefficient matrix compared to the off-diagonal elements. In sire models diagonal elements are generally quite large, because each sire has many daughters with records. This is not the case for animal models. In the IAM, the diagonal element consists only of the contribution of the inverse of the relationship matrix, plus the individual's own records. Thus, many more iterations will be required in the IAM, as compared to sire models in which the diagonal elements are generally much greater than the off-diagonal elements.

3.10 Grouping individuals with unknown ancestors

Although it is possible to include ancestors in the IAM, the original animals will have unknown parents. The animal model mixed model equations as given in {3.24} would assume that these individuals are a random sample from a "base population". However, this is generally not the case. The "founder" individuals are also selected, and generally are not from the same generation.

Thompson (1979) developed a strategy account for unknown parents by assuming "phantom" parents, which are then grouped based on common characteristics of the individuals with unknown parents, such as age. These "genetic group" effects are considered fixed effects, and are computed via the relationship matrix. The genetic evaluation of each individual is then computed as the sum of his genetic group and additive genetic effects. A single individual may have contributions from several group effects if his ancestors have phantom parents from several groups. Westell *et al.* (1988) developed an algorithm to directly compute the genetic evaluation of each individual from the mixed model equations.

3.11 The reduced animal model

Consider an IAM with only a single record per animal. In that case it is not possible to estimate a permanent environmental effect, since this effect will be completely confounded with the random residual. The analysis model can now be rewritten as follows:

$$Y_{ijkl} = H_i + \tfrac{1}{2}S_j + \tfrac{1}{2}D_k + M_{ijkl} + e_{ijkl} \qquad \{3.25\}$$

where S_j is the effect of sire j of individual l, D_k is the effect of dam k, M_{ijkl} is the remainder of the additive genetic effect for individual l not included in the sire and dam effects, and e_{ijkl} is the random residual.

As note above, for a specific individual, the variance of the sire effect is one-quarter of the additive genetic variance. Similarly, the variance of the dam effect is also one-quarter of the genetic variance. Therefore, for any specific individual with the same two parents, the effects of the sire and dam will not explain one-half of the genetic variance. This effect was therefore termed the "Mendelian sampling" effect (Quaas and Pollock, 1980). That is, the specific genetic component passed to individual l that differentiates this individual from his full sibs.

For individuals with no progeny, the Mendelian sampling for the variance matrix of the M effect will be $\mathbf{I}\sigma_m^2$, where σ_m^2 is the variance of Mendelian sampling. The covariances will be zero for individuals without progeny. Individuals with progeny will pass on part of their M effects to their progeny, and there will therefore be a positive covariance between the M effects of parents and the sire or dam effects of their progeny. For individuals without progeny, the M and residual effects will be completely confounded, and the model can be revised as follows.

$$Y_{ijkl} = \tfrac{1}{2}H_i + \tfrac{1}{2}S_j + D_k + \varepsilon_{ijkl} \qquad \{3.26\}$$

where $\varepsilon_{ijkl} = M_{ijkl} + e_{ijkl}$.

Thus only the H, S, and D effects are included in the model for individuals without progeny. That is, these individuals can be absorbed into the equations of their sires and dams, as shown by Quaas and Pollock (1981). They called this model the "reduced animal model" (RAM). If the number of individuals without progeny included in the analysis is relatively large, compared to the number of individuals with progeny, then there can be a substantial reduction in the total number of equations in the model. For individuals without progeny this can be also be considered a "gametic" model; because the effects included in the model are the contributions of the paternal and maternal gametes to each progeny.

3.12 Maximum likelihood estimation with mixed models

In a mixed model that includes both fixed and random effects, the likelihood function is the joint density function integrated over the random effects (Titterington *et al.*, 1985). We will illustrate this based on the simple mixed model described in Equation {3.1}. The statistical density function for this model assuming unrelated sires will be:

$$f(Y_{ijk}) = \prod^{J} \{ f(s_j) \prod^{IK} f(y_{ijk}) \} \quad \{3.27\}$$

where $f(Y_{ijk})$ is the density function for individual k, $\prod$ represents a multiplicative sum, $f(s_j)$ represents the density function for sire j, which is the normal density function with a mean of zero, and a variance of σ_s^2, $f(y_{ijk})$ represents the normal density function for daughter k of sire j, which has a mean of $s_j + h_i$, and a variance of σ_e^2. The likelihood function is then computed by integrating with respect to the random sire effects as follow:

$$L = \prod^{J} \int \{ f(s_j) \left[\prod^{IK} f(y_{ijk}) \right] \} ds_j \quad \{3.28\}$$

The ML parameter solutions are those values of the fixed effects, and variances that maximize the likelihood function. There are no simple algorithms for deriving ML parameter solutions for large mixed model systems.

3.13 Estimation of variance components, analysis of variance type methods

In order to solve the mixed model equations given in Equations {3.5} the variances of the random effects must be known. In practice these variance components must be estimated from the same data. Variance component estimation will be considered here in only very general terms. For a detailed discussion of methodology for estimating variance components see Searle *et al.* (1992).

Various methods have been proposed to estimate variance components. These methods can be grouped into "analysis of variance" type methods, and "maximum likelihood" type methods. In analysis of variance type methods variance components are estimated by first computing solutions for the fixed and random effects. The variance components are then estimated by their expectations, which are functions of the solutions.

The most important of these methods is Henderson's Method III, which first computes solutions for all effects under a completely fixed model (Henderson, 1984). These solutions are then used to derive expectations for the variance components based on reductions in sums of squares. Variance component estimates derived by Henderson's method III are unbiased, but are not guaranteed to lie with the parameter space. It is possible to obtain negative variance components, or genetic or environmental correlations outside the range of –1 to 1. This problem will be considered below in more detail in Section 3.16.

The estimated variances for the residual and the random effects in the general mixed model, $\hat{\sigma}_e^2$ and $\hat{\sigma}_u^2$, are computed as follows:

$$\hat{\sigma}_e^2 = \frac{y'y - R(b,u)}{N - r - t + 1} \quad \{3.29\}$$

$$\hat{\sigma}_u^2 = \frac{R(u|b) - \hat{\sigma}_e^2(t-1)}{tr[Z'Z - Z'X(X'X)^- X'Z]} \quad \{3.30\}$$

where N is the number of observations, r is the rank (the number of levels) of the fixed effects, t is the rank of the random effects, "tr" signifies the trace of a matrix, and $(X'X)^-$ is a "generalized" inverse of $X'X$. The trace of a square matrix is the sum of the diagonal elements. For an explanation of generalized inverses see Searle (1971). R(b,u) and R(u|b) are reductions of sums of squares, and are computed as follows:

$$R(b,u) = y'[X \; Z] \begin{bmatrix} X'X & X'Z \\ Z'X & Z'Z \end{bmatrix} \begin{bmatrix} X' \\ Z' \end{bmatrix} y \quad \{3.31\}$$

and:

$$R(b|u) = R(b,u) - y'Z(Z'Z)^{-1}Z'y \quad \{3.32\}$$

3.14 Maximum likelihood estimation of variance components

The current method of choice for variance component estimation is restricted maximum likelihood (REML). This method is by necessity iterative, because the formula used to estimate the variance components are functions of the mixed model solutions, which are computed based on the previous estimates of the parameter values. REML differs from standard maximum likelihood in that account is taken of the fact that the estimates of the fixed effects are not equal to their parameter values. This will be explained below. We will first describe maximum likelihood estimation of variance components, and then describe the modifications required for restricted ML estimation. The derivation given here closely follows Lynch and Walsh (1998). For a more detailed explanation see Searle *et al.* (1992).

As in the previous chapter, ML estimates are derived by constructing the likelihood function (the joint density function of the observations), differentiating the log of this function with respect to the parameters, setting these differentials equal to zero, and solving for the parameter values in the resultant system of equations. For the mixed model, the parameters are the variance components and the fixed effects. The statistical density function for a single observation from the mixed model was given in Equation {3.4}. The likelihood function is the joint density of all observations after integrating over the random effects.

As noted previously, the distribution of y in the mixed model is multivariate normal. The likelihood function for a sample from a univariate normal distribution was given in Equation {2.19}. Accounting for the fact that the means and variances in the mixed model can be different for each observation, this likelihood becomes:

$$L = \prod_{}^{N} \left[\frac{e^{-(y_i-\mu_i)^2/2\sigma_i^2}}{\sqrt{2\pi\sigma_i^2}} \right] \qquad \{3.33\}$$

where N is the sample size, and μ_i and σ_i^2 are the mean and variance for observation i.

For any series of values, x_1 to x_n, $\prod \exp(x_i) = \exp\sum(x_i)$, where exp[.] denotes [.] to the power of e. Therefore, after removing constants from the multiplicative sum, Equation {3.33} becomes:

$$L = (2\pi)^{-N/2} (\prod \sigma_i^2)^{-\frac{1}{2}} \exp\left[-\sum (-(y_i-\mu_i)^2/2\sigma_i^2)\right] \qquad \{3.34\}$$

Since $\prod \sigma_i^2 = |V|$, where $|V|$ is the determinant of V (Searle, 1982), Equation {3.34} can be written in matrix notation as follows:

$$L = (2\pi)^{-N/2} |V|^{-\frac{1}{2}} \exp\left[-\tfrac{1}{2}(y - X\beta)'V^{-1}(y - X\beta)\right] \qquad \{3.35\}$$

As noted in Equation {3.3}, for the mixed model:

$$V = ZGZ' + R = Z(A\sigma_u^2)Z' + I\sigma_e^2 \qquad \{3.36\}$$

The natural log of the likelihood function is as follows:

$$\text{Log } L = -(N/2)\ln(2\pi) - \tfrac{1}{2}\ln|V| - \tfrac{1}{2}(y - X\beta)'V^{-1}(y - X\beta) \qquad \{3.37\}$$

In theory, ML estimates can now be derived by differentiating the right-hand side of Equation {3.37} with respect to β, σ_u^2, and σ_e^2; and setting these derivatives equal to zero. However, the ML solutions for β are themselves functions of the variance components. Therefore an iterative solution will be necessary. Differentiating {3.37} with respect to β gives:

$$\partial (\log L)/\partial \beta = -2X'V^{-1}(y - X\beta) \qquad \{3.38\}$$

Setting this derivative equal to zero, and solving for β gives:

$$\hat{\beta} = (X'\hat{V}^{-1}X)^{-1} X'\hat{V})^{-1}y \qquad \{3.39\}$$

where $\hat{\beta}$ and $\hat{V}$ are the estimates of β and V. Equations {3.39} are the generalized least-squares solutions given in the previous chapter, except that V is replaced by $\hat{V}$. As noted above, these solutions are functions of the estimates of the variance components. Differentiating Log L with respect to the variance requires the derivatives of $|V|$ and V^{-1}. For any square matrix, M, the derivatives of $|M|$ and M^{-1} with respect to a scalar x are computed as follows (Searle, 1982):

$$\partial (\ln|M|)/\partial x = \text{tr}(M^{-1}\partial M/\partial x) \qquad \{3.40\}$$

$$\partial M^{-1}/\partial x = M^{-1}(\partial M/\partial x)M^{-1} \qquad \{3.41\}$$

Using these equations, the derivative of log L with respect to σ_i^2, the vector of variance components is:

$$\partial (\log L)/\partial \sigma_i^2 = -\tfrac{1}{2}\text{tr}(V^{-1}V_i) + \tfrac{1}{2}(y - X\hat{\beta})'V^{-1}V_iV^{-1}(y - X\hat{\beta})$$
$$+ \tfrac{1}{2}(\hat{\beta} - \beta)'X'V^{-1}V_iV^{-1}X(\hat{\beta} - \beta) \qquad \{3.42\}$$

where $V_i = \partial V/\partial \sigma_i^2 = I$ for $\sigma_i^2 = \sigma_e^2$ and $V_i = Z'AZ$ for $\sigma_i^2 = \sigma_u^2$. Setting these equations equal to zero, $\beta = \hat{\beta}$, and rearranging, this equation becomes:

$$\text{tr}(\hat{V}^{-1}V_i) = (y - X\hat{\beta})'\hat{V}^{-1}V_i\hat{V}^{-1}(y - X\hat{\beta}) \qquad \{3.43\}$$

For σ_e^2 Equation {3.43} becomes:

$$\mathrm{tr}(\hat{\mathbf{V}}^{-1}) = (\mathbf{y} - \mathbf{X}\hat{\boldsymbol{\beta}})'\hat{\mathbf{V}}^{-1}\hat{\mathbf{V}}^{-1}(\mathbf{y} - \mathbf{X}\hat{\boldsymbol{\beta}})$$ {3.44}

and for σ_u^2 Equation {3.43} becomes:

$$\mathrm{tr}(\hat{\mathbf{V}}^{-1}\mathbf{ZAZ'}) = (\mathbf{y} - \mathbf{X}\hat{\boldsymbol{\beta}})'\hat{\mathbf{V}}^{-1}\mathbf{ZAZ'}\hat{\mathbf{V}}^{-1}(\mathbf{y} - \mathbf{X}\hat{\boldsymbol{\beta}})$$ {3.45}

Equations {3.44} and {3.45} are functions of both $\hat{\boldsymbol{\beta}}$ and $\hat{\mathbf{V}}^{-1}$, which appears on both sides of these equations. Furthermore, $\hat{\mathbf{V}}^{-1}$ is a non-linear function of the variance components. Thus iterative solutions are required to solve these non-linear equations. The methods described in the previous chapter for iteration of non-linear equations can be used.

3.15 Restricted maximum likelihood estimation of variance components

The problem with standard ML estimation can be explained by considering the maximum likelihood estimation (MLE) of the variance for a normal distribution derived in the previous chapter. This estimate is: $(1/N)\Sigma(y_i - \mu)^2$. Thus, the estimate of the variance is a function of μ, the actual mean, which is unknown. For standard estimation of variance from a sample this problem is solved by replacing μ by the sample mean, and dividing by N–1, instead of N. Dividing by N–1 accounts for uncertainty in the value of the true mean. In mixed model variance component estimation, a parallel problem is encountered in that MLE assumes that the fixed effect solutions are equal to the true values.

In REML this problem is solved by a linear transformation of the observations that removes the fixed effects from the model. Consider the general mixed model given in Equations {3.2}. Define a matrix $\mathbf{K}$ such that $\mathbf{KX} = 0$. Then:

$$\mathbf{y^*} = \mathbf{Ky} = \mathbf{KZu} + \mathbf{Ke}$$ (3.46)

Searle *et al.* (1992) show that $\mathbf{K}$ satisfies the following relationship:

$$\mathbf{P} = \mathbf{K'}(\mathbf{KVK'})^{-1}\mathbf{K}$$ {3.47}

where:

$$\mathbf{P} = \mathbf{V}^{-1} - \mathbf{V}^{-1}\mathbf{X}(\mathbf{X'V}^{-1}\mathbf{X})^{-1}\mathbf{XV}^{-1}$$ {3.48}

So that:

$$\mathbf{y^{*'}V^{*-1}y^{*}} = (\mathbf{y'K'})(\mathbf{KVK'})^{-1}\mathbf{K}(\mathbf{Ky}) = \mathbf{y'Py}$$ {3.49}

Substituting **Ky** for **y**, **KX** = 0 for **X**, **KZ** for **Z**, and **KVK'** for **V** in Equations {3.43} gives the following REML variance component estimators:

$$\text{tr}(\hat{\mathbf{P}}) = \mathbf{y'}\hat{\mathbf{P}}\hat{\mathbf{P}}\mathbf{y} \quad \{3.50\}$$

For σ_e^2 and:

$$\text{tr}(\hat{\mathbf{P}}\mathbf{ZAZ'}) = \mathbf{y'}\hat{\mathbf{P}}\mathbf{ZAZ'}\hat{\mathbf{P}}\mathbf{y} \quad \{3.51\}$$

for σ_u^2. As in the case of ML, these non-linear equations can only be solved by iteration. Estimates of REML variance components can be obtained by derivative-based and derivative-free methods (see Lynch and Walsh, 1998, for a detailed explanation).

3.16 The problem of variance components outside the parameter space

In the previous chapter we noted that ML estimators could be biased. However, an important advantage of ML (and REML) methods is that all parameters estimates must lie within the parameter space. At first glance this property seems trivial. However, for multitrait models, especially models with more than two traits, it is very unlikely that the matrix of variance component estimates derived by other methods, such as Henderson's method III, will in fact be a valid variance component matrix.

We first note that for a valid variance component matrix, all estimated variances must be positive, and all correlations, as estimated from the variance and covariances, must be within the range of –1 to 1. However, these conditions are not sufficient. A valid variance matrix must be positive definite, and at least positive semi-definite. That is, all the eigenvalues must be positive, or at least non-negative. Henderson (1984) gives an example of the three-trait "pseudo" variance matrix for which all the variances are positive, and all the correlations are in the permissible range. However, this matrix is not a valid variance matrix, because one of the eigenvalues is negative. The diagonal elements of the inverse of this matrix are negative. Therefore, if this matrix is used to compute the genetic variance matrix in the mixed model equations, the solutions for individuals that are related would be less similar than the solutions for unrelated animals!

It should be noted that even if the variance components are computed by a ML type method, this does not guarantee that functions of the variance components will also lie within the permissible parameter space. For example, in a sire model the heritability is generally estimated as four times the sire component of variance divided by the sum of all the variance components. Although heritability must be less than 1, there is no guarantee that the heritability estimate derived from REML estimates of the variance components will lie within the parameter space.

3.17 Summary

Analysis of mixed models is much more complicated than analysis of fixed models. These models are preferred for genetic analysis, first because they utilize information on genetic variance and genetic relationships among animals that cannot be utilized by fixed models. Second, random effect solutions are regressed towards the mean. That is, the variance of the solutions increase as a function of the quantity of information included in the analysis. This allows for accurate comparison of the genetic values of individuals with widely differing amounts of information. The opposite is true of fixed model solutions. Their variances decrease as the amount of information increases. Finally, for random effects, regressions of the true effect values on their predictors are equal to unity. These properties will be considered relative to estimation of QTL effects in Chapter seven.

Methods were presented to estimate the variance components of random effects based on ML and REML. The REML equations are non-linear, and are themselves functions of the parameter estimates. Therefore these equations can only be solved by iteration. If QTL effects are considered random, it will also be necessary to estimate their variance via REML.

Chapter four:

Experimental Designs to Detect QTL; Generation of Linkage Disequilibrium

4.1 Introduction

Generally both natural and commercial populations are at linkage equilibrium for the vast majority of the genome. Therefore, even if a segregating genetic marker is linked to a QTL segregating in the population with an effect on some trait of interest, in most cases no effect will be associated with the marker genotypes, because the QTL and marker alleles will be independently assorted. In analysis of inbred lines we are confronted with the opposite problem. That is, a significant effect associated with a genetic marker may be due to many genes throughout the genome, and not necessarily to genes linked to the genetic markers. Thus, to detect the effect of a single QTL in outbred populations it is necessary to generate linkage disequilibrium. In crosses between inbred lines it is necessary to devise an experimental design that isolates the effects of the chromosomal segments linked to the segregating genetic markers.

The statistical methods used to detect QTL have generally been "parametric". That is, they were based on assumptions as to the nature of the distributions of the observations. An exception is the sib-pair analysis of Haseman and Elston (1972). In Section 4.2 we will describe the "usual" assumptions underlying the methods used to detect QTL, the types of effects postulated, and the types of data sets used. Models for QTL detection and analysis based on crosses between inbred lines will be considered in Sections 4.3 and 4.4. Models based on segregating populations will be considered in Sections 4.4 to 4.7, and models based on information derived from additional generations will be considered in Section 4.8. Comparison of the expected contrasts for different experimental designs will be considered in Section 4.9, and the final section of this chapter will explain the gametic effect model, which can be used for complete population analyses

4.2 Assumptions, problems and types of effects postulated

A large number of experimental designs and statistical methodologies have been suggested to detect the individual genes affecting quantitative traits with the aid of genetic markers. All of the experimental designs postulated have several elements in common, and these will now be reviewed briefly. The putative QTL is assumed to be genetically linked to a marker, with recombination frequency of r. *A priori*, we will assume only two alleles segregating in the population for both the marker locus, M, and the QTL locus, Q. The marker locus genotypes will be denoted M_1M_1, M_1M_2, and M_2M_2. The QTL genotypes will be denoted Q_1Q_1, Q_1Q_2, and Q_2Q_2, with expected effects of a, d, and –a, respectively, on the quantitative trait. If an individual is heterozygous for both loci, half of the progeny will receive the allele M_1, and half M_2. M and Q are assumed to be linked with recombination frequency equal. The parental genotypes are: $M_1Q_1|M_1Q_1$, and $M_2Q_2|M_2Q_2$. Therefore, except for recombinants, those progeny that receive M_1 will also receive Q_1, while those individuals that receive M_2 will also receive Q_2. Thus, the effect of the QTL can be detected by comparing the mean of the progeny groups that receive the alternative alleles from the heterozygous parent. The various designs suggested differ in the methods used to create the parent heterozygous for both loci and the crosses performed.

Most theoretical and experimental studies that have dealt with the detection of linkage between QTL and genetic markers have not been careful to rigorously list the assumptions on which they based their analyses, although there are exceptions. A number of assumptions have been employed in most analyses, and we will first list these "usual" assumptions. We will then describe some of the ramifications of these assumptions, and also note the studies that attempted to remove or test some of these assumptions. The usual assumptions are:

1. Both the M and Q loci segregate according to Mendelian principles.
2. The residual variance for the quantitative trait has a normal distribution.
3. No selection for either markers or QTL.
4. Only a single segregating QTL is linked to each marker or marker pair.
5. The genetic markers do not have pleiotropic effects on the quantitative traits.
6. Only two QTL alleles are segregating in the population.
7. No interactions among QTL alleles (dominance).
8. No interactions between the QTL and other loci (epistasis).
9. No interactions between the QTL and other, non-genetic, factors.
10. The QTL has only an additive effect on the quantitative trait.

The first assumption refers to the generally accepted principles of Mendelian genetics, i. e., equal probability that either chromosome of a pair will be transmitted to the zygote, and random assortment of homologous chromosomes in meiosis. A large body of data supports the generality of these principles, although exceptions have been found in certain cases, for example meiotic drive. Equal viability of all genotypes and complete penetrance for the genetic marker have been generally assumed. (Genetic "penetrance" is defined as the probability that a genotype is expressed phenotypically.) In one test of these assumptions, five out of 10 genetic markers displayed significant deviations from the expected Mendelian ratios

(Weller et al., 1988), but this may be due to unequal viability of phenotypes.

Nearly all analyses have assumed that, except for the effect of the segregating QTL, the underlying distribution of the trait is normal. This assumption is required for both ANOVA and is generally made for ML analyses. A few early studies that did not require this assumption are those that used the method of moment estimation (Zhuchenko et al., 1979a), χ^2, and the sib-pair method (Haseman and Elston, 1972). These methods are non-parametric, and do not depend on the nature of the distribution. Recently additional non-parametric methods have been proposed, and methods have also been proposed specifically for traits with discrete distributions (Hackett and Weller, 1995). These methods will be discussed in Chapter six. Theoretically, ML could be employed if some underlying distribution other than the normal distribution was postulated, but this has rarely been done in practice. Methods to test for deviations from normality are available but are not powerful for samples of moderate size. Weller et al. (1988) tested 18 quantitative traits, and found a number of traits with significant skewness and kurtosis; one trait had significant kurtosis even though the distribution was symmetrical. Even if a trait does have a normal distribution when measured on one scale, measuring the trait on a different scale can result in a skewed distribution. Either a power or logarithmic transformation of the data can generally alleviate this problem. Both types of transformations were employed to obtain distributions with virtually zero skewness (Weller et al., 1988).

Similar to natural selection, artificial selection can distort Mendelian ratios. Also, if selection is practiced for both QTL and genetic markers, then the distributions of the two loci may display a dependency, even if the loci are not linked. Most studies have not accounted for artificial selection of the genetic markers and the quantitative traits.

Most studies that have attempted to map QTL have assumed that there was only a single QTL linked to the genetic marker. The assumption of a single QTL is quite difficult to test if the two QTL are tightly linked. Soller and Genizi (1978) employed the heuristic argument that if the number of detectable segregating QTL is low, and these loci are randomly distributed, then the probability of two loci being closely genetically linked will be low. It should also be noted that two tightly linked QTL will give results similar to a single locus for most experimental designs employed. Several studies have proposed analysis methods for several loosely linked QTL segregating on the same chromosome. These studies will be considered in Chapter six.

It has also generally been assumed that the genetic marker does not have a pleiotropic effect on the quantitative trait, although methods have been devised to test this assumption (Bovenhuis and Weller, 1994). Most studies have also assumed that only two QTL alleles were segregating in the test population. This assumption is not problematic for crosses between highly inbred lines, since each line should be homozygous for a single allele. It may, however, not be appropriate for analysis of populations that are either outbred or only moderately inbred. Fernando and Grossman (1989) proposed a model for outbred populations that estimates the variance due to a QTL. This model is not dependent on the number of QTL alleles segregating in the population, and will be discussed in detail in Section 4.10.

Most analyses have assumed that the effect of the QTL on the quantitative trait was additive. That is, the only effect of allele substitution is on the mean of the quantitative trait. A few studies have considered QTL variance effects, and a rather large number of significant effects have been found (Edwards *et al.*, 1987; Weller *et al.*, 1988; Zhuchenko *et al.*, 1979b). An effect on the trait variance can be considered a multiplicative effect. Only Zhuchenko *et al.* (1979b) considered higher order QTL effects. For example, if the effect of gene substitution is non-linear, then the QTL could affect both the skewness and kurtosis of the distribution.

If the mean QTL effect is small relative to the trait mean in the population, then a QTL with a multiplicative effect will give results similar to an additive QTL. For example assume three individuals with trait values of 90, 100, and 110, and that the effect of QTL allele substitution is an increase of the trait value by 10%. The trait values obtained by substitution of a single allele will be 99, 110, and 121 for these three individuals. Thus the QTL substitution effect measured on an additive scale are 9, 10, and 11, which are very close to the values that would be obtained by a QTL with an additive effect of 10 units.

Finally most analyses have ignored both within loci interactions (dominance), and between loci interactions (epistasis), even though significant dominance and epistasis effects have been found. Dominance effects in an F-2 design will also affect the within marker-genotype variance for the quantitative trait.

In Chapter two we considered the property of "robustness". That is, how well do analysis methods perform if they are based on incorrect assumptions? A few studies have addressed the question of robustness of QTL analysis methods. These studies have found that both type I and type II errors may be much larger than the assumed values. Martinez and Curnow (1992) found that a "ghost" QTL will be detected in a bracket between two markers if two QTL are located outside the bracket on either side. Kennedy *et al.* (1992) demonstrated that for a segregating population, estimates of QTL effects would be biased for a population under selection if polygenic variance is ignored in the analysis model. On the other hand, Darvasi (1990) found that analysis with a model that assumes equal variance among QTL genotypes yields reliable results even if this assumption is incorrect. Aparametric analysis methods that do not require the assumption of underlying normality will also be considered in Chapter six.

4.3 Experimental designs for detection of QTL in crosses between inbred lines

Most early analyses performed to detect QTL have been based on planned crosses, although studies on humans, large farm animals, and trees have used existing populations. An overview of the basic experimental designs that have been used to detect segregating QTL is given in Figure 4.1. These designs can be divided into designs that are appropriate for crosses between inbred lines, and those designs that can be used for segregating populations.

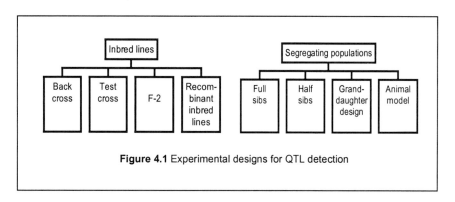

Figure 4.1 Experimental designs for QTL detection

We will first discuss the simpler case of crosses between inbred or haploid lines. As stated above, the first step is to cross two lines differing in genetic makers to produce heterozygous F-1 progeny. After this step the following progeny types have been considered for analysis:

1. Backcrossing (BC) the F-1 individuals to one of the parental strains.
2. F-2 individuals produced by self-breeding among the F-1 individuals, or intercrossing them.
3. Recombinant inbred lines produced by several generations of self-breeding individual F-2 progeny, or by brother-sister matings, where self-breeding is not possible (RILF).
4. Recombinant inbred lines produced from single backcross individuals, or brother-sister matings (RILB).
5. Doubled haploid (DH) lines produced by self-fertilizing DH derived from the F-1.
6. Testcross (TC) progeny produced by mating the F-1 individuals to a third inbred line.

More complicated designs can be considered, but these are basically variations of the designs listed above.

Biological, economic, genetic, and statistical considerations have been used to choose the experimental design. Biological considerations are that not all designs are possible with all species, for example, DH. For certain species with almost complete self-fertilization, it is much easier to produce large numbers of F-2 individuals, than either BC or TC, which require cross-fertilization. For outbreeding species, inbreeding can result in reduced fitness, due to the presence of recessive deleterious genes in the population.

The economic value of the possible crosses may be quite different. For example, if the goal is to introgress genes for a specific trait from a wild strain into a cultivar, the BC to the cultivar will have much greater economic interest than the F-2. Marker-assisted introgression will be discussed in detail in Chapter 16. The major reason for a TC-type analysis will also be the expected economic value obtained by crossing these three strains.

"Genetic" considerations refer to which genetic parameters will be estimable. For, example, dominance relationships cannot be estimated from either BC or TC analyses. "Statistical" considerations refer to selecting the design that maximizes power to detect QTL effects within the constraints imposed. For example, in the recombinant inbred and DH experimental designs, all individuals within the line will have the same genotype. Thus, it will be necessary to genotype only a single individual of each line, while the phenotypic performance of all individuals can be used to determine the QTL effect. Therefore, statistical power is increased per individual genotyped, but not per individual phenotyped. These considerations will be considered in more detail in Chapter eight.

4.4 Linear model analysis of crosses between inbred lines

Most statistical analyses of QTL effect have used a linear model. That is, the phenotype of each individual is modelled as a linear function of the marker genotypes, other "nuisance" variables that must be included in the model, and the residual, unexplained, variance.

We will consider the linear model in detail for by BC and F-2 designs. The BC design is illustrated in Figure 4.2. Two parental strains differing in both marker and QTL genotypes are mated to produce an F-1. It is generally assumed that the two parental strains are homozygous for alternate alleles of both loci. Thus all F-1 individuals will have the same heterozygous genotype. The F-1 is then mated to one of the parental strains. The genetic background for this cross is then three-quarters of the recurrent parent, and one-quarter of the other parent. The BC progeny are divided into two groups, based on their marker genotypes. As in all other experimental designs that will be considered, all loci not linked to the genetic marker under consideration should be randomly distributed among the marker genotype groups. With a single marker there are only two marker genotype groups for the BC design, and only a single contrast can be tested, the difference between the means of the two progeny marker genotype classes.

For the BC design, most studies have used simple variations of the following model:

$$Y_{ijk} = M_i + B_j + e_{ijk} \qquad \{4.1\}$$

where Y_{ijk} is the trait value for the kth individual of the jth "block" and the ith genotype, M_i is the effect of the ith marker genotype M_1M_2 or M_2M_2, B_j is the effect of the jth "block" and e_{ijk} is the random residual associated with each individual. The "block" effect represents all environmental effects that groups of individuals may have in common, such as row, field block, herd, season of growth, etc. (For simplicity, we have not included a "general mean" effect in the model. This effect can be considered included in the block effect. We will follow this convention for the other models considered below.) As noted above, both

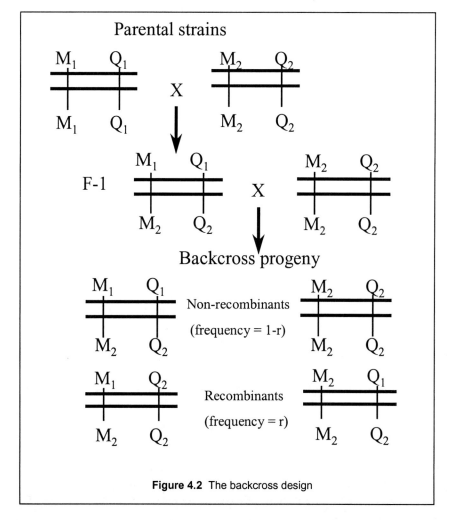

Figure 4.2 The backcross design

the marker and blocks are assumed to affect only the trait mean.

Significance of the genotype effect can be tested by two simple methods: analysis of variance (ANOVA), or a t-test of an "estimable" contrast. For ANOVA the ratio of the marker mean-squares to the residual mean-squares is computed. Under the null hypothesis of no segregating QTL this ratio will have a central F-distribution. A significant deviation of this statistic from the central F-distribution is indicative of a segregating QTL. For the t-test, the difference between the mean of two genotype classes is divided by the standard error of this contrast. Under the null hypothesis, this statistic will have a central t-distribution, with degrees of freedom equal to the total number of individuals included in the comparison minus two. The main advantages of linear model analysis are that they can be readily performed by most commonly used statistical packages, and significance and power can be computed analytically. The disadvantages are as follows:

1. The estimated effect is confounded with the effect of recombination between the QTL and the genetic marker, and is therefore a biased estimate of the actual QTL effect. This estimate is also not "consistent", as defined in Chapter two. No matter how large the sample, the estimate does not tend towards the true QTL effect.
2. Residuals are assumed to be normally distributed with equal variance. If this is not true, then tests of significance can yield incorrect results.
3. The independent variables are assumed to be uncorrelated. Therefore the method is inappropriate for multiple linked markers, which are of course correlated.
4. The method does not distinguish between a linked QTL and a pleiotropic effect of the genetic marker.

The QTL genotype probability given marker genotypes, and the expectations of the trait value for each marker genotype are given in Table 4.1. Assuming incomplete linkage between the QTL and the genetic marker, each BC marker genotype class will consist of two QTL genotypes, with frequencies of r and 1–r respectively. The expectation of the trait value for each marker genotype class is then computed as the sum of the conditional probabilities of each QTL genotype multiplied by its expectation. All expectations for all designs presented will be given relative to the mean of the two QTL homozygote genotypes.

The expectation for the contrast between the means of the marker genotype heterozygote and homozygote is computed as the difference between the expectations, and its value as shown in Table 4.1 is: $(1-2r)(d+a)$. The term: $1-2r$ will appear in most marker genotype contrasts. When $r = 0$, the contrast will be $d+a$, i. e. the complete QTL effect, and when $r = 0.5$, i. e. no linkage between the marker and the QTL, the value of the contrast will be zero. As noted above, for the BC design there is only one estimable contrast. Since this contrast is a function of a, d, and r, these parameters are confounded in the linear model BC analysis, and cannot be estimated separately.

Table 4.1 Backcross design genotype probabilities and quantitative trait expectations

Marker genotype	QTL genotype	QTL probability given marker genotype	Trait value	Marker genotype trait expectation
M_1M_2	Q_1Q_2	$1-r$	d	$d - r(d+a)$
	Q_2Q_2	R	$-a$	
M_2M_2	Q_2Q_2	$1-r$	$-a$	$-a + r(d+a)$
	Q_1Q_2	R	d	
Contrast $(M_1M_2 - M_2M_2)$				$(1-2r)(d+a)$

We will now consider the F-2 design illustrated in Figure 4.3. As in the previous case, two homozygous parents are crossed to produce a heterozygous F-1. The F-1 progeny are then selfed, or mated with each other to produce F-2 progeny. There are three marker genotypes in the F-2 progeny. Only the non-recombinant progeny types are shown. Unlike the BC design, recombination in either chromosome will effect the expectation of the trait value. The possible genotypes, their probabilities, and their expectations for the quantitative trait are given in Table 4.2.

In this design the probability of heterozygotes for the marker locus is 0.5, but most of the information with respect to QTL detection is in the homozygotes. As for the BC design, the marker-genotype class trait expectation is computed as the sum of the conditional probabilities of each QTL genotype multiplied by its expectation. For the F-2 design and incomplete linkage, all three QTL genotypes are possible for each marker genotype.

Significance of a segregating QTL can be tested by ANOVA including all three genotypes. In addition, several contrasts can be tested by t-test. The main contrast of interest is between the mean of the two homozygotes, and its value as given in Table 4.2 is $2a(1-2r)$. Note that, similar to the BC design, this contrast includes the term $1-2r$, but is not a function of d. However, a and r are still confounded.

Significance of the contrast between either marker homozygote and the heterozygote is also estimable, and can be tested by a t-test. The expectation of the difference between the M_1M_1 homozygote and the marker heterozygote is: $a(1-2r) - d(1-2r)^2$. This contrast is a confounded function of a, d, and r, and is therefore of little practical interest. However, significance of a dominance effect

Chapter four: Experimental Designs to Detect QTL 57

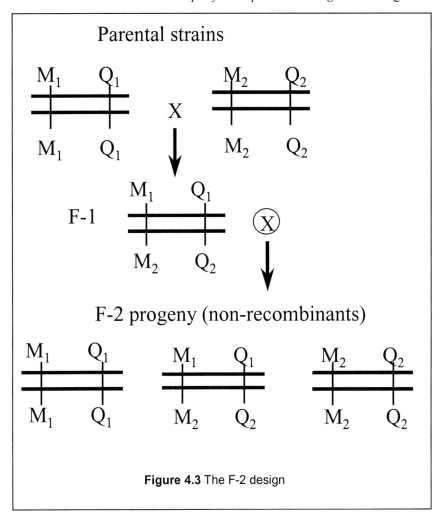

Figure 4.3 The F-2 design

can be tested as half the difference between the homozygote mean contrast and the heterozygote mean. This contrast will have a value of $-d(1-2r)^2$, and is thus also a function of $1-2r$, but is not dependent on a. Therefore, although it is possible to test for significance of additive and dominance effects, neither can be unbiasedly estimated by linear model analyses.

4.5 Experimental designs for detection of QTL in segregating populations - general considerations

For humans, most species of domestic animals, and fruit trees it is impractical to produce the inbred lines, which are the basis of the experimental designs described above. Instead experimental designs have been based on the analysis of families within existing populations. Three basic types of analyses have been proposed, the "sib-pair" analysis for analysis of many small full-sib families, the "full-sib" design for analysis of large full-sib families, and the "half-sib" or "daughter design" analysis for large half-sib families.

Table 4.2 F-2 design genotype probabilities and quantitative trait expectations

Marker genotype	Marker genotype probability	QTL genotype	QTL probability given marker genotype	Trait value	Marker genotype trait expectation
M_1M_1	1/4	Q_1Q_1	$(1-r)^2$	a	$a(1-2r)+$
		Q_1Q_2	$2r(1-r)$	d	$2dr(1-r)$
		Q_2Q_2	r^2	$-a$	
M_1M_2	1/2	Q_1Q_1	$r(1-r)$	a	$d(1-2r+2r^2)$
		Q_1Q_2	$1-2r+2r^2$	d	
		Q_2Q_2	$r(1-r)$	$-a$	
M_2M_2	1/4	Q_1Q_1	r^2	a	$-a(1-2r)+$
		Q_1Q_2	$2r(1-r)$	d	$2dr(1-r)$
		Q_2Q_2	$(1-r)^2$	$-a$	
Contrast $(M_1M_1 - M_2M_2)$					$2a(1-2r)$

Unlike crosses between inbred lines, not all markers will be "informative" in all progeny. A marker is considered informative if it can be unequivocally determined which parental allele was passed to the progeny (Da et al., 1999). Therefore if the genotyped parent is homozygous for the marker, it will not be informative in any of the progeny, because it will not be possible to determine which paternal allele was passed. Even if both parent and progeny are heterozygous, the marker still may not be informative. If only one parent is genotyped, and the progeny has the same genotype as its parent, the progeny could have received either allele from the sire or the dam. The expected frequency of individuals for which allele origin can be determined will be: $1-(p+q)/2$, where p and q are the frequencies of the two parental marker alleles.

Therefore, if only two marker alleles are present in the population, then half the daughters will have the same genotype as the sire, regardless of the allele frequencies among the dams. For multiallelic loci, such as microsatellites, p+q can be much less than one.

These calculations assume that the parent of interest is heterozygous, and the other parent was not genotyped. Planning an experiment, we can consider three situations of interest. First, it is possible to genotype either one or both parents. Second, if both parents are genotyped, it will be of interest to determine allele origin of either one or both of the progeny's alleles, depending on the experimental designs described below. The probability of obtaining a progeny for which allele origin of a single parent can be determined from a random mating is termed "polymorphism information content" (PIC) (Botstein *et al.*, 1980). The probability that allele origin of the progeny can be determined for both parents is termed the "proportion of fully informative matings" (PFIM) (Haseman and Elston, 1972). If both parents are genotyped, then PIC is computed as follows:

$$PIC_2 = 1 - \sum_{i=1}^{Na} p_i^2 - \sum_{i=1}^{Na-1} \sum_{j=i+1}^{Na} p_i^2 p_j^2 \qquad \{4.2\}$$

where PIC_2 = PIC with both parents genotype, Na is the number of marker alleles segregating in the population, and p_i is the frequency of allele i. If only a single parent is genotyped, then PIC is computed as follows:

$$PIC_1 = 1 - \sum_{i=1}^{Na} p_i^2 - \sum_{i=1}^{Na-1} \sum_{j=i+1}^{Na} p_i p_j (p_i + p_j) \qquad \{4.3\}$$

where PIC_1 = PIC with a single parent genotyped. For a given number of alleles, PIC will be maximum if the frequencies of all alleles is equal, that is: $p_1 = p_2 = \ldots = p_{Na} = 1/Na$. In this case, Equations {4.2} and {4.3} become:

$$PIC_2 = [(Na-1)^2(Na+1)]/Na^3 \qquad \{4.4\}$$

$$PIC_1 = [(Na-1)^2]/Na^2 \qquad \{4.5\}$$

For example with Na = 5, PIC_2 = 0.768, and PIC_1 = 0.64. PIC_2 will always be greater of equal to PIC_1.

PFIM is computed as follows (Gotz and Ollivier, 1992):

$$\text{PFIM} = \sum_{i=1}^{Na} \sum_{i=1}^{Na-1} p_i p_i \left[\left(\sum_{k=1}^{Na-1} \sum_{l=k+1}^{Na} 2p_k p_k \right) - 2p_i p_j \right] \quad \{4.6\}$$

with all alleles at equal frequency, this equation reduces to:

$$\text{PFIM} = [(Na-1)(Na-2)(Na+1)]/Na^3 \quad \{4.7\}$$

Using the same example of five alleles, PFIM = 0.576. PFIM will always be less or equal to both PIC_1 and PIC_2.

Records of uninformative progeny on heterozygous parents have generally been deleted. Although additional information can be extracted from these individuals (Dentine and Cowan, 1990), it will be considerably less than for individuals with known allele origin. With multiple linked markers, haplotypes consisting of several markers can be determined for each chromosomal segment. It will then be possible to determine parental origin of chromosomal segments with nearly complete certainty. Statistical methods that utilize this information will be considered in Chapter six.

4.6 Experimental designs for detection of QTL in segregating populations - large families

For large families, the full-sib and half-sib designs are most appropriate. We will first consider the half-sib or daughter design in detail. The daughter design, first proposed by Neimann-Soressen and Robertson (1961), has been used chiefly for dairy cattle in which a single sire can have hundreds or thousands of progeny with records on a number of quantitative traits, while each dam will have only a few progeny. The daughter design for a single family is illustrated in Figure 4.4. The daughters of a sire known to be heterozygous for a genetic marker are genotyped for the marker and scored for the quantitative trait. Since the dam genotypes are generally unknown and differ among individuals, the dam alleles for the marker locus and QTL are denoted M_x and Q_x, respectively.

If only progeny of a single parent are considered, then a marker-linked segregating QTL can be detected by analysis of the progeny records by the linear model given in Equation {4.1}, the only difference being that G_i now represents the allele substitution effect from the sire. If we assume that only the same two QTL alleles are present in the dam population, with frequencies of p and 1–p, then the trait value expectations for each progeny group can be computed, as shown in Table 4.3. The contrast between the two groups of progeny will be: $a(1-2r)+d(1-2r)(1-2p)$. If the frequency of the QTL two alleles is equal (p=0.5) then the contrast becomes: $a(1-2r)$, similar to the BC design. For the case of complete linkage (r=0) the contrast becomes: $a+d(1-2p)$. Defining the frequency

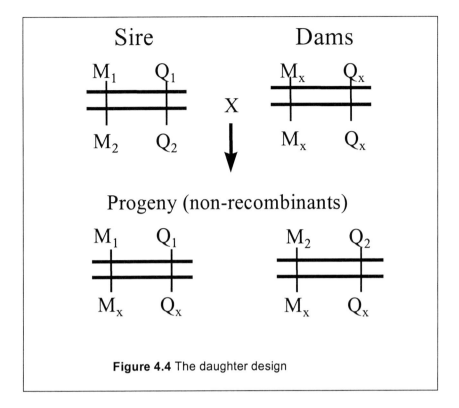

Figure 4.4 The daughter design

of the second allele as $q=1-p$, this formula becomes $a+d(q-p)$, which is the general formula for the effect of allele substitution (Falconer, 1981).

a, d, and p are confounded in a linear model analysis. It will be seen in Chapter six that with multiple families it is possible to estimate p by maximum likelihood. a and d are still confounded, unless the QTL alleles passed from the dams can also be identified, which is generally not possible for QTL.

Even if a QTL is segregating in the population, a specific parent may be homozygous for the QTL. Therefore, most studies have been based on analysis of number of heterozygous parents. In this case analysis by the model of Equation {4.1} can lead to incorrect conclusions. Even if several of the individuals analysed are heterozygous for a marker-linked QTL, the linkage relationships may be different for different individuals. Thus, summed over all progeny groups, there may be no effect associated with the segregating marker alleles. The appropriate linear model for the daughter design with multiple families is therefore as follows:

$$Y_{ijkl} = S_i + M_{ij} + B_k + e_{ijkl} \qquad \{4.8\}$$

where S_i is the effect of the ith parent, M_{ij} is the effect of the jth allele, nested within the ith parent, and the other terms are as defined above.

Table 4.3 Daughter design genotype probabilities and quantitative trait expectations

Paternal marker allele	Paternal QTL allele	Probability of paternal QTL allele	Maternal QTL allele	Probability of maternal QTL allele	Trait value	Marker genotype trait expectation
M_1	Q_1	1–r	Q_1	p	a	a(p–r) +
			Q_2	1–p	d	d(1–r–p+2rp)
	Q_2	R	Q_1	p	d	
			Q_2	1–p	–a	
M_2	Q_2	1–r	Q_1	p	d	a(r+p–1) +
			Q_2	1–p	–a	d(p+r–2rp)
	Q_1	r	Q_1	p	a	
			Q_2	1–p	d	

The progeny group inheriting sire allele M_1 and the group inheriting sire allele M_2 are compared. If the assumptions listed above hold, and if the distribution of dams between the two groups is random, then a difference between the two groups of progeny for the quantitative trait will be due to a QTL linked to M heterozygous in the sire. This assumes that marker allele origin can be determined for the daughters. Significance of a segregating QTL linked to the genetic marker can be tested by ANOVA. Under the null hypothesis of no segregating QTL the ratio of the marker allele effect mean-squares to the residual mean-squares should have a central F-distribution.

Actual analyses have generally been based on analysis of commercial populations, in which data are collected over many herds, and animal have multiple records. In this case the model of Equation {4.8} is not appropriate. This model does not accurately account for multiple records. Furthermore, if only a few cows are genotyped in each herd, it will not be possible to accurately estimate herd effects. Finally, this model assumes a random distribution of the dam additive genetic component, which may not be the case. Therefore, most studies that have analysed either the cows' yield deviations (VanRaden and Wiggans, 1991) or genetic evaluations, rather than phenotypic records. This question will be discussed in detail in Section 6.10.

Assuming that there are only two QTL alleles present with equal frequency in the population, and a Hardy-Weinberg distribution of genotypes, only half of the sires will be heterozygous for the QTL. Thus, the variance contributed by the A_{ij} term will be $a^2/8$. In addition to ANOVA, significance can be determined by a χ^2 test. The mean within-parent differences between the two progeny groups with opposing marker alleles are computed, and divided by their standard errors. Under the null hypothesis, the sum of squares of these statistics will have a χ^2 distribution, with degrees of freedom equal to the number of parents. Power as a function of sample size and QTL effect was estimated for both ANOVA (Soller and Genizi, 1978) and χ^2 (Weller et al., 1990).

We will briefly consider now analysis of large full-sib families. As with half-sib families, it will be possible that there are more than two QTL alleles segregating in the population. Thus, even within a single family, the two parents may be heterozygous for two different QTL alleles, and the four possible progeny QTL genotypes may each have a different value.

Similar to the half-sib design, not all progeny genotypes will be informative. In the "best" case the two parents have three or four different marker alleles, and the progeny can be divided into four different groups based on marker genotype. Significance can be determined by ANOVA considering the ratio of the parental allele effect to the residual. It will be possible to determine an allele substitution effect for each parent, but not an overall allelic effect. It will also be possible to estimate the total genetic variance associated with the genetic marker. An ANOVA analysis with marker effect nested within family is not appropriate for small full-sib families, such as in human populations, because of insufficient degrees of freedom. An alternative analysis strategy will now be described.

4.7 Experimental designs for detection of QTL in segregating populations - small families

Haseman and Elston proposed the sib-pair analysis method in 1972. This method is most appropriate for human populations in which many small full-sib families are available. The basic design is illustrated in Figure 4.5. In the simplest situation, the two parents have four different marker alleles denoted M_1, M_2, M_3, and M_4. We have also assumed that this locus is linked to a QTL also heterozygous in both parents. Three different sib-pairs are illustrated. For simplicity, only non-recombinants are shown. In sib-pair one, the two marker alleles of both individuals are identical by descent (IBD). Both individuals received the same two marker alleles from both parents. In sib-pair two, both sibs received allele M_1 from the father, but different alleles from the mother. Thus, one pair of alleles is IBD, while the other is not. In sib-pair three none of the marker alleles are IBD.

Assuming that the marker locus is linked to a segregating QTL, as illustrated in Figure 4.5, individuals with more marker loci IBD should also be more similar

64 *Quantitative Trait Loci Analysis in Animals*

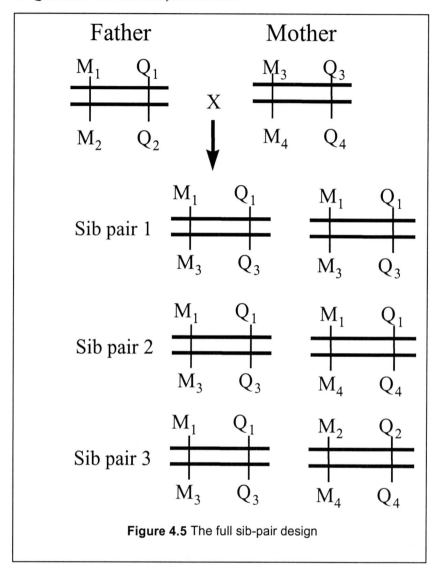

Figure 4.5 The full sib-pair design

for the quantitative trait. As in the case of large half-sib families, the analysis must take into account the family structure; a linked segregating QTL will not result in an overall marker genotype effect. Haseman and Elston (1972) therefore proposed the following statistical model. Define:

$$x_{1j} = \mu + g_{1j} + e_{1j}$$
$$x_{2j} = \mu + g_{2j} + e_{2j}$$

{4.9}

where: x_{1j} and x_{2j} are trait values for sibs 1 and 2 of family j, μ is the general mean, g_{ij} and e_{ij} are the direct QTL and residual effects for sib i.

We will first assume that QTL genotypes can be directly observed, and later consider analysis based on linked markers. For the previous models we considered the differences between genotypes means. With many small families this option is not viable. As noted above, some of the differences will be positive, and some will be negative. Therefore Haseman and Elston (1972) based their analysis on squared differences, which are always positive.

Let $Y_j = (x_{1j} - x_{2j})^2 = (g_{1j}+e_{1j}-g_{2j}-e_{2j})^2$. If the two sibs have both QTL alleles IDB then $g_{1j} = g_{2j}$ and $Y_j = (e_{1j}-e_{2j})^2$, which will be less than Y_j for sibs receiving different QTL alleles from their parents. With codominance or partial dominance, the expectation for Y_j for individuals receiving one allele IBD will be intermediate between individuals with zero or two allele IBD. Presence of a linked QTL can then be tested by the following regression:

$$Y_j = \alpha + \beta\pi_j \qquad \{4.10\}$$

where π_j is the fraction of marker alleles; 0, 1/2 or 1; IBD for sib-pair j; α is the y-intercept; and β is the regression, which will have a negative value. Presence of a linked segregating QTL can be tested by the value of β. Even with incomplete linkage between the marker and the QTL, this regression will still be negative. Under the null hypothesis, β should not be significantly different from zero.

Of course the expectation of β will depend on many factors, including recombination frequency between the QTL and the genetic marker, the number of QTL alleles segregating in the population, their frequencies, and dominance relationships among the alleles. Haseman and Elston (1972) were able to derive expectations for several simple cases of general interest.

First, still assuming complete linkage between the QTL and the genetic marker, we will also assume that there are only two QTL alleles segregating in the population with frequencies of p and q. We will further assume a Hardy-Weinberg distribution of genotypes, and that the population is at linkage equilibrium between the QTL and the genetic marker. As in the previous examples, the three QTL genotypes have expectations of a, d, and –a. Nine sib-pair combinations are possible for the three QTL genotypes. The expected frequencies of these combinations and their frequencies are given in Table 4.4.

The expectations for each value of π_j can be computed by multiplying the probabilities by the expectations of Y_j. These expectations are also given in Table 4.4. In the bottom line of the table, these expectations are given in terms of the additive genetic, and dominance variances contributed by the QTL, and residual variance, σ^2_e. The additive genetic variance, σ^2_a and dominance variance, σ^2_d are computed as follows (Falconer, 1981):

Table 4.4 The expected frequencies sib-pair QTL genotype combinations, and expectation of the squared differences (Y_j)

Sib-pair	Conditional probability (π_j)			Y_j
	0	½	1	
Q_1Q_1-Q_1Q_1	p^4	p^3	p^2	e_j^2
Q_2Q_2-Q_2Q_2	q^4	q^3	q^2	e_j^2
Q_1Q_2-Q_1Q_2	$4p^2q^2$	Pq	2pq	e_j^2
Q_1Q_1-Q_1Q_2	$2p^3q$	p^2q	0	$(a - d + e_j)^2$
Q_1Q_2-Q_1Q_1	$2p^3q$	p^2q	0	$(-a + d + e_j)^2$
Q_1Q_2-Q_2Q_2	$2pq^3$	pq^2	0	$(a + d + e_j)^2$
Q_2Q_2-Q_1Q_2	$2pq^3$	pq^2	0	$(-a - d + e_j)^2$
Q_1Q_1-Q_2Q_2	p^2q^2	0	0	$(2a + e_j)^2$
Q_2Q_2-Q_1Q_1	p^2q^2	0	0	$(-2a + e_j)^2$
$E(Y_j\|\pi_j)$	$e_j^2+4pq[a-(p-q)d]^2$ $+2pqd^2[1-(p-q)^2] =$ $\sigma_e^2 + 2\sigma_a^2+2\sigma_d^2$	$e_j^2+2pq[a-(p-q)d]^2$ $+2pqd^2[1-(p-q)^2] =$ $\sigma_e^2 + \sigma_a^2+2\sigma_d^2$	$e_j^2=\sigma_e^2$	

$$\sigma_a^2 = 2pq[a - (p-q)d]^2$$

$$\sigma_d^2 = 4p^2q^2d^2 \quad \{4.11\}$$

If there is a segregating QTL linked to the markers, $E(Y_j|\pi_j)$ will decrease monotonically with π_j unless $\sigma_a^2 = 0$. If $\sigma_d^2 = 0$, then $E(Y_j|\pi_j)$ can be described by the following linear function of π_j:

$$E(Y_j|\pi_j) = (\sigma_e^2 + 2\sigma_a^2) - 2\sigma_a^2 \pi_j \quad \{4.12\}$$

Thus $\alpha = \sigma_e^2 + 2\sigma_a^2$, and $\beta = -2\sigma_a^2$. Haseman and Elston (1972) show that with dominance, for large samples β tends to $-2\sigma_g^2$, where $\sigma_g^2 = \sigma_a^2 + \sigma_d^2$.

So far complete linkage between the QTL and the genetic marker was assumed. For incomplete linkage, but no dominance, and complete parental information, Haseman and Elston (1972) show that the expectation of β is equal to: $-2(1-2r)^2\sigma_a^2$. The algebra is rather complicated, and will not be presented here. "Complete parental information" means that the number of marker alleles IBD can be determined for each sib-pair. This will of course be the case for the example in Figure 4.5, in which the two parents have four different alleles. It will also be true if both parents are heterozygous, but have one allele in common. However, for any other combination of parental marker alleles, it will not be possible to determine the number of alleles IBD unequivocally for all possible sib-pair combinations. In these cases, Haseman and Elston (1972) demonstrate that π_j can be estimated as $f_{j2} + (1/2)f_{j1}$, where f_{j1} and f_{j2} are the probabilities that sib-pair j has one or two marker alleles IBD, respectively.

Note that unlike the previous models, the expectation for the different genotypic classes is now a function of the genetic variance, rather than a and d. In most realistic situations, the additive QTL effect will be less than the residual standard deviation. Thus, as we will show below, the sib-pair analysis method will have less statistical power than the other methods considered above.

Rather than a regression model, Y_j could also be analysed with the number of alleles IBD as a class effect. For incomplete dominance, the regression model will have greater power.

4.8 Experimental designs based on additional generations

All the designs considered so far are based on analysis of a single generation after production of the individuals heterozygous for both loci. Additional information can be obtained by analysis of further generations. We divide multi-generation designs into two categories: those in which future generations are scored for the quantitative traits and genotyped for the genetic markers; and those in which future generations are scored for the quantitative traits, but not genotyped for the markers. We will consider the latter case in detail, and then briefly consider the former case.

In many plant species, an F-3 progeny group can be readily produced from each F-2 individual. In the absence of selection or differential viability, the F-3 progeny group will have on the average the same frequency of alleles as the F-2 parent. Thus, the expected contrast will be equal to the F-2 design. However, the residual variance can be significantly reduced, because several F-3 trait phenotypes are scored for each F-2 genotype. All progeny of a specific F-2 individual will still share a common genetic component equal to half of the genetic variance, which will not be included in the residual variance. Thus, this design, and the grand-daughter design described below, are most useful for traits with low heritability.

For self-fertilizing plants it is possible to self-breed the F-2 or backcross progeny for several additional generations to produce recombinant inbred lines (RIL). Similar to the F-3 design, the residual variance is reduced, because many phenotypes can be obtained for a single genotype. An analysis based on RIL differs from the F-3 design in that instead of genotyping the F-2 parent, a single individual from each RIL is genotyped. Thus the effect associated with a genetic marker will be affected by recombination between the two loci in future generations. RIL will be considered in detail in Sections 6.13 and 8.3. RIL have the extra advantage that all individuals within the line are isogenic. Therefore it is possible to test the same genotype in different environments (Korol et al., 1998). Dominance cannot be estimated with RIL, because the QTL will be homozygous within each line.

For outcrossing species with limited female fertility, such as dairy cattle, genotypes can be determined on a sample of progeny of a heterozygous parent, and the quantitative traits can be scored on the grandprogeny (i. e. the progeny of genotyped offsprings of the heterozygous parent). This design is termed a "grand-daughter" design (Weller et al. 1990), as opposed to the "daughter" design described previously. The grand-daughter design is illustrated in Figure 4.6.

Sons of grandsires heterozygous for the genetic markers are genotyped, and the daughters of these sons, (i.e. the grand-daughters of the original grandsire) are scored for the quantitative traits. It is assume that both grandsire and son mates are random. This design is similar to the F-3 design in that the residual variance is reduced because many phenotypes are scored for each individual genotyped. However, the grand-daughter design differs from the F-3 design in that only half of the grand-daughters will receive the paternal allele. Therefore the expectation of the contrast between the grandprogeny groups is only half as large as for the daughter design. However, the much greater number of phenotypic records can more than compensate for the reduction in the contrast.

This design has the advantage that for certain species, especially dairy cattle, the commercial population has the appropriate population structure, and records on quantitative traits of interest are recorded by the industry. Furthermore, it may be logistically easier to obtain biological material from AI sires which are located at a few AI centers, rather than cows that are scattered over a large number of herds. A segregating marker-linked QTL can be detected with analysis by the following linear model:

$$Y_{ijklm} = GS_i + M_{ij} + SO_{ijk} + B_l + e_{ijklm} \qquad \{4.13\}$$

where GS_i is the effect of the ith grandparent, SO_{ijk} is the effect of the kth son with the jth marker allele, progeny of the ith grandparent, and the other terms are as defined for Equation {4.8}. As in the daughter design, a significant marker-allele effect will be indicative of a linked QTL. Significance of this effect can be tested by ANOVA, with the marker mean-squares in the numerator. However, this mean-squares will also include a component due to differences among sons. Thus, the denominator for the appropriate F-statistic will be a function of both the sons and residual mean-squares (Ron et al., 1994).

Alternatively, significance can be tested by a χ^2 analysis similar to the daughter design, as described by Weller et al. (1990). Increasing the number of grandprogeny will reduce the residual variation, but not between-progeny genetic variation. Thus, the advantage of the grand-daughter design is greater for low heritability traits.

Chapter four: Experimental Designs to Detect QTL 69

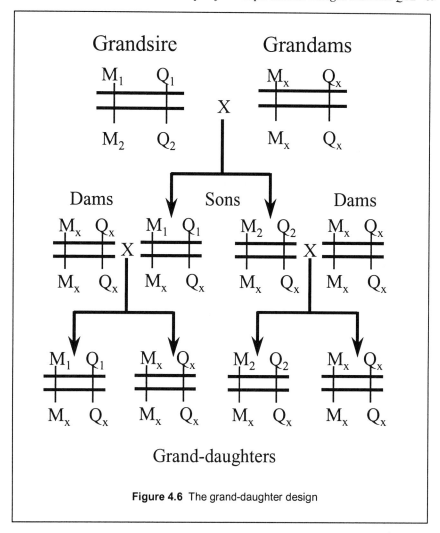

Figure 4.6 The grand-daughter design

Unlike the daughter design, it is not possible with the grand-daughter design to estimate dominance at the QTL. Even if the actual QTL alleles are identified, and both grandsires and grand-dams are genotyped, the expectation of the effect of the sons that are heterozygous for the QTL will still be midway between the two homozygous groups.

As noted above for the daughter design, the model of Equation {4.13} is generally not applied, because daughters have multiple records and it will not be possible to accurately estimate fixed effects. Generally either the genetic evaluations or the daughter-yield deviations (DYD) of the sons (VanRaden and Wiggans, 1991) will be analysed. In this case there is only a single record for each son, and the analysis model is as follows:

$$Y_{ijk} = GS_i + M_{ij} + e_{ijk} \quad \{4.14\}$$

where Y_{ijk} is the genetic evaluations or DYD for son k of grandsire i that received grandpaternal allele j, and the other terms are as defined in the previous equation. This model has been used very extensively in the literature, and will be considered in more detain in Section 6.10.

4.9 Comparison of the expected contrasts for different experimental designs

Although power of all the designs considered will be considered in more detail in Chapter eight, a comparison of the magnitude of the expected variance due to the QTL for various designs is given in Table 4.5. In all cases r=0 is assumed. For the segregating population designs, two segregating QTL alleles with equal frequency are assumed. Results are presented for the F-2 both for d=a, and d=0. Variances for all other designs were computed with d=0. Required sample sizes to achieve equal power are also given for a QTL with a substitution effect of 0.5. The magnitude of the substitution effect is critical only for the comparison of the full-sib design to the other designs.

Table 4.5 Expected variance due to the QTL, and required sample size for different designs

Design*	F-2 (d=a)	F-2	BC	Full-sibs	Half sibs	Grand-daughters
QTL Variance	$3a^2/2$	$a^2/2$	$a^2/4$	$a^4/8$	$a^2/8$	$a^2/32$
Required sample size†	1/3	1	2	16	4	16

*d = 0, unless otherwise indicated. a = 0.5.
† Relative to the F-2 design with d = 0.

Except for the full-sib design, the variance due to the QTL will be a function of a^2. Since the QTL effect will generally be small with respect to the residual standard deviation, the full-sib design will have a much smaller QTL variance than the other designs. With the exception of this design, the other designs are listed from the largest to the smallest QTL variance. As will be explained in Chapter eight, the variance due to the QTL is approximately inversely proportional to the sample size required to obtain a given power of QTL detection. Thus, the grand-daughter design will require approximately 16 times as many records to obtain the same power as the F-2 design with d=0.

If additional generations are both scored for the quantitative trait and genotyped, power of detection is not increased per individual genotyped, but accuracy of QTL mapping is increased, due to an additional generation of recombination. The advantage of additional generations with respect to QTL fine mapping will also be considered in detail in later Chapter ten.

4.10 Gametic effect models for complete population analyses

Mixed models including both fixed and random effects were considered in the previous chapter. In all the models considered above, the QTL was considered a fixed effect. Fernando and Grossman (1989) assumed that the QTL is a random effect with a known variance. They developed a method to estimate breeding values for all individuals in a population, including QTL via linkage to genetic markers, provided that the heritability and recombination frequency between the QTL and the genetic marker are known. Fernando and Grossman's method is based on Henderson's mixed model equations for the individual animal model (IAM).

The model of Fernando and Grossman (1989) is suitable for any population structure, and also can incorporate non-linked polygenic effects and other "nuisance" effects, such as herd or block. The model as described below assumes only a single record per individual, but can be readily adapted to a situation of multiple records per animal.

Each individual with unknown ancestors is assumed to have two unique alleles for the QTL, which are "sampled" from an infinite population of alleles. For each individual, they propose the following gametic model for the QTL, with separate effects for the sire and dam alleles:

$$y_i = B_i + v_i^p + v_i^m + u_i + e_i \qquad \{4.15\}$$

where B_i represents any fixed effects, v_i^p and v_i^m are the additive QTL effects received from the sire and dam, u_i is the random polygenic effect not explained by the genetic marker and e_i is the random residual. Assuming a single record per individual, this model can be written as follows in matrix notation:

$$y = XB + Wv_g + u + e \qquad \{4.16\}$$

where X and W are incidence matrices relating individuals to the specific block and gametic effects, and v_g is the vector of gametic additive genetic effects. The matrix **W** has rows equal to the number of records, and columns equal to twice the number of animals with records. Each row of **W** will have two non-zero elements corresponding to the two QTL allelic effect of each individual. An incidence matrix is not required for **u**, because each individual will have a different polygenic effect. Thus, an augmented set of mixed model equations with 2n additional equations, where n is the number of animals included in the analysis, can be constructed as follows:

$$\begin{bmatrix} X'X & X'W & X' \\ W'X & W'W + G_v^{-1}\sigma_e^2 & W' \\ X & W & I + G_u^{-1}\sigma_e^2 \end{bmatrix} \begin{bmatrix} B \\ v_g \\ u \end{bmatrix} = \begin{bmatrix} X'y \\ W'y \\ Y \end{bmatrix} \quad \{4.17\}$$

To solve these modified mixed model equations it is necessary to first construct G_v, and then invert both G_v and G_u. For animals that are not genotyped, the probability of receiving either allele from either parent will be equal. However, if both the parent and progeny are genotyped for a linked genetic marker, then the probability of receiving a specific parental allele for a QTL linked to the genetic marker will be a function of the progeny marker genotype and r. Based on these probabilities, Fernando and Grossman (1989) demonstrated how a variance-covariance matrix could be constructed for the QTL gametic effects. They further describe a simple algorithm to invert this matrix analogous to Henderson's method for inverting the numerator relationship matrix (Henderson, 1976). BLUP of **a**, the vector of additive genotypic values is estimated by: $W\hat{v} + \hat{u}$, where $\hat{v}$ and $\hat{u}$ and the estimates for **v** and **u**.

An additional advantage of this method is that by assuming random QTL effects, as opposed to fixed effects, the effects of the QTL with the largest estimates are not biased upwards (Georges et al., 1995; Smith and Simpson, 1986). This problem of bias with multiple QTL will be considered in detail in Chapters seven and eleven. This method has been extended to handle multiple markers and traits (Goddard, 1992). Cantet and Smith (1991) demonstrated that the number of equations could be significantly reduced by analysis of the reduced animal model (RAM), described in the previous chapter. These extensions of the Fernando and Grossman model will be considered in detail in Chapter seven.

Despite the attractive properties of this method, it has not as yet been applied to actual data. In addition to the huge computational requirements, this model assumes that both r and the variance due to the QTL are known *a priori*. With marker brackets the problem of estimating r is much less severe. Studies on simulated data demonstrate that although restricted maximum likelihood methodology can be used to estimate these parameters, they are completely confounded for a single marker locus (van Arendonk et al., 1994a). Methods to estimate the variance contributed by QTL with multiple markers were developed by Grignola et al. (1996a), and will also be considered in Chapter seven.

Furthermore, since each individual with unknown parents is assumed to have two unique alleles, the prediction error variances of the effects for any individual will be quite large, and therefore, not very informative. Finally, the assumption of a normal distribution of possible QTL allele effects may not be realistic. Simulation studies have attempted to estimate the effect of assuming only two QTL alleles segregating in the population if the actual number is greater (Grignola et al., 1996b).

4.11 Summary

Table 4.6 Summary of experimental designs for QTL detection

	Experimental designs*							
	Inbred lines				Segregating populations*			
Characteristics	BC	TC	F-2	RIL	FS	HS	GDD	GM
Power per trait record[†]	+++	+++	++	+	– –	–	– –	– – –
Power per genotyping	++	++	++	+++	– –	–	+	– – –
Power with high h^2	+	+	+	–	+	+	–	–
Power with low h^2	+	+	+	++	+	+	++	++
Dominance	No	no	yes	no	no	no	no	No
Use available records	No	no	no	no	some	some	some	all
Mating system	either	either	selfer	selfer	cross	cross	cross	cross

* BC = backcross, TC = testcross, RIL = recombinant inbred lines, FS = small full-sib families, HS = large half-sib families, GDD = grand-daughter design; GM = gametic model of Fernando and Grossman (1989).
[†] Power is graded from very high, +++, to very low, – – –.

The relative statistical power and other properties of the different experimental designs considered are summarized in Table 4.6. The optimal experimental design for a given situation will depend on the economic value of different strains, the relative cost of genotyping vs. scoring quantitative traits, what individuals are available for analysis, the type of mating prevalent in the species (self breeding vs. outbreeding), the relative fecundity of the two sexes, which individuals express traits and under what circumstances, and the possibility to exploit dominant genetic variance. The F-2 is the only design that can be used to estimate dominance directly. Although the inbred line designs have greater power both per individual genotyped and per individual phenotyped, they cannot be applied for analysis of human data or data from most farm animals. The statistical power of the various designs will be considered in more detail in Chapter eight.

Chapter five:

QTL Parameter Estimation for Crosses between Inbred Lines

5.1 Introduction

The main parameters that will be considered are means and variances of QTL genotypes, and recombination frequencies between the genetic markers and the QTL. From the previous chapter it should already be clear that estimation of QTL parameters is not trivial. The first problem encountered is that in nearly all cases of interest the variance due to the segregating QTL will be only a small fraction of the total phenotypic variance for the quantitative trait. As considered in detail in Chapter four, linkage between the genetic markers and QTL will be incomplete. Thus, recombination frequency must be included in the analysis, and consequently the analysis model will not be a linear function of the parameters. In crosses between inbred lines, all genetic factors not linked to the segregating markers will be randomly distributed, and can therefore be considered part of the residual variance.

In this chapter we will consider only the basic methods for QTL parameter estimation which are suitable for crosses between inbred lines. More advanced methods will be considered in Chapter six. In Section 5.2 we consider the moments method of estimation. In Sections 5.3 and 5.4 we will describe least-squared estimation, with focus on non-linear models. In Section 5.5 we will consider linear marker regression models, which give identical solutions to non-linear least-squares models, and can be solved analytically. In Section 5.6 we will explain the concept of marker information content for interval mapping. In Section 5.7 we will describe maximum likelihood (ML) QTL parameter estimation for crosses between inbred lines and a single marker, and in Section 5.8 we will describe test of significance for this analysis. In Section 5.9 we will consider ML models for QTL parameter estimation in crosses between inbred lines with two flanking markers, and in the following section we will discuss iterative methods for maximizing likelihood functions. Biases in estimation of QTL parameters with interval mapping will be considered in Section 5.11. In the last section we will consider the likelihood ratio test for single markers and interval mapping.

5.2 Moments method of estimation

This method is not currently in general use, and its interest can be considered purely historical. The method as proposed by Zhuchenko *et al.* (1979a) is based on the principle that even with recombination QTL parameters can be estimated by setting the empirical moments computed from the trait values to their expectations, computed as functions of the QTL parameters. The mth central moments of a sample, T^m, is computed as follows:

$$T^m = (1/N)\sum_{}^{N}(y - \bar{y})^m \quad \{5.1\}$$

where N is the sample size and $\bar{y}$ is the sample mean. The first central moment is equal to zero, and the second central moment is equal to the variance of the distribution. The statistics g_1 and g_2, which are used to estimate the skewness and kurtosis of the distribution, are derived from the third and fourth central moments, respectively.

Zhuchenko *et al.* (1979a) noted that for QTL detection in inbred lines with a single marker and incomplete linkage, the distributions of the marker genotypes will be skewed in opposite directions. This is illustrated in Figure 5.1 for one marker genotype of the backcross population described in Figure 4.1. As shown, assuming an underlying normal distribution, the marker genotype linked to the QTL with a negative effect on the mean will have positive skewness, while the genotype with the positive effect on the mean will have negative skewness.

In the previous chapter, it was demonstrated that the expectations for the marker genotype means could be computed as functions of the QTL genotype means and the recombination frequency. Similarly, the marker genotype variances and third moments can be computed as functions of the QTL genotype means, variances, and third moments. Assuming that the QTL genotypes have equal variances and third moments, we have a system of six equations: the two marker locus genotype means, the two variance, and the two third moments; with five unknowns: the two QTL genotype means, the residual variance and third moment, and the recombination frequency between the QTL and the marker loci. Although this system of equations will now be inconsistent, various techniques can be applied to obtain a solution.

The advantages of the moments method are that it is easy to apply, the estimates are unbiased, and no assumptions are made about the properties of the residual distributions. For example, it is not necessary to assume normality for the underlying distribution. The disadvantages are that parameter estimates outside the parameter space can be obtained, such as negative variance estimates, or recombination frequency outside the range of 0 to 0.5, and that not all information in the data is utilized. Zhuchenko *et al.* (1979b) applied several variations of this method to three tomato backcross (BC) populations scored for three markers and five quantitative traits. Most of the solutions obtained were outside the parameter space.

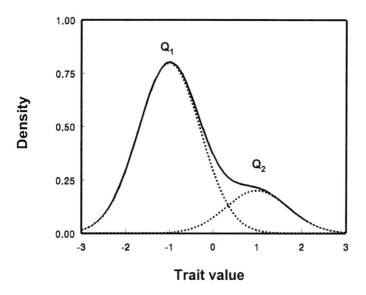

Figure 5.1 Distributions of quantitative trait value for marker genotype M_1M_2 from the backcross design illustrated in Figure 4.1. The allele Q_1 was linked to M_1 in the parental strain with 0.2 frequency of recombination. The effect of allele substitution was 2 standard deviations. The QTL genotype distributions are represented by dotted lines, and the marker genotype distribution by a solid line

5.3 Least-squares estimation of QTL parameters

As demonstrated in the previous chapter, the genotype means and variances and recombination frequencies cannot be described by a linear model of the trait values. Furthermore, as also noted in the previous chapter, within the context of least-squares estimation, genotype means and the recombination frequency between a QTL and a single marker are completely confounded, and cannot be estimated separately. With two markers flanking a QTL it is possible to derive separate estimates of genotype means and recombination frequencies, but it is not possible to construct a linear model that accurately describes the relationship between the observations and the QTL parameters, as will be explained below.

The non-linear least-squares method of QTL parameter estimation with two flanking markers was developed independently in 1992 by Haley and Knott, and by Martinez and Curnow. We will illustrate the method using the BC design, although the method has been adapted to most of the designs considered in the previous chapter with flanking markers. The BC design with two flanking markers is illustrated in Figure 5.2. For the BC progeny only the chromosome from the F-1 parent is shown. There are eight possible gametic haplotypes (including the QTL); two non-recombinants, four single recombinants, and two double recombinants. The following model can be defined:

$$Y_{ij} = \mu_1(1 - p_i) + \mu_2 p_i + e_{ij} \qquad \{5.2\}$$

where Y_{ij} is the production record of the jth individual with marker genotype i, μ_1

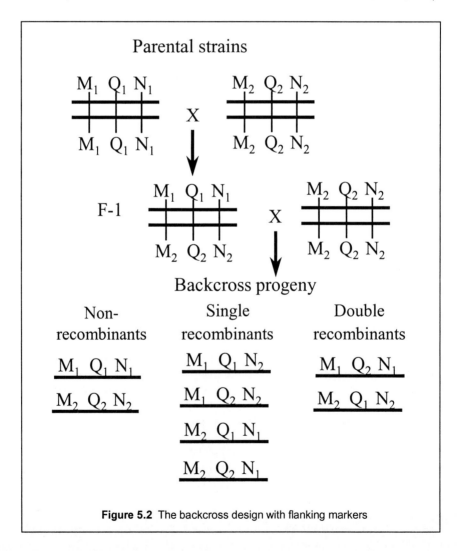

Figure 5.2 The backcross design with flanking markers

is the mean for individuals with genotype Q_1Q_2, μ_2 is the mean for individuals with genotype Q_2Q_2, p_i is the probability that an individual with marker genotype i has genotype Q_2Q_2, e_{ij} is the residual, and the other terms are as defined previously. This model can be simplified as follows:

$$Y_{ij} = \mu_1 + (\mu_2 - \mu_1)p_i + e_{ij} \qquad \{5.3\}$$

p_i is a function of the recombination parameters, and can be estimated for each of the four marker haplotypes as follows:

$$p_{m1n1} = r_1 r_2 / (1-R) \qquad \{5.4\}$$

$$p_{m1n2} = r_1(1-r_2)/R \qquad \{5.5\}$$

$$p_{m2n1} = r_2(1-r_1)/R \qquad \{5.6\}$$

$$p_{m2n2} = 1 - r_1 r_2 / (1-R) \qquad \{5.7\}$$

where R is the recombination frequency between the two markers, M and N; r_1 is the recombination frequencies between M and Q; and r_2 is the recombination frequency between Q and N.

If r_1 was known, it would be possible to substitute these values into Equation {5.3}, and then solve as a simple linear regression, with μ_1 as the y-intercept and $\mu_2 - \mu_1$ as the slope. Since r_1 is not known, Equation {5.3} can be considered as four separate equations, one for each marker haplotype. Assuming that R is known without error, it is possible to solve for r_2 in terms of R and r_1 for the assumed map function. For example, for the Haldane function (Haldane, 1919), which assumes zero interference:

$$R = r_1 + r_2 - 2r_1 r_2 \qquad \{5.8\}$$

$$r_2 = (R - r_1)/(1 - 2r_1) \qquad \{5.9\}$$

This still leaves with four equations, which are non-linear functions of the QTL means and r_1. The least-squares solution for this model, which is non-linear in r_1 for all three parameters, will be the values that minimize the residual sum of squares as a function of $RSS(r_1)$, computed as follows:

$$RSS(r_1) = \sum_{i=1}^{4} \sum_{j=1}^{n_j} [Y_{ij} - \hat{Y}_{ij}(r_1)]^2 \qquad \{5.10\}$$

where $\hat{Y}_{ij}(r_1)$ is the estimated value of Y_{ij} with recombination frequency of r_1

between the QTL and the first marker, and n_i is the number of individuals in marker class i.

The least-squares solutions can be derived by a non-linear least-squares algorithm, such as PROC NLIN of SAS (SAS, 1988). The appropriate SAS code is given in Figure 5.3. The appropriate ratio for the F-test is the model mean-squares divided by the residual mean-squares. The model sum of squares can then be computed as the total sum of squares less the residual sum of squares. In theory, the mean-squares are derived by dividing the sums of squares by their degrees of freedom. Under the null hypothesis of no segregating QTL, this ratio should have an approximate central F-distribution.

```
proc nlin ;
  R = 0.3 ;
  if m = 1 and n = 1 then p = r1*r2/(1-R) ;
  if m = 1 and n = 2 then p = r1*(1-r2)/R ;
  if m = 2 and n = 2 then p = (1-r1*r2)/(1-R) ;
  if m = 2 and n = 1 then p = r2*(1-r1)/R ;
  r2 = (r-r1)/(1-2*r1) ;
  parameters mu1= -.1 mu2 = .1 r1 = 0 to 0.3 by 0.05 ;
  model trait = mu1 + (mu2-mu1)*p ;
  bounds -0.3 < mu1 < 0.3 ;
  bounds -0.3 < mu2 < 0.3 ;
  bounds 0 < r1 < 0.3 ;
run ;
```

Figure 5.3 The SAS code for non-linear regression interval mapping for the BC design

As will be seen in Section 5.12, appropriate thresholds for QTL tests are quite problematic in most cases. The degrees of freedom for the model mean-squares should represent the number of additional parameters estimated in the model, relative to a model that does not assume a segregating QTL. Four parameters are estimated in this model, two QTL means, r_1, and the residual variance. This is two more than the null hypothesis of a single normal distribution for the quantitative trait, which postulates two parameters, a general mean and variance. However, with a marker bracket, the estimated QTL effect is highly correlated with its estimated location. As will be seen below, many studies have dealt with the question of the appropriate degrees of freedom for QTL effects estimated with linked markers. Most studies have found in simulation that the distribution of the test statistic under the null hypothesis of no segregating QTL is between the expected values for estimating one and two additional parameters. Appropriate tests of significance for the non-linear regression method will be considered in Chapter eight.

The main advantages of non-linear regression are that it can be performed by more statistical packages, and significance of the QTL effect can be tested by an F-test, which is more familiar to most researchers than a likelihood ratio test, discussed below. The disadvantage of this method is that it is applicable only in certain situations. It cannot be applied to estimate recombination frequency between a QTL and a single marker, or used to estimate QTL variance effects. These questions have been addressed by ML estimation (Weller, 1986; Bovenhuis and Weller, 1994).

5.4 Least-squares estimation of QTL location for sib-pair analysis with flanking markers

In Section 4.7 we showed that for the Haseman and Elston (1972) sib-pair analysis method with a single marker, the following linear relationship, given in Equation {4.10} is expected between the squared deviation between sib phenotypes and the fraction of marker alleles identical by descent (IBD) as follows:

$$Y_j = \alpha + \beta \pi_j \qquad \{5.11\}$$

where Y_j is the squared difference of phenotypes for sib-pair j, π_j is the fraction of marker alleles IBD, and $\alpha = \sigma^2_e + 2\sigma^2_a$; where σ^2_a is the additive variance due to the segregating QTL. With incomplete linkage between the QTL and the genetic marker, $\beta = -2(1-2r)^2 \sigma^2_a$.

With two flanking markers, regression equations similar to Equation {5.11} can be derived for each marker. The objective is then to use these two values for the fraction of marker alleles IBD to find the most likely QTL location. At this location, the fraction of alleles IBD, denoted $\hat{\pi}_q$, most closely reflects the fraction of alleles IBD for the QTL. $\hat{\pi}_q$ can be derived from the following function of the fractions of alleles IBD at the flanking markers (Fulker and Cardon, 1994):

$$\hat{\pi}_q = \alpha + \beta_1 \pi_1 + \beta_2 \pi_2 \qquad \{5.12\}$$

where π_1 and π_2 are the IBD values for the two flanking markers for family j, α is the y-intercept, and β_1, and β_2 are regression coefficients. The subscript, j, has been deleted for convenience. The regression coefficients can be derived as a solution to C = Vβ, where C is the covariance matrix between π-values for the flanking markers and $\hat{\pi}_q$, V is the variance matrix for the π-values for the flanking markers, and β is the vector of regression coefficients. Thus, the solutions for β can be derived from the following equations:

$$\begin{bmatrix} \mathrm{Cov}(\pi_1, \pi_q) \\ \mathrm{Cov}(\pi_2, \pi_q) \end{bmatrix} = \begin{bmatrix} \mathrm{Var}(\pi_1) & \mathrm{Cov}(\pi_1, \pi_2) \\ \mathrm{Cov}(\pi_1, \pi_q) & \mathrm{Var}((\pi_1)) \end{bmatrix} \begin{bmatrix} \beta_1 \\ \beta_2 \end{bmatrix} \quad \{5.13\}$$

For any two genetically linked locations on the chromosome, i and j, $\mathrm{Cov}(\pi_i, \pi_j) = (1-2r_{ij})^2/8$, where r_{ij} is the recombination frequency between the two genetic map locations, and $\mathrm{Var}(\pi) = 1/8$. The solutions for β_1 and β_2 can then be derived as: $\beta = V^{-1}C$, which gives the following solutions:

$$\beta_1 = [(1-2r_1)^2 - (1-2r_2)^2 (1-2R)^2]/[(1- (1-2R)^4] \quad \{5.14\}$$

$$\beta_2 = [(1-2r_2)^2 - (1-2r_1)^2 (1-2R)^2]/[(1- (1-2R)^4] \quad \{5.15\}$$

with all terms as defined previously. Note that these coefficients are only functions of R, r_1, and r_2. As in the previous section, r_2 is computed as a function of R and r_1, based on the assumed mapping function. To solve for α, we note that the mean of $\pi = \frac{1}{2}$, which yields the follow solution:

$$\alpha = (1 - \beta_1 - \beta_1)/2 \quad \{5.16\}$$

For short intervals, using the Morgan mapping function, which assumes complete interference, β_1 and β_2 can be approximately estimated as follows:

$$\beta_1 = r_2/R \text{ and } \beta_2 = r_1/R \quad \{5.17\}$$

Similar to the previous section, presence of a segregating QTL can be tested by the ratio of the model and residual sum of squares, based on Equation {5.12}. Under the null hypothesis, this ratio should have a central F-distribution. With a single marker, Haseman and Elston (1972) tested for the significance of the regression against the null hypothesis that the slope is equal to zero. Under the null hypothesis, the statistic $\hat{\beta}/SE(\beta)$ should have a t-distribution. Fulker and Cardon (1994) used this statistic, with $\hat{\beta}$ computed at the most likely QTL location. They used simulations to determine the distribution of the t-statistic under the null hypothesis of no QTL segregating within the marker bracket. They found that the test statistic was very close to the theoretical t-distribution. The length of the marker bracket over the range of 10 to 50 cM had virtually no effect on the empirical 0.05, 0.01, and 0.001 probability values under the null hypothesis.

In the previous chapter we noted that for the same magnitudes of QTL effect and sample sizes the sib-pair method is less powerful than crosses between inbred lines or half-sib designs, because this method is based on analysis of second ordered statistics. This is still the case with marker brackets, although for the same number of individuals genotyped, power is increased with marker brackets. Statistical power of different experimental designs will be considered in detail in Chapter eight.

As noted in the previous chapter, in many families will not be "fully informative". It will only be possible to compute π if at least three different marker alleles are present in the parents, and both parents are heterozygous. For regression with a single marker, Haseman and Elston (1972) showed that if π is not known with certainty, it can be replaced with its expectation. However, this conclusion was reached by Bayesian inference, and not by linear regression. Nevertheless, Fulker and Cardon (1994) obtained reasonable QTL parameter estimates using this approach with the multiple regression equation given in {5.12}.

5.5 Linear regression mapping of QTL with flanking markers

The non-linear least-squares method described in Section 5.3 can only be solved by iteration. This is also the case for the ML methods described in Sections 5.7 through 5.9. Whittaker et al. (1996) found that for crosses between inbred lines with linked markers, the same QTL parameter estimates can be obtained directly by a multiple regression of phenotypes on marker genotypes. As for the non-linear least-squares method, we will assume the Haldane (1919) mapping function throughout.

The regression model for the F-2 design assuming additivity with two linked markers is as follows:

$$Y_{ij} = \mu + \beta_m x_{mi} + \beta_n x_{ni} + e_{ij} \qquad \{5.18\}$$

where Y_{ij} is the trait value for individual j with marker genotype i, μ is the general mean, β_m and β_n are linear regression coefficients for markers 1 and 2, x_{mi} and x_{ni} are marker genotype indicator variables, and e_{ij} is the random residual.

x_{mi} and x_{ni} have values of 1 for individuals with genotypes M_1M_1 and N_1N_1, respectively; values of 0 for the marker heterozygotes; and values of -1 for individuals with genotypes M_2M_2 and N_2N_2, respectively. This is a simple multiple regression model with three parameters, μ, β_m, and β_n, and can be solved analytically. Thus significance of a segregating QTL can be tested by the ratio of model and residual mean-squares. Under the null hypothesis this ratio will have a central F-distribution with 2 degrees of freedom (df) in the numerator and N–3 df in the denominator.

Whittaker et al. (1996) showed that the residual sum of squares for this model is identical for the non-linear regression model given in Equation {5.3}. Furthermore, the same estimates for QTL effect and location can be derived as functions of β_m and β_n. Whittaker et al. (1996) prove the following equations for the F-2 design:

$$\beta_m = aE(g|x_m = 1, x_n = 0, r_1)$$

$$\beta_n = aE(g|x_m = 0, x_n = 1, r_1)$$

{5.19}

where a is the additive QTL effect, E(g|.) is the conditional expectation of g, and g is the QTL genotype with values of 1, 0, and −1 for QTL genotypes Q_1Q_1, Q_1Q_2, and Q_2Q_2, respectively. E(g|.) for all combinations of x_m and x_n values for the F-2 design are given in Table 5.1.

Table 5.1 $E(g|x_m, x_n, r_1)$ for the F-2 design

x_m	x_n	$E(g|x_m, x_n, r_1)$
1	1	$(1-r_1-r_2)/(1-R)$
1	0	$[r_2(1-r_2)(1-2r_1)]/R(1-R)$
1	−1	$(r_2-r_1)/R$
0	1	$[r_1(1-r_1)(1-2r_2)]/R(1-R)$
0	0	0
0	−1	$[r_1(1-r_1)(1-2r_2)]/R(1-R)$
−1	1	$(r_1-r_2)/R$
−1	0	$[r_2(1-r_2)(2r_1-1)]/R(1-R)$
−1	−1	$(-1-r_1-r_2)/(1-R)$

Assuming the Haldane (1919) mapping function, as given in Equation {5.9}, $r_2 = (R - r_1)/(1 - 2r_1)$. Selecting the appropriate values from Table 5.1, and solving for r_2, gives the following solutions for β_m and β_n:

$$\beta_m = a \frac{(R-r_1)(1-R-1-r_1)}{R(1-R)(1-2r_1)}$$

$$\beta_n = a \frac{r_1(1-r_1)(1-2R)}{R(1-R)(1-2r_1)}$$

{5.19}

Since R is assumed known, these are two equations with two unknowns, a, and r_1, with the following solutions:

$$r_1 = 0.5 - 0.5 \left[1 - \frac{4\beta_n R(1-R)}{\beta_n + \beta_m(1-2R)} \right]^{0.5}$$

{5.20}

$$a^2 = \frac{[\beta_m + \beta_n(1-2R)][\beta_n + \beta_m(1-2R)]}{1-2R}$$

{5.21}

Thus it is possible to analytically solve for both QTL location and additive effect. Whittaker et al. (1996) also note that r_1 depends only on the ratio of β_m and β_n, and both must have the same sign.

The BC design can be solved in a similar manner, and this method can also be used to estimate dominance effects in the F-2 design. Application of this model with multiple QTL and markers, and with only partially informative markers will be considered in the next chapter.

5.6 Marker information content for interval mapping, uninformative and missing marker genotypes

As noted previously, even for crosses between inbred lines, the allele passed from parents to progeny is known only at the marker location. Outside the marker intervals and between markers, there is uncertainty with respect to the progeny genotype, unless complete interference is assumed. With flanking markers, this uncertainty decreases as the recombination frequency between adjacent markers decreases. For example, consider Equation {5.2}. At the marker locations p_i is equal to either 1 or 0, with a mean of 0.5, and a variance of 0.25. At all other locations, p_i is between 0 and 1.

Kruglyak and Lander (1995b) proposed that the variance of p_i could be used to estimate the information content at each point along the genome. The information content is computed as $Var(p_i)/0.25$ (Spelman et al., 1996). Examples of expected information content with three different marker densities are plotted in Figure 5.4. At the marker locations information content is equal to unity for all three marker densities. Information content declines in the intervals between markers, with minimum information content at the midpoint between markers. Information content at the midpoint between markers decreases as marker spacing increases.

In crosses between inbred lines, all markers heterozygous in the parents will be completely "informative", as defined in Section 4.5. That is, allele origin for each of the progeny's two alleles can be determined without error. However, as noted in the previous section for the full-sib design, not all markers will be informative for all progeny. This will generally be the case for designs based on segregating populations, as discussed in detail in Section 4.5. Even in crosses between inbred lines, some marker geneotypes will generally be missing. Therefore information content will be different even at the marker locations (Spelman et al., 1996). With missing genotype non-linear least-squares estimation can be modified so that the probability of each QTL genotype is computed relative to the two closest informative markers (Knott et al., 1996; Martinez and Curnow, 1994). Equation {5.2} is modified as follows:

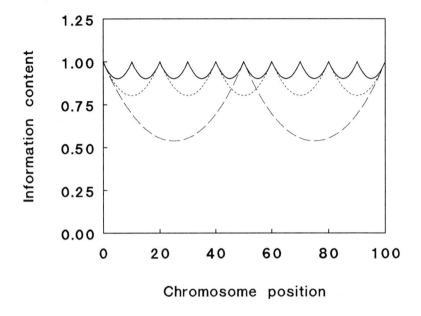

Figure 5.4 Information content as a function of chromosome position for three densities of evenly spaced markers. ——, 10 cM between adjacent markers; - - -, 20 cM between adjacent markers; — —, 50 cM between adjacent markers

$$Y_{ij} = \mu_1(1-p_{ij}) + \mu_2 p_{ij} + e_{ij} \quad \{5.22\}$$

where p_{ij} is computed separately for each individual, depending on which markers are informative.

Even if all markers to one side of the putative QTL location are uninformative in a specific individual, p_{ij} can still be calculated, based on the recombination frequency between the assumed QTL position and the single linked marker. Thus, only individuals without any markers in linkage to the putative QTL location will be discarded from the analysis.

In an F-2 design, it is possible to estimate both additive and dominance effects. Determination of the additive effect is based on the difference between the homozygotes, while determination of dominance is based on the difference between the heterozygotes and the midpoint of the homozygotes. Thus, information content can be different for the additive and dominance effect. With complete information, each homozygous individual will have a score of either 1 or –1 for the additive effect, with a variance of 0.5 in the complete sample, because only half the individuals will be homozygous. Heterozygous individuals will receive a value of 1 for the dominance effects, while homozygotes will receive a value of 0, again assuming that half of the individuals are homozygotes for the QTL. Thus the variance of the dominance effect will be 0.25 over the complete sample. Thus, Knott *et al.* (1998) proposed that information content should be computed as the variance of the additive effect, plus twice the variance of the dominance effect for the F-2 design. If more than half of the individuals are homozygous, then the information content can be slightly greater than unity. The marker information content will be considered again in Section 6.11.

5.7 Maximum likelihood QTL parameter estimation for crosses between inbred lines and a single marker

We will illustrate ML estimation of QTL parameters first for the BC design and a single QTL linked to a single genetic, as illustrated in Figure 5.1. We will assume that the residuals are normally distributed with equal variances. As will be seen below, ML is a more flexible technique than least-squares, and can handle many situations in which these assumptions do not hold. The statistical density function for a single individual of genotype M_1M_2 will be:

$$L = \frac{(1-r)e^{-(y-\mu_1)^2/2\sigma^2}}{\sqrt{2\pi\sigma^2}} + \frac{(r)e^{-(y-\mu_2)^2/2\sigma^2}}{\sqrt{2\pi\sigma^2}} \qquad \{5.23\}$$

where y is the trait value, σ is the standard deviation, μ_1 is the mean of individuals with the Q_1Q_2 genotype, μ_2 is the mean of individuals with the Q_2Q_2 genotype, and r is the recombination frequency between the marker and the QTL. Individuals with the M_2M_2 genotype will have the same likelihood, except that the QTL mean values will be reversed. The complete likelihood for a sample of individuals can be written as follows:

$$L = \prod^{N_1} [f(y_i, M_1M_2)] \prod^{N_2} [f(y_j, M_2M_2)] \qquad \{5.24\}$$

where $\prod$ represents the product of a series, $f(y_i, M_1M_2)$ and $f(y_j, M_2M_2)$ are the statistical densities for i^{th} and j^{th} observations with genotypes M_1M_2 and M_2M_2, respectively; and N_1 and N_2 are the number of individuals with the two genotypes, respectively.

To obtain the ML parameter estimates, the log of this function must be differentiated with respect to four parameters: μ_1, μ_2, σ, and r. The partial derivatives must then be equated to zero, and this system of four equations must be solved. This system of equations cannot be solved analytically. Iterative methods to derive solutions will be described below.

Alternatively, Equation {5.23} can be readily modified so that a different residual variance is assumed for each QTL genotype. In this case it is necessary to estimate five parameters, instead of four. The hypothesis of heterogenous variance can also be tested against the null hypothesis of homogenous variance by the log likelihood ratio of the heterogenous and homogenous variance maximum likelihoods.

For the F-2 design described in Figure 4.2, each genotype will consist of a mixture of three normal distributions for the two QTL homozygotes and the QTL heterozygote. The probabilities of each of the three QTL genotypes within each marker genotype are given in Table 4.2. Thus, it will be necessary to estimate at least five parameters, the three QTL means, r, and the residual variance. This model can also be modified so that a separate residual variance is assumed for each QTL genotype. In this case is necessary to estimate seven parameters: three means, three variances, and r (Weller, 1986). These examples give some indication of the flexibility of ML estimation.

5.8 Maximum likelihood tests of significance for a segregating QTL

Linkage of the genetic marker to a segregating QTL can be tested by a normal test based on the matrix of prediction error variances, or by a likelihood ratio test. In the case of the normal test, the null hypothesis for the BC design is $\mu_1 - \mu_2 = 0$. The test statistic will be $\mu_1 - \mu_2$ divided by its standard error. The standard error of this difference will be the standard errors of μ_1 and μ_2, less twice the standard error of the covariance. These standard errors can be computed from the matrix of second differentials, as described in Section 2.9. Under the null hypothesis, the test statistic will have a t-distribution, but for a relatively large sample, the normal distribution is a good approximation of the t-distribution.

For the likelihood ratio test, the test statistic is one-half the natural log of the ratio of likelihood in Equation {5.22} at convergence, to the maximum likelihood obtained with r fixed to 0.5, i. e. no linkage between the QTL and the genetic marker. As noted in Chapter two, this statistic will be asymptotically distributed as a central χ^2 statistic. The degrees of freedom are the number of parameters fixed in the null hypothesis, but are allowed to "float" in the alternative hypothesis. For models of QTL analysis, the distribution of the test statistic under the null hypothesis will be between a χ^2 distribution with one and two df. The recombination frequency and the estimated QTL effect, $\mu_1 - \mu_2$, are highly correlated. Therefore, fixing r = 0.5 also implies fixing $\mu_1 = \mu_2$ (Jansen, 1994).

5.10 Estimation of QTL parameters by the expectation-maximization algorithm

Expectation-maximization (EM) is based on computation of first derivatives of a function of log L. EM is generally considered the method of choice, because it is guaranteed to converge to a local maximum, provided that one exists within the parameter space. The rate of convergence, however, may be very slow. The principle behind EM is to consider two sampling densities, one based on the complete data specification (unknown), and the second based on the incomplete data specification (known).

The EM algorithm consists of two steps: the estimation step, in which the sufficient statistics are estimated for the complete-data density function, and the maximization step, in which this function is maximized with respect to the parameters. As noted in Section 2.13, a "sufficient statistic" is a statistic derived from the sample, which contains all the information in the sample relevant to the parameter being estimated. Lander and Botstein (1989) employed a partial EM algorithm that solved for QTL means and variances for a fixed recombination frequency. This procedure was then repeated for a range of recombination values to obtain the r_1 value which resulted in ML.

Jansen (1992) derived complete EM equations, which are suitable for a wide range of QTL models. For each individual i, the likelihood function can be written as $f(y_i,m_i)$, where y_i and m_i are the quantitative trait value and marker genotype for individual i. The joint likelihood over all individuals will be $\prod f(y_i,m_i)$ as given above. By the general product rule of probability:

$$L = \prod^I f(y_i,m_i) = \prod^I p(m_i) \prod^I f(y_i|m_i) \quad \{5.30\}$$

where I is the total number of individuals, $p(m_i)$ is the probability of genotype m, and $f(y_i|m_i)$ is the density of the trait value given the marker genotype for individual i. Setting the log of L to zero gives:

$$0 = \frac{\partial(\log L)}{\partial \theta} = \sum^I \frac{\partial[\log p(m_i)]}{\partial \theta} + \sum^I \frac{\partial[\log f(y_i|m_i)]}{\partial \theta} \quad \{5.31\}$$

After some complicated algebra based on the general product rule of probability, Equation {5.31} can be expressed as follows (Jansen, 1992):

$$0 = \frac{\partial(\log L)}{\partial \theta} = \sum^I \sum^Q p(q|y_i,m_i) \frac{\partial[\log p(q|m_i)]}{\partial \theta} + \sum^I \sum^Q p(q|y_i,m_i) \frac{\partial[\log f(y_i|q_i)]}{\partial \theta} \quad \{5.32\}$$

5.9 Maximum likelihood QTL parameter estimation for crosses between inbred lines and two flanking markers

The likelihood function for the BC design with two flanking markers, as shown in Figure 5.2, is described as follows (Lander and Botstein, 1989):

$$L = \prod^{n_{M_1N_1}} f_{M_1N_1} \prod^{n_{M_1N_2}} f_{M_1N_2} \prod^{n_{M_2N_1}} f_{M_2N_1} \prod^{n_{M_2N_2}} f_{M_2N_2} \quad \{5.25\}$$

where $n_{M_1N_1}$, $n_{M_1N_2}$, $n_{M_2N_1}$, $n_{M_2N_2}$ are the number of individuals with genotypes M_1N_1/M_2N_2, M_1N_2/M_2N_2, M_2N_1/M_2N_2, and M_2N_2/M_2N_2, respectively, and $f_{M_1N_1}$, $f_{M_1N_2}$, $f_{M_2N_1}$, and $f_{M_2N_2}$ are the density functions for the four possible marker genotypes. Since all individuals received an M_2N_2 chromosomal segment from the recurrent parent, only the chromosomal segment received from the F-1 is indicated. The density functions for the possible marker genotypes are computed as follows:

$$f_{M_1N_1} = (1-a)f(Q_1) + af(Q_2) \quad \{5.26\}$$

$$f_{M_1N_2} = (1-b)f(Q_1) + bf(Q_2) \quad \{5.27\}$$

$$f_{M_2N_1} = (1-b)f(Q_2) + bf(Q_1) \quad \{5.28\}$$

$$f_{M_2N_2} = (1-a)f(Q_2) + af(Q_1) \quad \{5.29\}$$

Assuming again the Haldane mapping function (zero interference), $R = r_1 + r_2 - 2r_1r_2$. In this case, $a = r_1r_2/(1-R)$ and $b = r_1(1-r_2)/R$. $f(Q_1)$ and $f(Q_2)$ are the normal density functions for each observation with standard deviations of σ, and means of μ_1 for the Q_1Q_2 genotype and μ_2 for the Q_2Q_2 genotype. Thus, the likelihood can be computed by calculating the appropriate density function for each individual, depending on its marker genotype, and multiplying.

Assuming zero interference, ML estimates are derived for only four parameters, r_1, σ, μ_1 and μ_2. Theoretically the ML values for these four parameters can be derived by computing the partial derivatives of the likelihood function, or its log, with respect to these four parameters. These four functions are then set equal to zero, and this system of four equations is then solved for four unknowns. In practice this non-linear system of equations cannot be solved analytically. It can be solved either by the derivative-free or second derivative methods described in Sections 2.11 and 2.12. These methods are quite straightforward, and need not be described here in detail. The expectation-maximization algorithm described briefly in Section 2.13 requires additional explanation, and will now be elaborated within the context of interval mapping.

where, Q is the total number of QTL genotypes, p(q|m$_i$) is the probability of QTL genotype q conditional on marker genotype m$_i$, f(y$_i$|q) is the density of trait value y$_i$ conditional on QTL genotype q, and p(q|y$_i$,m$_i$) is the probability of QTL genotype q conditional on trait value y$_i$ and marker genotype m$_i$.

The differential in the first expression of the right-hand side of Equation {5.32} is a function only of the recombination parameters r or r$_1$, and the differential in the second expression is a function only of QTL genotype means and variances. Using the values of p(q|y$_i$,m$_i$) from the current iteration, solutions can be derived for the parameters by setting each term equal to zero. In many of the designs considered, these equations can now be easily solved for the current values of p(q|y$_i$,m$_i$). The "estimation" step consists of computing p(q|y$_i$,m$_i$) using the current values of q for each individual. For example, for the BC design and a single marker, p(q=Q$_1$|y$_i$,m$_i$) for the M$_1$M$_2$ genotype is computed as follows:

$$ (q=Q_1|y_i,m_i) = \frac{e^{-(y_i-\mu_1)^2/2\sigma^2}}{(1-r)e^{-(y_i-\mu_1)^2/2\sigma^2} + (r)e^{-(y_i-\mu_2)^2/2\sigma^2}} \quad \{5.33\} $$

p(q=Q$_2$|y$_i$,m$_i$) is similarly computed with μ_2 in the numerator instead of μ_1. Thus, the sum of p(q=Q$_2$|y$_i$,m$_i$) and p(q=Q$_2$|y$_i$,m$_i$) of each individual are equal to unity, and these can be considered weighting factors for the differentials in Equation {5.27}.

The maximization step consists of solving Equation {5.32}. The first term is a weighted non-linear regression, and is a function only of the recombination parameter, r. For the BC design, log [p(q|m$_i$)] is equal to either log r or log (1–r), with derivatives of 1/r or –1/(1–r), respectively. The second term is a weighted linear regression, and is a function only of QTL means and variances. For the BC design, assuming a normal distribution, the QTL means and variances can be estimated as the trait means and variances weighted by p(q|y$_i$,m$_i$) for each combination of individual by genotype. Other "nuisance" factors, such as block or herd can readily be incorporated as part of the second term, which can be solved as a general linear model for traits with a normal distribution.

With marker brackets the first term is somewhat more complicated, but will still be a function of only a single parameter, r$_1$, assuming zero interference, and that R is known. This method can also be readily applied to analyse multiple QTL brackets. Algorithms are described in Jansen (1992). This method can also be applied even if the within-QTL genotype distribution of the quantitative trait is not normal, provided it is possible to compute the differential of log f(y$_i$|q), as will be described below for the case of discrete traits.

5.11 Biases in estimation of QTL parameters with interval mapping

As noted in Chapter two, ML estimators can be biased. Mangin *et al.* (1994) showed that not only is the ML estimate of QTL location biased, it is also not consistent. That is, as the sample size tends towards infinity, the estimate of QTL location does not necessarily tend towards the true value. This is because the information matrix is not positive-definite as the QTL effect tends towards zero. Therefore it is not possible to construct the classical Taylor expansion as the QTL effect approaches zero.

In addition, both the ML model described in the Section 5.8 and the non-linear regression method described in Section 5.4 assume a single segregating QTL between two flanking markers. If this is not the case, then estimates of both QTL effect and location will be biased. These biases have been shown to be especially significant in at least two important cases:

1. A QTL located near, but outside a marker interval.
2. Two QTL located within a marker interval.

In the first case, the estimates of QTL effect are unbiased only at the marker locations. At all other points within the interval, the estimated effect will be inflated. Thus, likelihood profiles with estimated QTL effects computed as a function of QTL location tend to be concave. It is therefore likely that a likelihood maximum will be found within the interval, even though the QTL is located outside the interval (Martinez and Curnow, 1992).

In the second case, a single "ghost" QTL will be found between the two true QTL. This will happen even if three adjacent intervals are analysed, with one QTL in each of the outer intervals, and no QTL segregating in the middle interval (Martinez and Curnow, 1992). Some of these problems can be alleviated with multiple linked markers. Analysis methods will be considered in Chapter six.
However, if the two QTL are relatively close, it will be not be possible to distinguish two separate loci, unless both the effects and samples size are very large.

For analyses based on segregating populations, markers can vary in information content, as noted in Section 5.5. In this case estimated QTL location will be biased towards marker brackets with greater information (Knott and Haley, 1992),

In addition to the problem of bias, neither a likelihood ratio test, nor an F-test for non-linear regression correctly tests the question of whether there is a QTL segregating in the marker bracket (Zeng, 1993, 1994). Neither statistic is independent of QTL that may be segregating outside the marker bracket. These problems can be solved by composite interval mapping, which will also be discussed in the following chapter.

5.12 The likelihood ratio test with interval mapping

As noted above, it is not clear what is the correct number of df to test for a segregating QTL by a likelihood ratio test. Even in the simplest case of a BC design with a single marker, it can be argued that it is sufficient to fix only a single parameter, r. If recombination between the genetic marker and the QTL is fixed at 0.5, then the magnitude of the putative segregating QTL is immaterial; it is by definition unlinked with the genetic marker (Simpson, 1986). However, it can also be argued that in fact both the QTL effect and the recombination frequency are fixed. Similarly with interval mapping it is not clear whether both the QTL location parameter and the QTL effect are fixed in the reduced model.

This question of the appropriate degrees of freedom for ML models was investigated by simulation by Jansen (1994) and Baret *et al.* (1994). Jansen (1994) simulated a BC population. Under the null hypothesis of no segregating QTL in the marker bracket, the cumulative distribution of the likelihood ratio was nearly midway between the theoretical χ^2 distributions with 1 and 2 df. Baret *et al.* (1994) simulated a daughter design assuming complete linkage between the QTL and a genetic marker. The empirical 5% threshold for the least-squares test statistic was very close to the theoretical central F-value. However, the empirical 5% threshold for LRT statistic was around 2.7. Multiplying by two gives a value of 5.4, which is more than the 5% χ^2 value of 3.84 with 1 df, but somewhat less than the 5% χ^2 value of 5.99 with 2 df.

Kadarmideen and Dekkers (1999) simulated the distribution of the following likelihood ratio test statistic (LR) under the null hypothesis for linear and non-linear regression models with a marker bracket:

$$LR = N\log(RSS_r/RSS_f) \qquad \{5.34\}$$

where N is the sample size and RSS_r and RSS_f are residual sums of squares when fitting only a general mean, and when fitting the "full" model, including a segregating QTL, respectively.

If all simulations were included, the distribution of the test statistic was between the χ^2 distributions with 1 and 2 df for the non-linear regression model, but nearly equal to the χ^2 distribution with 2 df for the linear regression model. However, if those simulations for which the putative QTL location was outside the marker bracket were deleted, then the distribution of the test statistic was nearly identical to the χ^2 distribution with 2 df for both models. For the linear regression model, the sign of the two regression coefficients must be the same to obtain a QTL location within the marker bracket. They explain these results as follows. In the non-linear regression model two parameters are estimated if the putative QTL lies within the marker bracket. However if the assumed QTL position is outside the marker bracket, then it is not possible to estimate its location, and the only parameter estimated is the effect associated with the closer marker. These questions will be considered again in the next chapter for more complicated models.

In addition to the problem of the distribution of the test statistic under the null hypothesis, segregating QTL outside the marker interval will also affect the test statistic, as noted above for linked QTL located outside the marker bracket. Even unlinked segregating QTL will slightly affect the distribution of the test statistic (Jansen, 1994).

Another difficulty in applying a likelihood ratio test is that statistical power to detect a segregating QTL cannot be computed analytically. In order to estimate the power of the test, it is necessary to determine the distribution of the test statistic under the assumption that the alternative hypothesis is correct. It would seem that under the alternative hypothesis, the log of the likelihood ratio should have an approximately non-central χ^2 distribution, with the non-central parameter determined by the expected ratio of the likelihoods for the alternative and null hypotheses. The expectation of the likelihood for the alternative hypothesis will be a function of both the QTL effect and its location relative to the genetic markers. Lander and Botstein determined that for the situation of complete linkage, the expectation of the log of the likelihood ratio, ELOD, will be:

$$\text{ELOD} = 0.5N\log(1 + \sigma_v^2/\sigma_e^2) \qquad \{5.35\}$$

where N is the sample size, σ_v^2 is the variance due to the QTL and σ_e^2 is the residual variance. For the backcross design, $\sigma_v^2 = a^2/4$. Although Lander and Botstein (1989) gave their formula in terms of the base 10 log, it will also apply to natural base logarithms. Power of likelihood ratio tests will be considered in Chapter eight.

5.13 Summary

In this chapter we considered various methods for QTL parameter estimation of crosses between inbred lines, emphasizing maximum likelihood, which although not trivial to apply, can be applied to many models which are not amenable to solution by other methods. Unlike other estimates derived by other methods, ML estimates must be within the parameter space. Least-squares models give nearly identical results to ML, and can be applied using standard statistical packages, such as SAS, but are much more limited as to possibilities of model specification. Unlike either non-linear regression or ML, marker regression models can be solved analytically, and significance of the QTL effect can be directly tested by the mean-squares ratio.

We presented an EM method to maximize likelihood functions for a wide range of models. EM is guaranteed to converge to a local maximum, provided one exists within the parameter space. Although the local maximum found may not be the global maximum, multiple likelihood maxima is generally not a problem for the models considered.

Estimates can be biased, especially if the assumptions of the analysis model are incorrect. Appropriate statistics to test for a segregating QTL are problematic for both analysis methods, and statistical power can only be estimated by simulation.

Chapter six:

Advanced Statistical Methods for QTL Detection and Parameter Estimation

6.1 Introduction

In the previous chapter we described the basic methods for QTL parameter estimation, which are applicable to crosses between inbred lines. Maximum likelihood estimation is the most flexible method, and was described in most detail. In this chapter we will consider more advanced methods for QTL parameter estimation that must be applied to other experimental designs. In the analysis of inbred lines, all genetic factors not linked to the segregating markers will be randomly distributed, and can therefore be considered part of the residual variance. However, this will not be the case for segregating populations, and it will be necessary to account for polygenic variance not linked to the genetic markers. Furthermore, if the analysis is based on field data there will usually be confounding "nuisance" variables, such as herd or block. Parameter estimates may be biased if these factors are not included in the analysis model. Finally, most analyses will include multiple traits and markers, which creates further complications. Although non-linear regression has also been applied to experimental designs for segregating populations, this method is more limited than maximum likelihood (ML).

Estimation of higher order QTL effects will be considered in Sections 6.2 and 6.3. In Section 6.4 we will introduce the problems related to simultaneous analysis of multiple marker brackets. Sections 6.5 to 6.8 deal with "composite interval mapping". Section 6.9 describes marker regression analysis with multiple markers and QTL. In Sections 6.10 and 6.11 we will consider the basic problems of QTL analysis from segregating populations, and present the solutions that have been proposed. In Section 6.12 we will discuss ML analysis of the daughter design with a single marker, and in Section 6.13 we will consider methods for ML analysis of additional complex pedigrees. In Section 6.14 we will consider non-linear regression estimation for complex pedigrees. In Section 6.15 we will consider ML with random effects included in the analysis model. In the last three sections we will describe methods for estimation of QTL effects on categorical traits.

6.2 Higher order QTL effects

In Section 4.2 we presented a list of "usual" assumptions, which are generally employed in QTL parameter estimation. The last three assumptions were:

8. No interactions between the QTL and other loci (epistasis)
9. No interactions between the QTL and other, non-genetic, factors.
10. The QTL has only an additive effect on the quantitative trait

Studies that have attempted to test or remove these assumptions will be considered in detail in this section. The first assumption, Mendelian segregation of both markers and QTL will not be considered in detail. Models that include dominance (assumption 7) have already been considered in the previous chapter. Models that remove the remaining assumptions will be considered in the remaining sections of this chapter.

The final assumption was first considered in detail by Zhuchenko *et al.* (1979a, 1979b). Using the moments method of estimation they postulated that the different QTL genotypes could have different residual variances. They also considered the possibility that the residual variance was skewed, and that skewness was different for different QTL genotypes.

Weller (1986) considered a ML model in which a separate residual variance was estimated for each QTL genotype, and was able to derive estimates for both QTL main and variance effects. In the F-2 design used in this study, this increases the number of parameters that must be estimated from five to seven: three QTL means, three residual variances, and a QTL location parameter. Weller *et al.* (1988) analysed 180 marker-by-trait combinations, and found significant variance effects in more than 10% of the combinations. In a few cases the variance effects were significant even when QTL main effects were not. Variance effects cannot be estimated by non-linear least-squares.

6.3 QTL interaction effects

In the backcross design, estimation of an interaction effect entails only a single parameter, in addition to the parameters that must be estimated for each of the two QTL. This is illustrated by the example given in Table 6.1 for the expected effects in a backcross design with two loci. Genotype effects are given relative to the general mean. The expected genotype means without epistasis are listed in the top part of the table.

Without an interaction, the mean for each specific two-QTL genotype is equal the sum of the mean effects of each genotype for each locus. With epistasis this is no longer the case, as shown in the bottom part of the table. For the example with epistasis, the effect of genotype AaBb is equal to –15.

However, if the mean value of one of the four genotypes is changed, the three other genotypes must be changed accordingly to obtain the same main effect for each locus. Thus the interaction term has only a single degree of freedom. Therefore, in the backcross design including two QTL and an interaction term, it is necessary to estimate seven parameters: a general mean, an effect for each QTL, an interaction effect, location parameters for the two QTL, and the residual variance. However, for the F-2 design, the interaction term has four degrees of freedom. Thus it is necessary to estimate at least 12 parameters: a general mean, an additive and dominance effect for each QTL, four interaction effects, two QTL location parameters, and a residual variance.

Table 6.1 Expected effects in a backcross design with two loci without and with epistasis (an interaction)

Epistasis	Genotypes	Genotypes Aa	Aa	Mean Effects
Without	Bb	−12.5	2.5	−5.0
	bb	−2.5	12.5	5.0
With	Bb	−15.0	5.0	−5.0
	bb	0.0	10.0	5.0
Mean effects		−7.5	7.5	0

Weller et al. (1988) applied a model including the main effects of two QTL and an interaction term. They found a number of significant QTL interactions, but only QTL combinations with main effects for both loci were tested. Eshed and Zamir (1996) analysed the complete tomato genome for QTL affecting five quantitative traits using chromosomal segment substitution lines. The background parent was *Lycopersicon esculentum* (common tomato), and the donor parent was *L. pennellii*. Fifty substitution lines, each containing a single chromosomal segment from *L. pennellii* on the background of the *L. esculentum* genome, were analysed. Of 250 line-by-trait combinations, 81 were significantly different from the control isogenic line ($p<0.05$). The different substitution lines were then crossed to produce lines differing from the control each in two chromosomal segments. For those cases in which both *L. pennellii* chromosomal segments gave significant effects in the same direction, the effect estimates for the double substitution lines were consistently less than the sum of the effect estimates in the single chromosomal segment substitution lines. Of 46 cross-by-trait combinations, there was a significant interaction between the effects of the two chromosomal segments. Eshed and Zamir (1996) proposed that these results were due to epistasis. Although this result seems to indicate that interactions among QTL are quite prevalent, an alternative explanation will be presented in Section 11.7.

For animals and humans it is very difficult to address the question of QTL-by-environment interactions. For plants, this question can be addressed by generation of recombinant inbred lines (RIL), as described in Chapter four. All individuals within each RIL are isogenic. Thus, it is possible to grow identical genetic material in different environments. If the RIL are the product of a backcross or F-2 between two inbred lines, it is possible to estimate a QTL effect in each environment by growing samples of individuals from the same RIL in different environments. Thus it is possible to estimate a main QTL effect and a QTL-by-environment interaction for each environment tested. If a large number of QTL are analysed in many different environments, then the total number of parameters analysed can be quite large.

Korol *et al.* (1998) proposed that the number of parameters include in the model can be significantly reduced be expressing the interaction effects as a polynomial function of the mean trait value in each environment. They also assumed that the residual variance could be different in different environments, and also expressed the residual variances as a function of the mean trait value in each environment. This method was tested on both simulated and actual data from an experiment with barley. An alternative approach, also suggested by Korol *et al.* (1998), is to consider the interaction as a random effect. Thus no additional parameters are added, but it is necessary to know or estimate the interaction variance component.

6.4 Simultaneous analysis of multiple marker brackets

In the previous chapter we noted that a separate analysis of each individual marker bracket might result in biased estimates for the QTL parameters. Furthermore, neither the likelihood ratio test nor the F-test correctly tests for whether a QTL is segregating in the marker bracket. Martinez and Curnow (1992) considered a situation in which four linked markers are analysed by interval mapping. If two QTL are segregating, one between the first and second marker, and the second between the third and fourth markers, a "ghost" QTL will be detected in the middle bracket. Furthermore, the effect of this ghost QTL will be greater than the effect of the two actual QTL.

With several linked markers distributed across a chromosome, Martinez and Curnow (1992) proposed estimating QTL parameters for each adjacent pair of marker brackets using a model that postulates one QTL located between each pair of markers. We will consider only the BC design in detail, which is the simplest for analysis. As in the previous chapter we will consider only the haplotype derived from the F-1 parent, because the other haplotype will be the same for all BC progeny.

With three linked markers and two postulated segregating QTL, one within each marker bracket, there are four possible QTL haplotypes for the BC design. Denoting the two QTL, A and B, the possible QTL haplotypes are AB, Ab, aB, and aa. The non-linear regression model is:

$$Y_{ij} = \mu_1 p_{1i} + \mu_2 p_{2i} + \mu_3 p_{3i} + \mu_4 p_{4i} + e_{ij} \qquad \{6.1\}$$

where μ_1, μ_2, μ_3, and μ_4 are the four means for the four possible genotypes, and p_{1i}, p_{2i}, p_{3i}, and p_{4i} are the corresponding probabilities, given the haplotypes for the three segregating markers. Note that this model does not assume additivity between the two QTL, as explained in Section 6.3. If additivity is assumed, it is necessary to estimate only the additive effects of each QTL and a general mean.

Denoting: $p_{1i} = 1 - p_{2i} - p_{3i} - p_{4i}$, this model can be re-parameterized as follows:

$$Y_{ij} = \mu_1 + (\mu_2 - \mu_1)p_{2i} + (\mu_3 - \mu_1)p_{3i} + (\mu_4 - \mu_1)p_{4i} + e_{ij} \qquad \{6.2\}$$

$$Y_{ij} = \beta_1 + \beta_2 p_{2i} + \beta_3 p_{3i} + \beta_4 p_{4i} + e_{ij} \qquad \{6.3\}$$

Thus it is necessary to solve for four QTL effect parameters: β_1, β_2, β_3, and β_4. p_{2i}, p_{3i}, and p_{4i} will be functions of the two QTL location parameters, one for each marker interval. This complete model can then be tested against submodels that assume a QTL in only one of the two intervals. Martinez and Curnow (1992) found that this model was able to generate unbiased QTL parameter estimates when either a single QTL was located in the analysed chromosomal segment, or when a single QTL was segregating in each bracket, provided that there were no segregating QTL outside the analysed chromosomal segment.

However, Whittaker et al. (1996) demonstrated that in the case considered, three linked markers with a postulated QTL in each bracket, the solution obtained is not unique. That is, the effects of the two QTL will be confounded. This problem will be considered again in Section 6.9. Furthermore, the proposed analysis will still give biased estimates for the case considered at the beginning of the section: three marker brackets with QTL segregating in the two outlying brackets. With multiple linked markers, Martinez and Curnow (1992) propose estimating QTL affects jointly for each pair of brackets, but incrementing the markers by one for each analysis. Thus, the middle brackets will be analysed twice. Radically different parameter estimates derived from the two analyses of each intermediate bracket will be indicative of a ghost QTL.

Even if the two analyses are not radically different, it is still not clear how the results of the two analyses should be combined. To account for these factors, Jansen and Stam (1994) and Zeng (1993, 1994) proposed multiple regression QTL models. Jansen and Stam (1994) proposed modifying the non-linear regression model presented in the previous chapter. First consider the general linear model given in Equation $\{2.3\}$:

$$y = X\theta + e \quad \{6.4\}$$

where **y** is a vector of records, **X** is an incidence matrix, and θ is a vector of effects. If all effects are class effects, then **X** will be a matrix of zeros and ones. This model is appropriate for simultaneous estimation of multiple QTL if the QTL genotype of each individual is known without error for all segregating QTL. This, of course, is never the case. In the non-linear regression model described in the previous chapter, the coefficients of either zero or one in the **X** matrix are replaced by the probabilities of each possible QTL genotype for each individual. These probabilities are estimated based on marker genotypes and the assumed QTL location.

Jansen and Stam (1994) proposed expanding the non-linear regression model to consider simultaneously multiple marker intervals. At least two additional parameters must be estimated for each additional interval included in the model. Therefore, this model is mathematically tractable, provided that the number of intervals considered is not too large.

6.5 Principles of composite interval mapping

Rather than simultaneously analysing all marker brackets with potential QTL, Zeng (1993, 1994) proposed the following general model to test for a QTL in the marker interval between markers i and i+1:

$$y_j = b_o + b^* x_j^* + \sum_{k \neq i, i+1}^{t} b_k x_{jk} + e_j \quad \{6.5\}$$

where t is the total number of markers considered, y_j is the trait value for individual j, b_o is the general mean, b^* is the effect of the putative QTL located in the interval between markers i and i+1, x_j^* is the indicator variable of individual j for this interval, b_k is the partial regression coefficient of the phenotype for the kth marker, x_{jk} is the known indicator variable for marker k for individual j, and e_j is the random residual. x_j^* has a value of either 1 or 0, with probabilities $p_j^*(1)$ and $1 - p_j^*(1)$, respectively. As for single bracket interval mapping, $p_j^*(1)$ will be a function of the individual's genotype and QTL location within the marker bracket. Thus it is necessary to solve for two unknowns for each marker interval: QTL effect and location within the marker bracket.

Although all other markers are included as cofactors, this model only estimates QTL location and effect for the putative QTL located between markers i and i+1.

6.6 Properties of composite interval mapping

The following properties have been established for this model:

1. Assuming additivity of QTL effects, as explained in Section 6.3, the expected partial regression coefficient of the trait on a marker depends only on those QTL which are located in the interval bracketed by the two neighbouring markers, and is unaffected by the effect of QTL located in other intervals.
2. Conditioning on unlinked markers in the multiple regression analysis will reduce the sampling variance of the test statistic by controlling some residual genetic variation, and thus will increase the power of QTL mapping
3. Conditioning on linked markers in the multiple regression analysis will reduce the chance of interference of possible multiple linked QTL on hypothesis testing and parameter estimation, but with a possible increase of sampling variance.
4. Two sample partial regression coefficients of the trait value on two markers in a multiple regression analysis are generally uncorrelated, unless the two markers are adjacent markers. Even when the two intervals are adjacent, the correlation between the two test statistics is usually very small (Zeng, 1993).

6.7 Derivation of maximum likelihood parameter estimates by composite interval mapping

The likelihood function for Equation {6.5} is given by:

$$L = \prod_{j=1}^{N} [p_j(1)f_j(1) + p_j(0)f_j(0)] \quad \{6.6\}$$

where N is the sample size, $p_j(1)$ is the probability that $x_j^* = 1$, $p_j(0) = 1 - p_j(1)$, $f_j(1)$ and $f_j(0)$ specify a normal density function for y_j with a means of $b_o + b^* + \sum b_k x_{jk}$, and $b_o + \sum b_k x_{jk}$, respectively, and variances of σ^2. Maximum likelihood (ML) estimates of the parameters b^*, b_k's, and σ^2 can be derived as solutions to the following equations:

$$\hat{b}^* = (Y - X\hat{B})'\hat{p} / \hat{c} \quad \{6.7\}$$

$$\hat{B} = (X'X)^{-1}X'(Y - \hat{p}\hat{b}^*) \quad \{6.8\}$$

Chapter six: Advanced Statistical Methods 103

$$\hat{\sigma}^2 = (Y - X\hat{B})'(Y - X\hat{B}) - \hat{c}\,\hat{b}^{*2}]/N \quad \{6.9\}$$

where Y is the vector of records, $\hat{B}$ is the vector of estimates of the b_k values, X is the N by t–1 matrix of x_{jk} values, $\hat{p}$ is a vector with elements $\hat{p}$ specifying the ML estimates of the posterior probability that $x_j^* = 1$:

$$\hat{p}_j = p_j(1)\hat{f}_j(1)/[p_j(1)\hat{f}_j(1) + p_j(0)\hat{f}_j(0)] \quad \{6.10\}$$

and

$$\hat{c} = \sum_{j=1}^{N} \hat{p}_j \quad \{6.11\}$$

Equations {6.7} through {6.10} are themselves functions of the parameter estimates. Parameter estimates can be derived iteratively by the expectation/conditional maximization (ECM) algorithm (Meng and Rubin, 1993). In each step the algorithm consists of one estimation step, Equation {6.10}, and three conditional maximization steps, which are equations {6.7}, {6.8}, and {6.9}. Each equation is solved in turn using the parameter values estimated at the current iteration.

The ECM algorithm differs from the standard expectation maximization (EM) algorithm described in the previous chapter in that there are multiple conditional maximization steps. Like the standard EM algorithm, the ECM algorithm is guaranteed to converge to a local maximum, provided that there is a maximum within the parameter space. The ECM algorithm should be more efficient, because the inverse of the coefficient matrix, $(X'X)^{-1}$ is independent of the parameter estimates, and therefore has to be computed only once.

If many markers are genotyped, and a putative QTL is assumed in each interval, then it is necessary to solve this system of equations for each interval. Zeng (1994) suggest a stepwise approach. Intervals with the smallest effects can be tested first, and non-significant regions can be deleted from the model. If several closely linked markers are genotyped, Zeng suggested discarding some of the markers to obtain brackets of approximately 15 cM. QTL mapping with a saturated genetic map will be considered in Chapter ten.

6.8 Hypothesis testing with composite interval mapping

Presence of a QTL between markers i and i+1 can be tested by a likelihood ratio test of the complete model, and a model with b* set to zero. The likelihood function under the null hypothesis is:

$$L_o = \prod_{j=1}^{N} f_j(0) \qquad \{6.12\}$$

with the standard ML fixed linear model parameter estimates of:

$$\hat{B}_o = (X'X)^{-1}X'Y \qquad \{6.13\}$$

$$\hat{\sigma}_o^2 = (Y - X\hat{B}_o)'(Y - X\hat{B}_o)/N \qquad \{6.14\}$$

where $\hat{B}_o$ and $\hat{\sigma}_o^2$ are the estimates of σ^2 and B under the null hypothesis (no segregating QTL within the interval tested), respectively. This test is independent of the effects of QTL located outside the interval and adjacent intervals, provided that there are no epistasis effects among loci. Epistasis among QTL even in non-adjacent intervals can still cause bias in the test statistic. Furthermore, most studies have estimated QTL effects conditionally on the significant tests. In this case the estimates of QTL effects will still be biased.

6.9 Multi-marker and QTL analysis by regression of phenotype on marker genotypes

In Section 5.5 we considered the method of regression of phenotypes on marker genotype as proposed by Whittaker *et al.* (1996) for the case of a single QTL within a marker bracket. In this case the regression model for the F-2 design assuming additivity given in Equation {5.18} is:

$$Y_{ij} = \mu + \beta_m x_{mi} + \beta_n x_{ni} + e_{ij} \qquad \{6.15\}$$

Where μ is the general mean, β_m and β_n are linear regression coefficients for markers 1 and 2, x_{mi} and x_{ni} are marker genotype indicator variables, and e_{ij} is the random residual. x_{mi} and x_{ni} have values of 1 for individuals with genotypes. With multiple QTL and multiple marker brackets the model becomes:

$$Y_{ij} = \mu + \sum_{m=1}^{M} \beta_i x_{ij} + e_{ij} \qquad \{6.16\}$$

where β_i is the regression coefficient for marker i, x_{ij} is the indicator variable for the marker genotype for this marker, and M is the number of markers. As in the case of two markers, analytical solutions are derived for the marker regression coefficients, and these coefficients can be used to directly derive estimates of the

QTL effects and map locations, as explained in the previous chapter. Unlike the methods considered above, no iteration is required, and the solutions are equivalent to the solutions obtained by non-linear least-squares, although not exactly equivalent to solutions obtained by ML.

As noted in Section 6.4 QTL effects will be confounded if there are two segregating QTL in adjacent marker brackets. However, if linked QTL are separated by at least two markers, each QTL affects only the two adjacent markers. Equations {5.20} and {5.21} can be used to derive estimates of QTL location and effect for the F-2 design, assuming additivity. Similar equations were derived for the F-2 design, accounting for dominance, and the backcross (BC) design (Whittaker *et al.,* 1996).

If many markers are included in the analysis, Whittaker *et al.* (1996) propose a two-step procedure. In the first step, all markers are included in the analysis. In the second step the regression analysis is repeated, deleting markers with non-significant coefficients. Significance can still be tested by an F-test, but there is no uniformly "best" method to determine which markers should be deleted for the second analysis. "Stepwise" regression methods can be used, and are available in many statistical packages. They also note that, unless two QTL are segregating in adjacent marker brackets the sign of the coefficients of the two markers bracketing a QTL must be the same. Since QTL locations relative to genetic markers are not known *a priori*, this means that a marker adjacent to a segregating QTL must have the same sign as either the marker to the left or to the right, and that the QTL will be located between markers with the same sign.

In the case of the F-2 design with dominance effects in the model, QTL effects in adjacent intervals are no longer confounded, and additive, dominance, and location parameters can be estimated for both loci (Whittaker *et al.*, 1996).

6.10 Estimation of QTL parameters in outbred propulations

Analysis methods for outbred populations was reviewed recently by Hoeschele *et al.* (1997). The analysis models described in the previous chapter assumed that all effects on the trait value other than the segregating QTL are included in the residual. As noted previously, in the analysis of most experimental data and all field data, it will be necessary to account for systematic environmental effects and other "nuisance" effects, such as age or sex. In addition, individuals may have multiple records which are partially correlated. Finally, for models with complicated pedigree structure, such as daughter or grand-daughter designs, individuals with common marker genotypes can also have a common polygenic component of variance. In Chapter three, we noted that generally polygenic effects are considered random. As noted previously, the model of Fernando and Grossman (1989) that can potentially handle all of these factors, but has several significant deficiencies.

Solutions may be biased if there is a non-random distribution of other effects, such as herd effects. In addition, if outbred populations of animals or humans are analysed, there will generally be a non-random distribution of polygenic effects. For a random effect, it is generally assumed that the effect of each individual is randomly sampled from a continuous sample. However, if the analysis is based on a small group of preselected individuals, several studies have suggested that the polygenic effect should be considered fixed.

Kennedy et al. (1992) considered the effect of ignoring polygenic effects in QTL analysis of outbred populations in detail. They assumed a simple mixed model consisting of a fixed QTL effect and a random genetic effect. They further assumed that for each individual, QTL genotype was determined without error. In the mixed model analysis, it is possible to test a null hypothesis, such as **K'q** = 0, where **q** is the vector of QTL effects, and **K** is a matrix of coefficients. For example, if all three QTL genotypes are determined, the following **K'** matrix can be used to test the hypothesis of no difference among the genotypes:

$$\mathbf{K'} = \begin{bmatrix} 1 & -1 & 0 \\ 0 & 1 & -1 \end{bmatrix} \qquad \{6.17\}$$

Under the null hypothesis, $Q/(f\sigma_e^2)$ has a central F distribution (Henderson, 1984), where f is the rank of **K**, σ_e^2 is the residual variance, and **Q** is computed as follows:

$$\mathbf{Q} = (\mathbf{K'q})(\mathbf{K'C_{11}K})^{-1}(\mathbf{K'q}) \qquad \{6.18\}$$

where C_{11} is the quadrant of the inverse of the coefficient matrix pertaining to the QTL effects, as described in Chapter three. Kennedy et al. (1992) estimated σ_e^2 by Henderson's method III, as described in Chapter three.

Kennedy et al. (1992) found that even with random selection, type I errors for a standard fixed model ignoring polygenic effects were inflated if the polygenic effects were distributed non-randomly. This will be the situation in all commercial animal populations. QTL effect estimates ignoring polygenic effects were unbiased if the QTL did not affect the selection criterion, but were biased if the QTL affected the trait under selection. If polygenic effects were included in the model, then estimates of QTL effects were unbiased, even with selection on the trait affected by the QTL.

Designs based on analysis of additional generations were first described in Section 4.8. In the grand-daughter design sons of a heterozygous grandsire are genotyped but the records of their daughters, the grand-daughters of the original sire are analysed. Testing for a segregating QTL by ANOVA is somewhat more problematic for the grand-daughter design, because the sons that are genotyped pass a common polygenic effect to their daughters. As noted in Equation {4.13}, segregating marker-linked QTL can be detected with analysis by the following linear model:

$$Y_{ijklm} = GS_i + M_{ij} + SO_{ijk} + B_l + e_{ijklm} \quad \{6.19\}$$

where Y_{ijklm} is the production record of cow m, daughter of sire k, GS_i is the effect of the ith grandparent, M_{ij} is the effect of the jth allele, nested within the ith grandsire, SO_{ijk} is the effect of the kth son with the jth marker allele, progeny of the ith grandparent, B_l represents other fixed effects, and e_{ijklm} is the residual. Significance of the QTL effect can be tested by ANOVA, with the marker mean squares in the numerator. Under the null hypothesis of no segregating QTL, these mean squares will be a function of the variance among son effects, not the variance among individual records. Thus, the error term for the appropriate F-statistic will be the sire effect, defined as a random variable (Ron et al., 1994).

6.11 Solutions for analysis of field data from segregating populations

In the previous section we showed that unbiased estimates could be derived for QTL effects, if these effects are included in a general mixed model analysis that accounts for both other systematic fixed effects and polygenic effects. In most cases this is not a practical solution, because only a very small fraction of the population is genotyped for the QTL. Analysing only the genotyped individuals is not a viable option, because inclusion of all records is required to estimate genetic relationships, and "nuisance" factors, such as herd or block. Second, the effect estimated will be biased by recombination, as noted in the previous chapter. Thus, alternative methods of analysis have been proposed.

For the grand-daughter design, several studies have suggested analysing either estimate breeding values (EBV) (Andersson-Elkund et al., 1990; Cowan et al., 1992) or daughter yield deviations (DYD) (Hoeschele and vanRaden, 1993b) based on mixed models that include repeat records and fixed nuisance effects. DYD are the daughter record means of each son adjusted for systematic environmental effects and merits of mates (VanRaden, and Wiggans, 1991). The EBV or DYD are then analysed by a linear model including only the effects associated directly with the genetic markers. EBV derived from a mixed model will be regressed, and therefore estimates of QTL effects derived as described will be biased. In addition, the variances of either EBV or DYD will be a function of the quantity of information on the son. Thus, these studies have proposed to weight the evaluations by some function of their reliabilities. In the mixed model equations the coefficient matrix is multiplied by the inverse of the residual variance matrix. Therefore, for DYD, for which the variance decreases as the number of daughters increases, weighting by the repeatabilities is approximately correct. However, for mixed model EBV, which *increase* in variance as the number of progeny increases, the effect of weighting by the repeatability has an effect opposite to that desired. Sons with few daughters are multiplied by a smaller factor, even though their variance is less.

Israel and Weller (1998) proposed a complete mixed model analysis of the population with a fixed genotype effect for all individuals, including individuals that were not genotyped. For these individuals the coefficients of the genotype effect are the probability of each possible QTL genotype, based on allele frequencies in the population, and known genotypes of relatives. This method was able to derive almost unbiased estimates of QTL effects on simulated data for both daughter and grand-daughter designs, assuming complete linkage between the QTL and the genetic markers. In the daughter design, the cows' EBV and their yield deviations (VanRaden and Wiggans, 1991) both underestimated the simulated QTL effects. Likewise for the grand-daughter design, the sons' EBV and DYD underestimated simulated QTL effects. As expected the underestimate was greater for EBV.

The methods described so far in this chapter were based on linear model analyses and assumed complete linkage between the QTL and the genetic markers. Various studies have also attempted to estimate recombination frequencies for outbred populations, and derived unbiased estimates of QTL effects. As with crosses between inbred lines, both ML and non-linear regression techniques have been applied.

An additional problem in the analysis of segregating families is the question of whether different families should be analysed jointly or separately. In crosses between inbred lines, if each individual phenotyped is also genotyped, then the polygenic effect of each individual is completely confounded with the other factors that make up the random residual associated with each individual. This is not the case with the daughter design where all daughters of a sire have a common polygenic effect. The common polygenic effect will not affect QTL genotype estimates computed within a family. The common polygenic effects can then be considered part of the general mean.

Analysing DYD in a grand-daughter design, Georges *et al.* (1995) use ML to derive QTL parameter estimates for each family separately. This model is parallel to the BC design, except that not all grandsires are informative for all markers and marker phase of the grandsires must be estimated from the sons' genotypes. Because each family is analysed separately, it is not necessary to estimate a common polygenic effect for each family, or to estimate QTL allele frequencies in the population. The disadvantages of this method are as follows:

1. All of the QTL parameters are computed separately for each family. Thus, if the same QTL are segregating in different families this information is not utilized to estimate either the allelic effects or QTL location over all families.

2. The total number of comparisons is increased by a factor of the number of families. Questions related to multiple tests will be considered in detail in Chapter eleven.

Knott *et al.* (1994, 1996) assumed that the QTL location was the same for all families, but estimated a separate QTL substitution effect for each family. This model is amenable to analysis by non-linear regression; and in common with the method of Georges *et al.* (1995), does not require estimation of a common family polygenic effect. The disadvantage is that all families are assumed to be heterozygous for the QTL, which will generally not be the case. Mackinnon and Weller (1995) proposed a joint ML analysis across families assuming that only two QTL alleles were segregating in the population. Thus some of the families are assumed to be homozygous for the QTL. This model does require estimating a within-family polygenic effect, and the QTL allelic frequencies. The actual number of segregating QTL alleles in the population is not known, and may be greater than two. These two methods will be discussed in detail in the following sections. At present there is no completely satisfactory method for QTL parameter estimation of complex pedigrees.

6.12 Maximum likelihood analysis of QTL parameters for the daughter design with linkage to a single marker

We will first describe ML parameter estimation for segregating populations, beginning with the daughter design and a single marker linked to the putative QTL. Analyses of daughter and grand-daughter designs are complicated by the fact that marker and QTL linkage phase can be different in each family, and the number of QTL alleles segregating in the population is unknown. Furthermore, as noted previously, unlike crosses between inbred lines polygenic effects are not random with respect to marker genotypes, because each family has a common sire.

If only two QTL alleles are assumed, it is possible in the daughter design to estimate both additive and dominance effects. In the grand-daughter design it is only possible to estimate allele substitution effects, since grand-daughters are not genotyped. The allele substitution effect is defined as: $\alpha = a + d(p_1 - p_2)$, where a and d are the QTL additive and dominance effects and p_1 and p_2 are the frequencies of the two QTL alleles.

Mackinnon and Weller (1995) used ML to estimate QTL parameters for the daughter design. They assumed that only two QTL alleles were segregating in the population, that the distribution of the QTL alleles throughout the population was random, and that only sires heterozygous for the genetic marker were included in the analysis. Thus, four sire genotypes are determined with respect to the QTL and the genetic marker; homozygotes for Q_1Q_1 or Q_2Q_2, the heterozygote with Q_1 linked to M_1, and the heterozygote with Q_1 linked to M_2. Thus, in addition to the parameters that were estimated for the BC design, it is also necessary to solve for the relative frequency of the two QTL alleles among the sires. The likelihood for the model of Mackinnon and Weller (1995) is as follows:

$$L = \prod_{k=1}^{K} \sum_{v=1}^{4} P_v \prod_{i=1}^{3} \prod_{l=1}^{L_i} \sum_{j=1}^{3} p_{j|i,v} f(y_{ikl} - \mu_j) \quad \{6.20\}$$

where K is the number of sires, P_v is the probability of sire QTL genotype v, $p_{j|i,v}$ is the probability of progeny QTL genotype j conditional on the combination of sire QTL genotype v and progeny marker genotype i, L_i is the number of daughters with marker genotype i, y_{ikl} is the trait value for progeny l of sire k, with marker genotype i, μ_j is the mean for progeny QTL genotype j, and $f(y_{iklm} - \mu_j)$ is the normal density function for progeny m of sire k, conditional on QTL genotype j.

P_v was computed based on the assumed Hardy-Weinberg distribution of QTL genotypes among the sires. $p_{j|i,v}$ will be dependent on which marker and QTL alleles were passed from both the sire and the dam. As noted above, only sires heterozygous for the marker were included in the analysis, but dams could have any marker genotype, including alleles not present in the sires. For progeny with the paternal marker genotype, it is not known which allele was received from the sire, and which allele was received from the dam. Thus, $p_{j|i,v}$ is a function of marker allele frequency among the dams. Even if there are numerous marker alleles segregating in the population, to compute $p_{j|i,v}$ it is necessary to define only three marker genotype classes for the progeny: those that receive M_1 but not M_2, those that receive M_2 but not M_1, and those that receive both paternal alleles. Mackinnon and Weller (1995) derived formula for $p_{j|i}$, based on the assumption that the marker allele frequencies in the dam population were known. These probabilities are given in Table 6.2, with minor modifications to account for the possibility of multiple marker alleles in the dam population. As noted previously, if there are multiple alleles in the population, it will be possible to determine unequivocally marker allele origin in the progeny, unless the progeny received the same heterozygous genotype as the sire.

Assuming that QTL genotype does not affect the variance, it is necessary to estimate six parameters, the three QTL genotype means, the residual variance, the recombination frequency between the marker and the QTL, and the frequency of the Q_1 allele. With large samples, reasonable estimates can be derived for all parameters (Mackinnon and Weller, 1995). With this model it is also possible to determine the relative likelihood of each possible sire QTL genotype. Mackinnon and Weller (1995) found that the simulated genotype generally had the highest likelihood. For relatively large QTL effects relative to the polygenic variance, this statistic could be used to correctly determine the sire QTL genotype.

Table 6.2 Progeny QTL genotype probabilities conditional on sire marker-QTL genotype and their own marker genotype ($p_{j|i,v}$)*

Progeny QTL genotype			Progeny marker genotype	Sire genotype
Q_1Q_1	Q_1Q_2	Q_2Q_2		
P	1 – p	0	M_1M_x	M_1Q_1/M_2Q_1
P	1 – p	0	M_1M_2	
P	1 – p	0	M_2M_y	
p(1 – r)	1 – p – r + 2pr	(1 – p)r	M_1M_x	M_1Q_1/M_2Q_2
tpr+(1–t)p(1–r)	t(p+r–2pr) +(1–t)(1–p–r+2pr)	t(1–p–r+rp) +(1–t)(1–p)r	M_1M_2	
Pr	p + r – 2pr	1 – p – r + pr	M_2M_y	
Pr	p + r – 2pr	1 – p – r + pr	M_1M_x	M_1Q_2/M_2Q_1
tp(1–r)+(1–t)pr	t(1–p–r+2pr) +(1–t)(p+r–2pr)	t(1–p)r +(1–t)(1–p–r+rp)	M_1M_2	
p(1 – r)	1 – p – r + 2pr	(1 – p)r	M_2M_y	
0	P	1 – p	M_1M_x	M_1Q_2/M_2Q_2
0	P	1 – p	M_1M_2	
0	P	1 – p	M_2M_y	

* p = probability of QTL allele Q_1Q_1, r = recombination frequency between M and Q, t = relative frequency of the allele M_1 among M_1 and M_2 alleles in the population of dams, M_x = any marker allele other than M_2, M_y = any marker allele other than M_1.

6.13 Maximum likelihood estimation of QTL parameters from other complex pedigrees

Mackinnon and Weller (1995) modified their model to include a fixed polygenic sire effect. In this case the normal density function becomes $f(y_{iklm} - \mu_j - g_k)$, where g_k is the polygenic effect of sire k on his daughters. This increases the number of parameters that must be estimated by the number of sires. Bovenhuis and Weller (1994) modified this model to include a direct effect of the marker genotype in addition to a linked QTL.

Song and Weller (1998) developed a method to simultaneously estimate QTL and sire polygenic effects for the daughter design, based on the EM algorithm of Jansen (1992). They assumed a fixed sire polygenic effect and only two QTL alleles segregating in the population. This method was tested on simulated data with a QTL bracketed by two markers. They estimated the same parameters as Mackinnon and Weller (1995), including the sire polygenic effect. QTL location was estimated accurately in all cases. The QTL substitution effect was underestimated for relatively small effects ($\alpha=0.5$ phenotypic standard deviations). For larger effects it was possible to determine accurately sire QTL genotype by the method of Mackinnon and Weller (1995), but this determination was often incorrect for $\alpha=0.5$.

6.14 Non-linear and linear regression estimation for complex pedigrees

Knott et al. (1994, 1996) proposed that the non-linear regression method could also be used to estimate QTL effects for multiple pedigrees. As noted previously, they assumed that the QTL location was the same for all families, but estimated a separate substitution effect for each family. The analysis model is as follows:

$$Y_{ijk} = \mu_{1i}(1 - p_{ij}) + \mu_{2i}p_{ij} + e_{ijk} \qquad \{6.21\}$$

where Y_{ijk} is the trait record for individual k of family i with marker genotype j, μ_{1i} and μ_{2i} are the means for progeny that received paternal QTL alleles 1 and 2 in family i, p_{ij} is the probability that a progeny of sire i with marker genotype j received paternal QTL allele 1, and e_{ijk} is the random residual. Although QTL location is assumed to be the same in all families, p_{ij} must be computed separately for each individual, because it will depend on which markers are informative in each progeny of each family. As noted also by Martinez and Curnow (1994) even if all markers to one side of the putative QTL location are uninformative in a specific individual, p_{ij} can still be calculated based on the recombination frequency between the assumed QTL position and the single linked marker. Thus, only individuals without any markers in linkage to the putative QTL location will be discarded from the analysis.

There are two main advantages of this method. First, data across families is combined to estimate QTL location. This is especially important in daughter and grand-daughter designs, because, as noted above, only some of the markers analysed will be informative in each pedigree. Second, since an individual substitution effect is computed within each family, it is not necessary to estimate a common polygenic effect for each family. The main disadvantage of this method, as noted previously, is that each family is considered to be heterozygous for two different QTL alleles.

Knott et al. (1996) compared QTL parameter estimation by non-linear regression to the ML method described in the previous two sections, and to least-squares estimation using the individual markers (Weller et al., 1990). They simulated a QTL with two alleles of equal frequency, no dominance, and an additive effect of 1.09. They assumed a grand-daughter design analysis, in which the estimated effect is one half of the additive effect, as explained in Section 4.8. For the grand-daughter design only a substitution effect can be estimated, which simplifies the likelihood function proposed by Mackinnon and Weller (1995). They further assumed that the sons' "records" (DYD or genetic evaluations) were adjusted for the grandsire family mean. Thus only three parameters are estimated: the QTL allelic frequency, the substitution effect, and the residual variance. They assumed marker intervals of 10, 20 and 50 cM on a 100 cM chromosome, and equal allelic frequencies for the marker alleles. The number of marker alleles simulated was either two or four. They considered both analyses in which dam were or were not genotyped. When dams are genotyped, the frequency of informative progeny is increased, as explained in Section 4.5.

Even though this model is in accordance with the ML assumption of two alleles with equal frequency, power by ML and non-linear least-squares were almost equal, while power was lower for least squares on the individual markers. Statistical power and parameter confidence intervals will be considered in more detail in Chapter eight.

Kadarmideen and Dekkers (1999) proposed that the linear regression model described in Sections 5.5 and 6.9 could also be applied to the half-sib design. The two problems that must be solved as considered above, are that not all markers are informative in all families, and data must be accumulated across families. For analysis of a single half-sib family with partially informative markers they showed that Equation {5.18} could be modified as follows:

$$Y_j = \mu + \beta_m p_{mj} + \beta_n p_{nj} + e_j \qquad \{6.22\}$$

where p_{mj} and p_{nj} are the probabilities that individual j received one of the two paternal alleles. (No subscript i is required, because the alternative allele of each marker has an implied coefficient of zero.) p_{mj} and p_{nj} are computed based on all available information, such as recombination frequencies, known parental genotype phase, and population allelic frequencies. If the paternal allele is known without error, then p_{mj} and p_{nj} are equal to either one or zero, and this model is the same as the half-sib linear regression model. To apply this model to multiple families, Kadarmideen and Dekkers (1999) propose two solutions:

1. Computing the regression coefficients as nested within a family. In this case a separate QTL effect and location will be estimated in each family.
2. A random regression model, with estimated variances at markers expressed in terms of a genetic model of a single QTL will multiple alleles. It is not clear how this model can be applied in practice, since the variance due to the QTL is unknown.

114 Quantitative Trait Loci Analysis in Animals

In Section 5.5 we showed how marker information content could be computed for all points within marker brackets. For complex pedigrees computation of marker information content will depend not only on the chromosomal location, relative to the markers, but also on the information content of each marker. However, several studies have noted that with standard interval mapping, the estimated QTL position will be biased towards more informative markers (Haley *et al.*, 1994; Spelman *et al.*, 1996).

6.15 Maximum likelihood estimation with random effects included in the model

As noted in the previous chapter, polygenic breeding values are generally considered random effects in genetic evaluation models. In Section 6.12 we presented a ML model for analysis of the daughter design that included a fixed polygenic family effect. Estimating the sire effect as fixed can be justified, because each sire will have many progeny, and those sires with many daughters are generally not a random sample from the population. However, the granddaughter design is more problematic than the daughter design, because a common sire effect is nested within the grandsire QTL, and will therefore affect QTL estimates within families. Furthermore, nearly all AI sons will be included in the analysis. Therefore the distribution will be much closer to a random sample.

Only fixed effects should be estimated by maximum likelihood estimation, while random effects should be "removed" by integration (Titterington *et al.*, 1985). This will be illustrated using the daughter design model of Equation {6.18}. The likelihood function, modified to include a polygenic sire effect is:

$$L = \prod_{k=1}^{G} \int \{f(g_k - \mu_g, \sigma_g^2) \sum_{v=1}^{4} P_v \prod_{i=1}^{3} \prod_{l=1}^{L_i} \sum_{j=1}^{3} c_{jli,v} f(y_{ikl} - \mu_j - g_k, \sigma_e^2)\} dg_k \quad \{6.23\}$$

where $f(g_k - \mu_g, \sigma_g^2)$ represents the normal density function for the sire effects. This function has a mean of μ_g and a variance of σ_g^2, which will be equal to one-quarter of the genetic variance. $f(y_{ikl} - \mu_j - g_k, \sigma_e^2)$ represents a normal density function with a mean of $\mu_j + g_k$ and a variance of σ_e^2, and the other terms are as defined above. σ_e^2 includes the residual variance, and three-quarters of the genetic variance not explained by the segregating QTL. The likelihood function is the joint density of the observations integrated over g_k, the polygenic sire effect, which is now assumed to be random.

Although the integral cannot be solved analytically, it can be approximately solved by summation for each sire. Thus, the likelihood value can be approximately computed for any combination of parameter values. However, this model still does not include "nuisance" fixed effects, such as herd-year-season effects, which would have to be included in any analysis of field data. Therefore, it is not surprising that ML solutions have not been computed on actual data. For the grand-daughter design it is necessary to include normal density distribution terms for both the sire and grandsire, and integrate over both terms, if the analysis is based on the actual production records.

6.16 Maximum likelihood estimation of QTL effects on categorical traits

Nearly all QTL analyses have assumed normal distributions for the quantitative traits. As noted in the previous chapter, if the trait distribution is continuous, it will generally be possible to transform the trait values so as to obtain an approximately normal distribution. Kruglyak and Lander (1995a) proposed a non-parametric approach, based on a statistic Z_W, which generalizes the non-parametric Wilcox rank-sum test to interval mapping. In this method, rather than analyse the actual phenotypic scores, the dependent variable is the rank of each value, which by definition has a uniform distribution. The Z_W statistic for the BC design is computed as follows:

$$Z_W(s) = Y_W(s)/\{[Y_W(s)]^2\}^{1/2} \quad \{6.24\}$$

where s is the assumed QTL location, and $Y_W(s)$ for a BC design, as illustrated in Figure 5.2, is computed as follows:

$$Y_W(s) = \Sigma(N + 1 - 2 \text{ (rank i)}E[x_i(s)|\ y_1, y_2,...y_n] \quad \{6.25\}$$

where $x_i(s)$ is either 1 or –1, depending on the QTL genotype of progeny i, Q_1Q_1 or Q_1Q_2, and N is the sample size. This expectation can be computed based on the assumed values for the recombination parameter. For the BC design, the probabilities that $x_i(s)$ is either 1 or –1 will be: $r_1(1-r_2)/R$ and $(1-r_1)r_2/R$, if the individual is a recombinant for the flanking markers; and $r_1r_2/(1-R)$ and $(1-r_1)(1-r_2)/(1-R)$, if the individual is a non-recombinant, where R is the recombination frequency between the two markers, and r_1 is the recombination frequency between one of the markers and the QTL. r_2, the recombination frequency between the QTL and the other marker is computed as a function of R and r_1, based on the assumed mapping function, as described in Section 5.3. Since the mean of $Y_W(s) = 0$, $Y_W(s)^2$ is equal to the variance of $Y_W(s)$. $Y_W(s)^2$ is computed as follows (Kruglyak and Lander, 1995a):

$$Y_W(s)^2 = \sum_{i=1}^{N} (N + 1 - 2i)^2 \{E[x_i(s)|\ y_1, y_2,...y_n]\}^2 \qquad \{6.26\}$$

The sum of $(N + 1 - 2i)^2$ will be equal to $(N^3 - N)/3$, while the second term will be a function of the specific experimental design. For the half-sib design this equation becomes:

$$Y_W(s)^2 = \left[\frac{N^3 - N}{3}\right]\left[\frac{(r_1 - r_2)^2}{R} + \frac{1 - (r_1 + r_2)^2}{1 - R}\right] \qquad \{6.27\}$$

The value of r_1 that maximizes $Z_W(s)$ gives the most likely QTL location. Once r_1 is estimated, the QTL genotype means can then be estimated from Equation 5.2, with p_i assumed known. In this case, Equation 5.2 is a linear model. For any location s on the genome, $Z_W(s)$ is asymptotically distributed as a standard normal variable with a mean of 0 and a variance of 1. Thus significance of a segregating QTL can be evaluated by a t-test of $Z_W(s)$.

If several individuals have the same phenotypic score, then these individuals can be ranked randomly. Alternatively, these individuals can be assigned the average rank, but the gain achieved by this procedure is small. For the F-2 design, $x_i(s)$ will have values of -1, 0 and 1, for QTL genotypes of Q_1Q_1, Q_1Q_2, and Q_2Q_2.

Coppieters et al. (1998) modified this method for analysis of the daughter and grand-daughter designs. In this case, a Z_w statistic is computed for each half-sib family, and significance is tested by the sum of squares of the Z_w scores, as first proposed by Neimann-Soressen and Robertson (1961) for analysis of the daughter design. This statistic should have a χ^2 distribution, with degrees of freedom equal to the number of families analysed. $x_i(s)$ is now equal to 1 if the progeny inherited one of the sire QTL alleles, and -1 if the progeny inherited the other allele. As proposed by Knott et al. (1996) the expectations were computed using the closest informative markers for each progeny for each possible QTL location. This complicates computation of the variance of Y_W, which must be calculated separately for each family by simulating all possible offspring, and calculating a frequency weighted mean of $\{E[x_i(s)|\ y_1, y_2,...y_n]\}^2$.

The Wilcox rank-sum test was less powerful than the regression method of Knott et al. (1996) if the residual variance had a univariate normal distribution. However, power was greater with the rank-sum test if this was not the case. Thus, as originally proposed, the rank-sum test is more robust to deviations from the assumptions of the parametric methods.

6.17 Estimation of QTL effects with the threshold model

The Wilcox rank-sum test described in the previous section is not applicable if the trait is scored with only a few categories. A "worst case" situation is when the quantitative trait has a dichotomous distribution with one phenotype at a much higher frequency. This situation is common for disease traits and survival data.

The threshold model is based on the assumption of an underlying normal distribution for the trait, which is not observed. Along the distribution are threshold points. All individuals with values for the continuous trait between two thresholds display the same discrete phenotype. Factors affect the displayed phenotype by shifting the mean of the underlying trait. Gianola and Foulley (1983) considered application of the threshold model to analysis of polygenic variance in detail.

Hackett and Weller (1995) derived an ML model suitable for categorical traits. They assumed a threshold model with an underlying logistic distribution, and solved using the method of Jansen (1992). The logistic distribution yields results very similar to the normal distribution, but is more mathematically tractable. We will assume a vector of fixed effects, β, acting additively on the underlying continuous variable, and an incidence matrix of $\mathbf{X}$. Assume that there are k–1 thresholds and thus k observed categories for the quantitative trait. The cumulative probability up to category j, P_j, is then computed as follows:

$$P_j = \frac{e^{(\tau_j - \mathbf{X}\beta)}}{1 + e^{(\tau_j - \mathbf{X}\beta)}} \qquad \{6.28\}$$

where τ_j is the jth threshold on the scale of the continuous variable. This model can be rewritten as a generalized linear model with the logit link function as follows:

$$\log[P_j/(1 - P_j)] = \tau_j - \mathbf{X}\beta \qquad \{6.29\}$$

It is now possible to apply the EM algorithm of Jansen (1992) as described in Equation {5.31}, with:

$$p(q|y_i, m_i) = \frac{e^{(\tau_j - \mathbf{X}\beta)}}{1 + e^{(\tau_j - \mathbf{X}\beta)}} - \frac{e^{(\tau_{j-1} - \mathbf{X}\beta)}}{1 + e^{(\tau_{j-1} - \mathbf{X}\beta)}} \qquad \{6.30\}$$

∂[log f(y$_i$|q$_i$)]/∂θ can be derived by solving the general linear model of Equation {6.29}, and p(q|m$_i$) is a simple function of the recombination parameters: R for a single marker, or r$_1$ and r$_2$ for marker brackets.

This model was compared on simulated data to a model which assumed that the categorical trait scores had a normal distribution. The threshold model was able to estimate recombination parameters more accurately than the normal model, especially when the trait was score with only two categories. Comparison of QTL effects is not straightforward since the scales of the two models cannot be compared directly. In the threshold model QTL effects are estimated on the underlying scale, which is not directly observed.

6.18 Estimation of QTL effects on disease traits by the allele-sharing method

In Section 4.7 we considered the sib-pair method of Haseman and Elston (1972), which is the most appropriate design for detection of QTL in humans. Disease traits are generally scored dichotomously, either the syndrome is observed or it is not. Generally the effect of an individual gene on a disease syndrome is phrased in terms of "penetrance", defined as the fraction of individuals carrying the disease genotype that actually display the syndrome. If the penetrance is low, the unaffected individuals will add very little information with respect the QTL analysis. Even if both the parent and progeny are carriers, chances are that neither will display the affected phenotype. Therefore the "allele-sharing" analysis method was developed based on analysis of only affected individuals.

The allele-sharing method is based on the assumption that if a genetic marker is linked to a QTL affecting expression of the disease, two related individuals will have a higher than expected probability of sharing the same marker allele, identical by descent (IBD). For example, the probability that a grandparent and its grandchild with have the same allele by chance is one half. Similarly the probability that two half-sibs will have the same allele IBD is also one half, while for first cousins the probability is one-quarter. If the two related individuals both display the disease phenotype, and the marker locus is linked to a QTL affecting the disease, then it is more likely that both individuals carry the same marker allele IBD. (Of course this method can only be applied effectively to highly polymorphic markers. Otherwise there will be a significant probability that the two individuals may both have the same allele, but not IBD.)

With the allele-sharing method significance of linkage can be determined by a χ^2 test, comparing the expected numbers of relative pairs with and without common alleles, based on their relationships, to the observed numbers. Alternatively, these values for a specific marker can be expressed as a LOD score (Risch, 1990) as follows:

$$LOD(m) = N_s(m)\log[p_m/p_e] + [N - N_s(m)]\log[(1 - p_m)/(1 - p_e)] \quad \{6.31\}$$

where LOD(m) is the LOD score (log base 10 of the likelihoods ratio) for marker m, $N_s(m)$ is the number of relative pairs which share a common marker allele IBD, p_m is the observed probability of allele sharing, p_e is the expected probability of allele sharing, and N is the total number of relative pairs included in the analysis.

If multiple linked markers are genotyped, it is also possible to test for allele sharing for all points within the marker interval, similar to interval mapping for continuous traits. Similar to the situation with large half-sib families considered in Sections 6.12 to 6.14, not all markers will be informative for all relative pairs. Power of detection is increased if information from all linked markers is used to determine whether the two relatives share a common haplotype (Kruglyak and Lander, 1995b).

6.19 Summary

In this chapter we considered methods for QTL parameter estimation for more complex models. Bias estimates will result if polygenic effects and other nuisance effects, such as herd, are not included in the analysis model. Thus most studies have been based on analysis of either genetic evaluations or DYD, both of which are problematic. Another major problem encountered with analysis of complex pedigrees is that the number of segregating QTL alleles is not known. Most models have therefore either assumed two alleles or an infinite number of alleles. Although we again emphasized maximum likelihood, non-linear regression and linear regression on marker genotypes were also considered. ML is clearly the most flexible method. The disadvantages are that it may be difficult to apply technically in certain cases, and it is also relatively difficult to test significance and estimate confidence intervals. Also, prior knowledge is ignored in ML estimation. There is no completely satisfactory method at present for analysis of QTL data from large complex families, such as commercial dairy cattle populations.

In the last three sections of this chapter we considered several analysis methods that have been proposed for traits with categorical distributions. In this case the assumption of a normal distribution of residuals is clearly incorrect. However, if the number of categories is not too low, and no single category includes most of the observations, the gain obtained by removing the assumption of normality will be minimal.

Chapter seven:

Analysis of QTL as Random Effects

7.1 Introduction

In the previous two chapters we described the methods for QTL parameter estimation, which are applicable to crosses between inbred lines and segregating populations. Maximum likelihood estimation is the most flexible method, and was described in most detail. Although the previous chapter considered models with both fixed and random effects, in both chapters QTL effects were considered to be fixed effects. As first noted in Chapter in four, in contrast with crosses between inbred lines the number of QTL alleles segregating in outbred populations is unknown. In Chapter four we presented the model of Haseman and Elston (1972) for analysis of full-sib families, and the model of Fernando and Grossman (1989) that can be applied to any outbred diploid population. In the former model, the segregating QTL can be considered to be either a fixed or random effect, while in the latter model the QTL must be considered to be random.

In this chapter we will describe analyses methods that consider QTL as random effects. Generally for random effects the objective is to estimate the variance due to the effect, rather than the effects of specific alleles, although both questions will be addressed with respect to the model of Fernando and Grossman. General methods for estimating variance components were described in Chapter three, and these methods, specifically maximum likelihood (ML) and restricted maximum likelihood (REML), will be applied to estimation of the variance due to segregating QTL.

In Chapter eleven we will consider whole genome scans for multiple QTL. If QTL effects are estimated by a fixed model, and all effects greater than specified threshold are deemed "significant", the substitution effects in the selected group will be overestimated. This was first noted by Smith and Simpson (1986), and will be discussed in detail in Chapter eleven. Unlike estimates derived from fixed models, random estimates of effects are "shrunken" or regressed towards the mean based on prior knowledge. It should therefore be possible to derive unbiased estimates of QTL effects if the QTL are estimated as random effects.

In Section 7.2 we will describe methods to estimate QTL variance for the Haseman-Elston sib-pair model. In Sections 7.3 to 7.8 we will describe how the model of Fernando and Grossman can be expanded to handle multiple QTL with marker brackets. In Sections 7.9 and 7.10 we will discuss estimation of variance components for the Fernando-Grossman model. We will discuss Bayesian QTL parameter estimation in Sections 7.11 to 7.13, and in Section 7.14 we will briefly discuss estimation of QTL parameters by Gibbs sampling.

7.2 ML estimation of variance components for the Haseman-Elston sib-pair model

In Section 4.7 we first considered the sib-pair experimental design proposed by Haseman and Elston (1972). In that section we derived methods to estimate the QTL effect as a function of the regression of the squared difference between sib-pair phenotypes on the fraction of alleles identical by descent (IBD). The QTL additive and dominance effects can be estimated, assuming that only two QTL alleles are segregating in the population. If the number of segregating QTL alleles is unknown, it is still possible by ML or REML to estimate the variance due to the QTL, and its location relative to linked genetic markers. The hypothesis of a segregating QTL linked to the genetic markers can also be tested against the null hypothesis of no segregating QTL by a likelihood ratio test.

Xu and Atchley (1995) proposed a ML method to test for a segregating QTL within a marker bracket for the Haseman-Elston model. Their model can accommodate any number of sibs within each whole-sib family, and accounts for polygenic variance, but assumes that the whole-sib families are unrelated. They assumed no other fixed effects in the analysis except a general mean, although the model can be easily expanded to include fixed effects. Since ML is used instead of REML, there will be a slight bias, as described in Chapter three. However, this bias will be minimal if the sample size is large, and the only fixed effect is the general mean.

The original model for the sib-pair analysis was given Equations {4.9}. As in the previous chapters we will denote recombination frequency between the two markers as R, and recombination frequency between each marker and the QTL as r_1 and r_2. We will now modify this equation for a single sib to include an additive polygenic effect as follows:

$$x_{ij} = \mu + a_{ij} + g_{ij} + e_{ij} \quad \{7.1\}$$

where: x_{1j} is the trait values for sibs i of family j, μ is the general mean, a_{ij}, g_{ij} and e_{ij} are the additive polygenic, QTL, and residual effects for sib i. All effects, except the general mean are considered random. Thus:

$$\text{Var}(x_{ij}) = \sigma^2 = \sigma_A^2 + \sigma_V^2 + \sigma_e^2 \quad \{7.2\}$$

where σ^2 is the total variance, and σ_A^2, σ_V^2, and σ_e^2 are the polygenic, QTL and residual variance components.

As noted above, the model assumes that individuals from different full-sib families are unrelated. This assumption is not required if the analysis is based on the regression model given in Equation {4.10}. With this assumption the only non-zero covariance will be among full-sibs from the same families. Full sibs have one-half of their genes IBD. Therefore the covariance between a sib-pair from family j will be $\pi_j \sigma_v^2 + \frac{1}{2}\sigma_A^2$ where π_j is the fraction of marker alleles IBD for the sib-pair from family j. π_j is unknown, but as noted in Chapter four, it can be replaced by its expectation. For a QTL bracketed by two markers, this expectation, $\hat{\pi}$, can be computed as follows (Fulker and Cardon, 1994):

$$\hat{\pi}_j = \alpha + \beta_1 \pi_{j1} + \beta_2 \pi_{j2} \qquad \{7.3\}$$

where π_{j1} and π_{j2} are the IBD values for the two flanking markers, and:

$$\beta_1 = [(1-2r_1)^2 - (1-2r_2)^2 (1-2R)^2]/[(1-(1-2R)^4] \qquad \{7.4\}$$

$$\beta_2 = [(1-2r_2)^2 - (1-2r_1)^2 (1-2R)^2]/[(1-(1-2R)^4] \qquad \{7.5\}$$

$$\alpha = (1 - \beta_1 - \beta_2)/2 \qquad \{7.6\}$$

The likelihood function for a mixed model analysis, assuming a normal distribution of residuals, is given in Equation {3.35}, and will be repeated here:

$$L = (2\pi)^{-n/2} |V|^{-\frac{1}{2}} \exp\left[-\frac{1}{2}(y - X\beta)' V^{-1} (y - X\beta)\right] \qquad \{7.7\}$$

where V is the variance matrix, β is the vector of fixed effects, and X is the incidence matrix. If the only fixed effect included in the model is the mean, the likelihood function for a single family, L_i, with k full-sibs will be:

$$L_i = (2\pi\sigma^2)^{-k/2} |C_i|^{-\frac{1}{2}} \exp\left[-[1/(2\sigma^2)](y_i - 1\mu)' C_i^{-1} (y_i - 1\mu)\right] \qquad \{7.8\}$$

where y_i is the vector of records of length k of the sibs from family i, 1 is a vector of 1s, and $C_i = V/\sigma^2$ is a k × k matrix with 1s on the diagonal, and off-diagonal elements of: $[\hat{\pi}_j \sigma_v^2 + \frac{1}{2}\sigma_A^2]/\sigma^2$. The log of the likelihood over all families is then:

$$\text{Log } L = \sum (\log L_i) \qquad \{7.9\}$$

with the summation over all the families.

This likelihood can then be maximized as a function of the three variance components: σ_A^2, σ_v^2, and σ_e^2, and μ, and a recombination parameter, either r_1 or r_2. As in most other studies, Xu and Atchley (1995) assumed that recombination frequency between the markers was known without error. Thus, for a given map function, r_2 can be computed as a function of r_2 and R. Similar to interval mapping, as proposed by Lander and Botstein (1989), Xu and Atchley (1995) maximized Log L for the first four parameters, over the range of possible QTL locations. For each analysis, the QTL location was assumed known. The final ML parameter estimates were the set of estimates that give the highest likelihood as a function of the assumed QTL location. At each assumed QTL location, Xu and Atchley (1995) used a two-step iterative algorithm. At each iteration, they first solved for μ and σ^2, using the current values for h_V^2 and h_A^2, where $h_V^2 = \sigma_V^2/\sigma^2$ and $h_A^2 = \sigma_A^2/\sigma^2$. They then used a simplex algorithm to solve for h_V^2 and h_A^2.

Significance of a segregating QTL was tested by a likelihood ratio test, as described in Section 5.7. In this case the null hypothesis is $h_V^2 = 0$. As noted in Chapter five, although only one parameter is fixed in the null hypothesis, this also "fixes" the QTL location, since under the null hypothesis there is no segregating QTL. The empirical distribution of the test statistic with six markers equally spaced on a chromosome of 100 cM was between the theoretical χ^2 distributions with 1 and 2 degrees of freedom (df). For high values of the test statistic, which are the values of interest for rejecting the null hypothesis, the empirical distribution approached the theoretical χ^2-distribution with 2 df. The power and accuracy of this method to detect a segregating QTL will be considered in the following chapter.

7.3 The random gametic model of Fernando and Grossman, computing G_v

As explained in Chapter four, Fernando and Grossman (1989) proposed a random gametic QTL model suitable for analysis by a set of modified individual animal model equations. This model can handle any population structure. Furthermore, "nuisance" effects, such as herd or block, can also be included in the analysis. The model assumes that each individual with unknown ancestors contributes two different QTL alleles to the population. The allelic effects are assumed to be sampled from a normal distribution of allelic effects with a known variance. The QTL is further assumed to be codominant with respect to the trait analysed. We will first consider the original Fernando-Grossman model, which postulated a single QTL linked to a single marker locus.

As noted in Section 4.10, this model requires computation of the variance matrix among the QTL gametic effects, G_v. Fernando and Grossman (1989) demonstrated how this matrix can be constructed by first considering the allele passed to each progeny from its sire. As in the previous chapters we will denote the QTL alleles Q, and the marker alleles M, with recombination frequency of r between these two loci. Assume that individuals o and o' with sires s and s' received QTL alleles Q^p_o and $Q^p_{o'}$ from their sires, where the superscript signifies the allele origin (paternal or maternal), and the subscript signifies which allele was received. The covariance between the additive QTL effect of o and o', $\text{Cov}(v^p_o, v^p_o{}')$ is computed as follows:

$$\text{Cov}(v^p_o, v^p_o{}') = \sigma_v^2 \, P(Q^p_o \equiv Q^p_o{}') \quad \{7.10\}$$

where σ_v^2 is the additive variance of the QTL allele, and $P(Q^p_o \equiv Q^p_o{}')$ is the probability that these two alleles are IBD. In this model the QTL alleles of individuals with unknown parents are sampled from a distribution with a known variance. The two QTL alleles can be IBD in one of three ways:

1. One of the two individuals is a descendent of the other.
2. Q^p_o is IBD to the paternal QTL allele of the sire of o', and o' received allele $Q^p_s{}'$ (the paternal allele of s').
3. Q^p_o is IBD to the maternal QTL allele of the sire of o', and o' received allele $Q^m_s{}'$ (the maternal allele of s').

If marker information is available, the conditional probability that o' inherits $Q^p_s{}'$ given that o' inherits $M^p_s{}'$ is equal to $1 - r$. Assuming that o and o' are not ancestor and descendent, $P(Q^p_o \equiv Q^p_o{}')$ can be computed recursively as follows:

$$P(Q^p_o \equiv Q^p_o{}') = P(Q^p_o \equiv Q^p_s{}')(1-r) + P(Q^p_o \equiv Q^m_s{}')r \quad \{7.11\}$$

if o' received marker allele $M^p_s{}'$, and:

$$P(Q^p_o \equiv Q^p_o{}') = P(Q^p_o \equiv Q^p_s{}')r + P(Q^p_o \equiv Q^m_s{}')(1-r) \quad \{7.12\}$$

if o' received marker allele $M^m_s{}'$. If no marker information is available, then $r = (1-r) = 0.5$. Thus, $\mathbf{G_v}$ can be constructed in tabular fashion, beginning with the individuals with unknown parents. As we noted previously, $\mathbf{G_v}$ will be a symmetric matrix with rows and columns equal to twice the number of individuals included in the analysis, because each individual has two QTL alleles. The individual, o, will have two rows and columns, one each for the allele inherited from the sire and the allele inherited from the dam. The diagonal elements of $\mathbf{G_v}$ will be equal to σ_v^2. Denoting element ij of $\mathbf{G_v}$ as $g_{i,j}$, the off-diagonal elements of the row i corresponding to the paternal alleles of o, $g^p_{i\,o,j}$, are computed as follows:

$$g^p_{i\,o,j} = (1 - \rho^p_o) g^p_{i\,s,j} + \rho^p_o g^m_{i\,s,j} \quad \{7.13\}$$

for $j = 1 \ldots i^p_o - 1$, where $\rho^p_o = r$, if o inherits paternal marker allele M^p_s, or $\rho^p_o = 1 - r$ if o inherits paternal marker allele M^m_s. $g^p_{i\,s,j}$ and $g^m_{i\,s,j}$ are the elements of $\mathbf{G_v}$ corresponding to the paternal and maternal QTL effects of the sire of o in column

j. Row elements corresponding to the maternal allele of o are computed similarly. If no marker information is available along the path from sire to offspring then: $(1 - \rho^P_o) = \rho^P_o = 0.5$. An example to compute $\mathbf{G}_v$ from a list of progeny, their parents, and their marker genotypes is given in Fernando and Grossman (1989).

7.4 Computing the inverse of $\mathbf{G}_v$

In order to solve the mixed model equations presented in Equations {4.17}, there is no need to actually compute $\mathbf{G}_v$, if its inverse can be computed directly from the marker and relationship information. Fernando and Grossman (1989) presented an algorithm to directly compute $\mathbf{G}_v^{-1}$, similar to the algorithm of Quaas (1988) to compute the inverse of the numerator relationship matrix. The effect of the paternal allele of individual o, v^P_o, can be computed from the following linear model:

$$v^P_o = (1 - \rho^P_o)v^P_{s,} + \rho^P_o v^m_s + \varepsilon^P_o \qquad \{7.14\}$$

where ε^P_o is a residual effect. The maternal effect can be computed similarly. Fernando and Grossman proved that the residuals in this model have a diagonal variance matrix. That is, all covariances between residuals are zero. Thus in matrix notation, the vector of QTL effects, $\mathbf{v}$, can be written as follows:

$$\mathbf{v} = \mathbf{\Lambda v} + \boldsymbol{\varepsilon} \qquad \{7.15\}$$

where $\boldsymbol{\varepsilon}$ is the vector of residuals, and $\mathbf{\Lambda}$ is a matrix relating the QTL effects of parents to progeny. If the parents of o are known, then the row will contain two non-zero elements corresponding to $(1 - \rho^P_o)$ and ρ^P_o. If the parents are unknown, then all elements of the corresponding row will be zero. This equation can then be written as follows:

$$\mathbf{v} = (\mathbf{I} - \mathbf{\Lambda})^{-1}\boldsymbol{\varepsilon} \qquad \{7.16\}$$

The variance of $\mathbf{v}$ can then be computed as follows:

$$\mathbf{G}_v = (\mathbf{I} - \mathbf{\Lambda})^{-1}\mathbf{G}_\varepsilon(\mathbf{I} - \mathbf{\Lambda}')^{-1} \qquad \{7.17\}$$

Inverting gives:

$$\mathbf{G}_v^{-1} = (\mathbf{I} - \mathbf{\Lambda}')\mathbf{G}_\varepsilon^{-1}(\mathbf{I} - \mathbf{\Lambda}) \qquad \{7.18\}$$

Since $\mathbf{G}_\varepsilon$ is diagonal, $\mathbf{G}_v^{-1}$ can be computed as follows:

$$\mathbf{G}_v^{-1} = \sum_{j=1}^{2n} \mathbf{q}_j \mathbf{q}_j' d_j \qquad \{7.19\}$$

where $\mathbf{q}_j$ is the column j of the matrix $(\mathbf{I} - \Lambda)$ and d_j is the diagonal element for row j of $\mathbf{G}_\varepsilon^{-1}$.

Element j of $\mathbf{q}_j$ is equal to unity. $\mathbf{q}_j$ will have two additional elements, corresponding to the parents of j equal to $-(1-\rho^p_o)$ and $-\rho^p_o$. Since $\mathbf{G}_\varepsilon$ is diagonal, d_j will be equal to the reciprocal of the diagonal elements of $\mathbf{G}_\varepsilon$. The diagonal elements of $\mathbf{G}_\varepsilon$ for the paternal and maternal QTL alleles of o will be: $2\sigma_v^2(1-\rho^p_o)\rho^p_o(1-F_s)$ and $\sigma_v^2(1-\rho^m_o)\rho^m_o(1-F_d)$, where F_s and F_d are the inbreeding coefficients of the sire and dam, respectively. If the sire or dam are not inbred, but marker information is available, then the coefficients become $2\sigma_v^2(1-r)r$. If there is no marker information, then the coefficients are $\sigma_v^2/2$. If the dam or sire is unknown, the appropriate coefficient becomes σ_v^2. Specific rules to compute the elements of $\mathbf{G}_v^{-1}$ from a list of parents and progeny are given in Fernando and Grossman (1989).

7.5 Analysis of the random gametic model by a reduced animal model (RAM)

As noted above, the original model of Fernando and Grossman (1989) assumed a single QTL linked to a single genetic marker, and that recombination frequency between the two loci and the variance due to the QTL were known without error. Clearly these assumptions are not realistic. Therefore several studies have proposed modified forms of this model that more clearly reflect the actual situation in field data.

The number of equations in the original Fernando-Grossman model will be greater than three times the number of individuals included in the analysis. For a large population, this system of equations can only be solved by iteration, and convergence will not be rapid. Cantet and Smith (1991) proposed that the number of equations could be significantly reduced by application of the "reduced animal model" of Quaas and Pollak (1980). In the RAM equations of individuals without progeny are absorbed into the equations of their parents. Thus equations are constructed only for individuals with progeny. With the possibility of multiple records per individual, and individuals without records, the linear model given in Equation {4.16} becomes

$$\mathbf{y} = \mathbf{XB} + \mathbf{Zu} + \mathbf{Wv_g} + \mathbf{e} \qquad \{7.20\}$$

with **Z** as the incidence matrix for the polygenic effects, and the other terms as described previously. To apply the RAM, the data and effects are partitioned into records pertaining to parents and to non-parents. The model can then be expressed as follows:

$$\begin{bmatrix} y_p \\ y_n \end{bmatrix} = \begin{bmatrix} X_p \\ X_n \end{bmatrix} \beta + \begin{bmatrix} Z_p & 0 \\ 0 & Z_n \end{bmatrix} \begin{bmatrix} u_p \\ u_n \end{bmatrix} + \begin{bmatrix} W_p & 0 \\ 0 & W_n \end{bmatrix} \begin{bmatrix} v_p \\ v_n \end{bmatrix} + \begin{bmatrix} e_p \\ e_n \end{bmatrix} \quad \{7.21\}$$

where the subscripts "p" and "n" refer to parents and non-parents, respectively. As explained by Quaas and Pollak (1980) the polygenic breeding value of an individual without parents can be expressed as the mean of the parental value, plus a residual representing Mendelian sampling of the parental genomes, as follows:

$$u_n = Pu_p + \phi_n \quad \{7.22\}$$

where **P** is a matrix relating non-parental to parental breeding values. Each row of **P** contains at most two values of 0.5 for the sire and dam. All other elements are zero. ϕ_n is the deviation of the progeny polygenic value from the mean of the parental values. The expectation of ϕ_n is equal to zero, and its variance will be a function of the number of parents included in the analysis, as explained by Quaas and Pollak (1980). Similarly for the QTL effects, the non-parental effects can be expressed in terms of the parental effects as follows:

$$v_n = Fv_p + \varepsilon \quad \{7.23\}$$

where **F** is a matrix that relates the QTL additive effects of non-parents to parents, as shown above, and ε is a vector of residuals for progeny effects not explained by the parental effects. Since each animal received two QTL alleles, there will be an element in ε for both the paternal and maternal allele of each individual. Each row of **F** contains two non-zero elements, which are equal to the probability that each paternal allele was passed to the progeny. If marker information is available for both individuals then these values are either r or 1 – r, as explained above.

The model in Equations {7.21} can then be rewritten as follows:

$$\begin{bmatrix} y_p \\ y_n \end{bmatrix} = \begin{bmatrix} X_p \\ X_n \end{bmatrix} \beta + \begin{bmatrix} Z_p \\ Z_nP \end{bmatrix} u_p + \begin{bmatrix} W_p \\ W_pF \end{bmatrix} v_p + \begin{bmatrix} e_p \\ e_n + Z_n\phi_n + W_n\varepsilon \end{bmatrix} \quad \{7.24\}$$

and only fixed effects and effects pertaining to parents are included in the model. The residual variance matrix is still diagonal, but similar to the RAM of Quaas and Pollak (1980) is no longer equal to an identity matrix times a scalar. The mixed model equations for this model are:

$$\begin{bmatrix} X_p'X_p+X_n'Q^{-1}X_n & X_p'Z_p+X_n'Q^{-1}Z_nP & X_p'W_p+X_n'Q^{-1}W_nF \\ Z_p'X_p+P'Z_n'Q^{-1}X_n & Z_p'Z_p+P'Z_n'Q^{-1}Z_nP+A_p^{-1}\lambda_A & Z_p'W_p+P'Z_n'Q^{-1}W_nF \\ W_p'X_p+F'W_n'Q^{-1}X_n & W_p'Z_p+F'W_n'Q^{-1}Z_nP & W_p'W_p+F'W_n'Q^{-1}W_nF+G_{vp}^{-1}\lambda_v \end{bmatrix}$$

$$\begin{bmatrix} \hat{\beta} \\ \hat{u}_p \\ \hat{v}_p \end{bmatrix} = \begin{bmatrix} X_p'y_p+X_n'Q^{-1}y_n \\ Z_p'y_p+P'Z_n'Q^{-1}y_n \\ W_p'y_p+F'W_n'Q^{-1}y_n \end{bmatrix} \qquad \{7.25\}$$

where $Q = I + Z_n'D_AZ_n\lambda_A + W_n'G_\varepsilon W_n\lambda_v$. D_A is a diagonal matrix that accounts for the polygenic variance of the progeny not explained by the parents, as described by Quaas and Pollak (1980), G_ε is computed as described in the previous section, $\lambda_A = \sigma_a^2/\sigma_e^2$, and $\lambda_v = \sigma_v^2/\sigma_e^2$. The matrices A_p and G_{vp} are the corresponding submatrices of A and G_v that refer to parents. Cantet and Smith (1991) also presented the mixed model equations for more than one QTL, and the formula to obtain back-solutions for non-parents.

7.6 Analysis of the random gametic QTL model with multiple QTL and marker brackets

Goddard (1992) extended this model to consider multiple markers and QTL. He assumed that there was at most a single segregating QTL within each marker bracket. Like Fernando and Grossman (1989), he assumed that the variance due to each QTL was known *a priori*, and that both the recombination frequencies between each pair of markers, and between either of the two markers and the QTL within the marker bracket were known. The model of Fernando and Grossman (1989) in matrix notation, expanded to include J QTL, each within a marker bracket becomes:

$$y = X\beta + \sum_{j}^{J} W_jv_j + u + e \qquad \{7.26\}$$

with all terms as defined previously. Similar to the matrix W in the previous section, the matrix W_j has rows equal to the number of records, and columns equal to twice the number of animals with records. Each row contains two 1s for the two alleles of QTL j for the particular individual, and zeros for the other elements. The vector v_j is of length twice the number of animals, and contains the effects of the two alleles of QTL j for each individual. The vector **u** is of length equal to the number of individuals with records.

This model assumes a single record per animal, although the equations can be readily modified for the case of multiple records. It will be further assumed that the base population is in linkage equilibrium with respect to the QTL included in the analysis. In this case the covariance between **u** and each $\mathbf{v}_j$ is zero. As in the standard animal model, the variance matrices of the polygenic additive effects and the residuals are still $\mathbf{A}\sigma_u^2$ and $\mathbf{I}\sigma_e^2$, respectively. Defining $\mathbf{v'} = [\mathbf{v}_1, \mathbf{v}_2, ...\mathbf{v}_J]$, the variance of **v** is block diagonal, with each block corresponding to one QTL. The mixed model equations after multiplication by σ_e^{-2} can then be constructed as follows:

$$\begin{bmatrix} \mathbf{X'X} & \mathbf{X'} & \mathbf{X'W}_1 & \mathbf{X'W}_2 & \cdots \\ \mathbf{X} & \mathbf{I}+\mathbf{A}^{-1}\gamma & \mathbf{W}_1 & \mathbf{W}_2 & \cdots \\ \mathbf{W}_1'\mathbf{X} & \mathbf{W}_1' & \mathbf{W}_1'\mathbf{W}_1+\mathbf{G}_1^{-1}\sigma_e^{-2} & \mathbf{W}_1'\mathbf{W}_2 & \cdots \\ \mathbf{W}_2'\mathbf{X} & \mathbf{W}_2' & \mathbf{W}_2'\mathbf{W}_1 & \mathbf{W}_2'\mathbf{W}_2+\mathbf{G}_2^{-1}\sigma_e^{-2} & \cdots \\ \cdots & \cdots & \cdots & \cdots & \cdots \end{bmatrix} \begin{bmatrix} \hat{\beta} \\ \hat{\mathbf{u}} \\ \hat{\mathbf{v}}_1 \\ \hat{\mathbf{v}}_2 \\ \cdots \end{bmatrix} = \begin{bmatrix} \mathbf{X'y} \\ \mathbf{Y} \\ \mathbf{W}_1'\mathbf{y} \\ \mathbf{W}_2'\mathbf{y} \\ \cdots \end{bmatrix}$$

{7.27}

where $\gamma = \sigma_e^2/\sigma_u^2$, and $\mathbf{G}_j = \text{var}(\mathbf{v}_j)$. Derivation of $\mathbf{G}_j$ for a QTL bracketed between two markers will be described in the next section.

7.7 Computation of the gametic effects variance matrix

Continuing the notation of Section 5.3, we will assume that a QTL, denoted Q, is bracketed between two markers, denoted M and N. Recombination frequency between the two markers will be denoted R. Recombination frequencies between M and Q, and Q and N will be denoted r_1 and r_2, respectively. As in Chapter five, zero interference will be assumed, and $R = r_1 + r_2 - 2r_1r_2$. Goddard (1992) provided a solution for this case, but the equations are considerably simplified if complete interference is assumed. In this case, $R = r_1 + r_2$. Results will be very similar if the marker brackets are relatively short. Only this situation will be presented here. As in the original model of Fernando and Grossman (1989), the elements of the **G** matrix are determined by the relationships between parents and progeny.

Assume a sire heterozygous for both genetic markers and the QTL, with haplotypes: $M_1Q_1N_1$ and $M_2Q_2N_2$. Relative to the genetic markers, the sire can pass four different haplotypes to his progeny. The effects of the paternal QTL gametes, Q_1 and Q_2, will be denoted v_{s1} and v_{s2}. The paternal gametic value of the progeny in terms of his sire can be written as follows:

$$\begin{bmatrix} v_{o11} \\ v_{o12} \\ v_{o21} \\ v_{o22} \end{bmatrix} = \begin{bmatrix} 1 & 0 \\ r_2/R & r_1/R \\ r_1/R & r_2/R \\ 0 & 1 \end{bmatrix} \begin{bmatrix} v_{s1} \\ v_{s2} \end{bmatrix} + \begin{bmatrix} \varepsilon_{11} \\ \varepsilon_{12} \\ \varepsilon_{21} \\ \varepsilon_{22} \end{bmatrix} \quad \{7.28\}$$

where v_{o11}, v_{o12}, v_{o21}, and v_{o22} are the QTL paternal gametic effects of progeny that received paternal haplotypes M_1N_1, M_1N_2, M_2N_1, and M_2N_2, respectively. ε_{11}, ε_{12}, ε_{21}, and ε_{22} are the deviations of each progeny's gamete from the haplotype mean. For the complete interference model: $\varepsilon_{11} = \varepsilon_{22} = 0$, because in these cases the progeny must have received the paternal haplotype intact. For the recombinant haplotypes the value of the paternal allele that the progeny received will be either v_{s1} or v_{s2}, which are different from the mean values. In matrix notation the general relationship described in equation {7.28} can be written as follows:

$$\mathbf{v} = \Lambda \mathbf{v} + \varepsilon \quad \{7.29\}$$

which is the same as Equation {7.15}. Each row of Λ still contains at most two non-zero elements, which sum to one. As for a single marker linked to the QTL, solving for $\mathbf{v}$ gives:

$$\mathbf{v} = (\mathbf{I} - \Lambda)^{-1} + \varepsilon \quad \{7.30\}$$

and:

$$\mathbf{G}^{-1} = (\mathbf{I} - \Lambda)[\text{var}(\varepsilon)]^{-1}(\mathbf{I} - \Lambda)' \quad \{7.31\}$$

Goddard (1992) proved that var(ε) is still diagonal for a marker bracket. Thus this matrix can be readily inverted, and the elements of $\mathbf{G}^{-1}$ can be computed from a list of parents and progeny with known marker genotype. A list of simple rules is presented in Goddard (1992).

As noted above, this method requires that the variance due to each QTL, and its location be known *a priori*. However, unlike the case of a QTL linked to a single marker, the recombination parameter is bounded, that is $0 < r_1 < R$. If the marker bracket is short, estimating r_1 as $R/2$ should result in a good approximation. Methods to estimate both r_1 and σ_v^2 will be considered below in Section 7.9. This method has not been applied to actual data.

7.8 The gametic effect model for crosses between inbred lines

We will now consider a cross between two inbred lines. Both lines are assumed to be homozygous for a different allele of each QTL under consideration. The F-1 progeny are backcrossed to one of the parental strains. Therefore only one $W_j v_j$ term is needed per locus, because the gametes from the other parent are identical. The only estimable QTL effect is the difference between the effects of the two alleles derived from the two parental strains. Consider a single QTL flanked by two markers. Using the reduced animal model described above, with progeny absorbed into the parental equations, the model for a single QTL can be simplified as follows:

$$y = X\beta + Pv + e^* \quad \{7.32\}$$

where $e^* = u + \varepsilon + e$. The elements of P for the four possible marker haplotypes: y_{11}, y_{12}, y_{21}, and y_{22} will be: -1, $-(1-2r_1/R)$, $(1-2r_1/R)$ and 1. An equivalent model for the four possible haplotypes can be described as follows:

$$\begin{bmatrix} y_{11} \\ y_{12} \\ y_{21} \\ y_{22} \end{bmatrix} = \begin{bmatrix} -1 & -1 \\ -1 & 1 \\ 1 & -1 \\ 1 & 1 \end{bmatrix} \begin{bmatrix} (1-r_1/R)v \\ vr_1/R \end{bmatrix} + e^* \quad \{7.33\}$$

$$= X\beta + W_2\theta_2 + e^* \quad \{7.34\}$$

and:

$$\text{Var}(\theta_2) = \begin{bmatrix} 1/3 & 1/6 \\ 1/6 & 1/3 \end{bmatrix} \sigma_v^2 \quad \{7.35\}$$

The proof of equation {7.35} is given in Goddard (1992). He also expanded this model to handle several linked marker brackets. In this case, the number of columns of W_2 will be twice the number of linked markers. Similarly, the number of elements for θ_2 will be equal to the number of markers. The variance matrix for θ_2 will have covariances of 1/6 between elements corresponding to adjacent markers, and variances of 1/3 for the extreme markers of the linkage group. Intermediate markers will have variances of 2/3. Zhang and Smith (1992, 1993) applied this model to simulated data, and these studies will be discussed in detail in Chapter fifteen.

7.9 REML estimation of the QTL variance and recombination for the model of Fernando and Grossman

Because the QTL effect is random in the model of Fernando and Grossman (1989), it is only necessary to solve for four parameters in addition to block effects: the QTL, polygenic, and residual variances, and the recombination frequency between the QTL and the marker locus. Since the analysis model will include both random and fixed effects, such as herd-year-season, REML should be used instead of ML, as noted above in Section 7.2. REML methodology was explained in general terms in Section 3.15.

Weller and Fernando (1991) presented formula to estimate the variance components and the recombination parameters via REML. Starting with the likelihood equation {3.35}, the likelihood for REML can be modified as follows:

$$L = (2\pi)^{-N/2} |C|^{-1/2} |V|^{-1/2} \exp\left[-\tfrac{1}{2}(y'y - \hat{\theta}'C\hat{\theta})\right] \quad \{7.36\}$$

where $\hat{\theta}$ is a vector of solutions for both the fixed and random effects, N is the number of individuals included in the analysis, C is the coefficient matrix, and $|.|$ signifies a determinant. $(2\pi)^{-N/2}$ is a constant, and can be deleted from the equation. V, the variance matrix includes the polygenic variance, the variance due to the QTL effects, and the residual. Expanding this matrix gives:

$$L \propto |C|^{-1/2} |G_v|^{-1/2} (\sigma_u^2)^{-N/2} (\sigma_e^2)^{-N/2} \exp\left[-\tfrac{1}{2}(y'y - \hat{\theta}'C\hat{\theta})\right] \quad \{7.37\}$$

where G_v is the variance matrix for the QTL effects, σ_u^2 is the polygenic variance component, σ_e^2 is the residual variance, and N is the sample size. Although r does not directly appear in {7.37}, G_v is a function of this parameter. The determinant of C can be obtained by sparse matrix techniques. As explained by Weller and Fernando (1991) the determinant of G_v is computed as follows:

$$|G_v| = \prod d_{ii} \quad \{7.38\}$$

where d_{ii} is the ith diagonal element of G_ε, as described in Section 7.4. Since each individual receives two alleles for the QTL, the multiplicative summation is over twice the number of individuals in the analysis. Of course iterative methods must be used to maximize this likelihood.

Van Arendonk et al. (1994a) used REML to estimate QTL variance and recombination frequency, but found that these parameters are confounded for a single marker in a grand-daughter design. They also presented methods to incorporate information from animals that were not genotyped.

7.10 REML estimation of the QTL variance and location with marker brackets

Grignola et al. (1996a) used the RAM to estimate variance components by REML for analysis of a livestock population. They applied the RAM (Cantet and Smith, 1991) to a QTL located within a marker bracket, as described by Goddard (1992). They further assumed that only non-parents had records, and that there was at most one record per individual. This model is appropriate to daughter or grand-daughter designs in which the number of sires is much less than the number of progeny, and only progeny have records. In the grand-daughter design, daughter yield deviations (DYD) are generally analysed, and therefore each son has only a single record.

The parameters estimated were the heritability, h^2, defined as the additive polygenic variance divided by the phenotypic variance, the fraction of the additive genetic variance explained by the QTL, v^2 and QTL location.

Following Meyer (1989), the log of the REML likelihood for the full animal model is as follows:

$$\text{Log } L(y;\theta) = -(N/2)\log(2\pi) \\ - 0.5\log|G| - 0.5(N - N_F - N_R)\log(\hat{\sigma}_e^2) - 0.5\log|C| - 0.5y'Py\hat{\sigma}_e^{-2} \quad \{7.39\}$$

where θ is the vector of parameters, G is the variance matrix for the random effects (u and v), N is the number of records, N_F is the rank of X, N_R is the number of random effects, C is the coefficient matrix for the animal model mixed model equations, reparameterized to full rank and with σ_e^2 factored out, and $P = V^{-1} - V^{-1}X(X'V^{-1}X)^{-1}XV^{-1}$, as defined in Equation {3.48}. V and $\hat{\sigma}_e^2$ are computed as follows:

$$\hat{\sigma}_e^2 = y'Py/(N - N_F) , V = \text{Var}(y)/\sigma_e^2 \quad \{7.40\}$$

For the RAM, equation {7.39} becomes after removing the constant:

$$\text{Log } L_{RAM} \propto - 0.5\log|G_{RAM}| \\ - 0.5(N - NF - NR_{RAM})\log(\hat{\sigma}_e^2) - 0.5\log|C_{RAM}| - 0.5y'Py\hat{\sigma}_e^{-2} \quad \{7.41\}$$

where the subscript "RAM" refers to those matrices that remain in the RAM mixed model equations. Similar to Xu and Atchley (1995), as described in Section 7.2, the likelihood was maximized with respect to h^2, v^2, and σ_e^2 with QTL location fixed. This procedure was repeated for a range of QTL values covering the marker bracket at 1 cM intervals. The final solution was set of parameters, including QTL location, which resulted in ML.

The null hypothesis of no segregating QTL within the marker bracket can be tested by a likelihood ratio test comparing the likelihood of the complete model as described to a restricted model with $v^2 = 0$. The empirical distribution of the test statistic under the null hypothesis was between the expected χ^2 distributions with 1 and 2 df, similar to both the results of Xu and Atchley (1995) for ML variance component estimation, and those presented in Chapter five for estimation of QTL parameters with a fixed model.

This method was tested on simulated grand-daughter design data with 20 grandsires, each with 100 sons. Thus, it is assumed that 2000 individuals were genotyped. Each son had 50 daughters, and DYD were generated and analysed. Three models were simulated with respect to the distribution of QTL effects:

1. A normal distribution model, in which the additive effects of each QTL allele for each grandsire was sampled from a normal distribution.
2. A multi-allelic model, in which 10 alleles of equal frequency with equal differences between the allelic effects were simulated.
3. A biallelic model, with equal frequency for the two alleles.

Although the first model is most appropriate to the Fernando-Grossman model, parameters were estimated with good accuracy for all three simulation models, if the QTL explained at least 12.5% of the additive genetic value. In the case of the biallelic model with heritability of 0.25, this is comparable to a QTL with a substitution effect of 0.25. As will be seen in the following chapter, power of detection for this design by a linear model analysis is close to 100%.

7.11 Bayesian estimation of QTL effects, determining the prior distribution

As explained in Section 2.14, Bayesian estimation is based on the joint density of a prior distribution of parameters and the likelihood function. Hoeschele and VanRanden (1993a) derived Bayesian estimates of QTL parameters for a grand-daughter design using simulated data, and compared the Bayesian estimates to ML estimates. Bayes Theorem, in general terms, was given in Equation {2.26} and will be repeated here with minor modification, for a continuous distribution:

$$f(\theta_1, \theta_2,...\theta_m | y_1, y_2,...y_n) = f(\theta_1, \theta_2,...\theta_m) f(y_1, y_2,...y_n | \theta_1, \theta_2,...\theta_m) \qquad \{7.42\}$$

where $f(\theta_1, \theta_2,...\theta_m | y_1, y_2,...y_n)$ is the "posterior" density function of the parameters, $f(\theta_1, \theta_2,...\theta_m)$ is the "prior" density function of the parameters, and $f(y_1, y_2,...y_n | \theta_1, \theta_2,...\theta_m)$ is the likelihood function.

In order to derive a prior distribution of QTL parameters, it is necessary to make assumptions about the relevant QTL parameters: the QTL genotype means and variances, the number of frequencies of QTL alleles, and the QTL location.

Hoeschele and VanRanden (1993a) simplified the analysis somewhat by employing the following assumptions:

1. For each QTL only two alleles are segregating in the population.
2. All QTL were assumed codominant. Strictly speaking this assumption is not required for a grand-daughter design, because only substitution effects are estimable, as noted in Chapter four.
3. The residual variance is independent of the QTL genotypes.

Under these assumptions, prior distributions must be derived for only three parameters, the QTL additive effect, the allele frequency, and QTL location. No prior assumptions are required with respect to the residual variance, which is also estimated, and the total additive genetic variance including the segregating QTL, σ_A^2, is assumed to be known without error.

Although the actual distribution of QTL effects is unknown, it is known that the total variance contributed by all QTL should be no larger than σ_A^2. Most simulation studies have assumed that polygenic variance is due to a few QTL with relative large effects, and numerous QTL with progressively smaller effects. Several mathematical models that generate this type of distribution have been proposed, and these models are reviewed in Chapter fifteen. Hoeschele and VanRaden (1993a) assumed a prior exponential distribution of QTL effects. The exponential distribution has the form:

$$f(a) = \lambda e^{-\lambda a} \qquad \{7.43\}$$

where a is the QTL additive effect, and λ is the parameter of this distribution. The statistical density of this distribution is maximum with a = 0, and is equal to λ. The expectation of the distribution, that is the expectation of a, is $1/\lambda$.

Although the additive effect can have a value from zero to infinity, Hoeschele and VanRaden (1993a) imposed lower and upper bounds. A lower bound was imposed, because very small QTL cannot be detected by the sample sizes generally considered. An upper bound was imposed for two reasons. First, a very large additive effect will lie outside the permissible parameter space, determined by σ_A^2. In this case the QTL will explain more than the total genetic variance, unless the allelic frequency is very low. Second, with values of λ that are appropriate for polygenic inheritance, the probability of sampling a very large effect tends towards zero, and can therefore be ignored. Therefore, the density function in Equation {7.43} must be divided by a constant to account for the extremes of the theoretical exponential distribution that are deleted from consideration. The value of this constant is: $e^{-\lambda a_l} - e^{-\lambda a_u}$, where a_l and a_u are the lower and upper limits of a.

As noted above, Hoeschele and VanRaden (1993a) assumed only two alleles for each QTL segregating in the population. Thus, it is necessary to determine a prior distribution for the allelic frequency for only one allele. Hoeschele and VanRaden (1993a) assumed a uniform distribution over the range of zero to unity, subject to two restrictions. First, the frequency of the less frequent allele must be high enough, so that at least one of the sires included in the analysis is heterozygous for the QTL. This will be considered again below. Second, the variance contributed by each QTL must be no greater than σ_A^2. Therefore, the joint distribution of the additive QTL effect, and allelic frequency, p, is:

$$f(a, p) = \begin{cases} k*f(a) & \text{if } 2p(1-p)a2 \leq \sigma_A^2 \\ 0 & \text{otherwise} \end{cases} \quad \{7.44\}$$

where k is the reciprocal of the integral of f(a, p) over the restricted space of a and p.

The prior distribution for the QTL location parameter was computed based on the assumption of a uniform distribution throughout the genome. Two situations must be considered, linkage between the QTL and the genetic markers, and non-linkage. In the case of a single marker, non-linkage can be defined as r=0.5, where r is the recombination frequency between the two loci. The joint prior density of a, p, and r can be represented as follows:

$$\text{Prior}(a, p, r) = \begin{cases} \text{Prob}(r=0.5) \\ [1 - \text{Prob}(r=0.5)]*f(a, p)*f(r) \end{cases} \quad \{7.45\}$$

where f(r) is the density of the distribution of r if the marker and QTL are linked. If r was measured in Morgans, then f(r) would have a uniform distribution. However, r is measured in recombination frequency, and, as shown in Chapter one, r is a non-linear function of genetic map length for the commonly used mapping functions, such as Haldane or Kosambi. If g(r) is the assumed mapping function, so that $\delta = g(r)$, where δ is the map distance between the QTL and the genetic marker, then:

$$f(r) = f[g(r)d\delta/dr]/\text{Prob}(\delta<\delta_r) \quad \{7.46\}$$

where δ_r is the maximum linkage distance at which linkage can be detected in the same map units as δ.

If the genome consisted of a single circular chromosome, then the probability of linkage would be: $(2\delta_r N_Q)/L_t$, where N_Q is the detectable number of segregating QTL and L_t is the total genome length, with both δ_r and L_t measured in genetic map units. For example, if $\delta_r = 1$ Morgan, and $N_Q = 10$, and $L_t = 30$ Morgans, then Prob(r=0.5) = 1 − 10/30 = 0.67. The detectable number of QTL, N_Q, was derived as follows:

$$N_Q = F*\sigma_A^2/E(V_Q) \quad \{7.47\}$$

where F is the fraction of the genome under analysis for QTL, and $E(V_Q)$ is the expected variance due to a single detectable QTL, which is computed as follows:

$$E(V_Q) = k\int_{a_l}^{a_u} f(a) \left\{ \int_0^{p_a} [2p(1-p)a^2]dp + \int_{1-p_a}^{1} [2p(1-p)a^2]dp \right\} da \quad \{7.48\}$$

where p_a is the appropriate value of p for each value of a.

As noted above, in the grand-daughter design, p will be estimated as the frequency of one of the QTL alleles within the sample of grandsires. The total number of alleles will be twice the number of grandsires, and at least one of the grandsires must be heterozygous for the QTL. Therefore, the lower and upper bounds for p are 1/2G and 1−1/2G, where G is the number of grandsires.

Setting a_l and a_u at approximately 0.2 and 1.1 genetic standard deviations, and 1/λ at 0.36 genetic standard deviations, $N_Q = 10$ for a complete genome scan of 10 grandsire families (Hoeschele and Vanraden, 1993a). With a heritability of 0.25, these limits for the additive effect are equal to 0.1 and 0.55 phenotypic standard deviations. More than 200 sons per sire will be required to obtain power > 0.5 to detect a QTL of 0.1 phenotypic standard deviation (Weller et al., 1990).

With a single marker, and a genome divided into chromosomes of differing lengths, Prob(r=0.5) will also depend on the length of the marked chromosome, and the position of the marker along the chromosome. If the marker is located at one end of the chromosome, then the length of the chromosomal segment for which a QTL can be detected is only δ_r, instead of $2\delta_r$. The final calculations for Prob(r=0.5)] and f(r), considering any possible marker location and genome and any mapping function, are rather complicated and are given in Hoeschele and Vanraden (1993a).

With a marker bracket, Equation {7.45} becomes:

$$\text{Prior}(a, p, r) = \begin{cases} 1 - \text{Prob}(0 < r_1 < R) \\ [\text{Prob}(0 < r_1 < R)]*f(a, p)*f(r_1) \end{cases} \quad \{7.49\}$$

where r_1 is the recombination frequency between one of the markers and the QTL, R is the recombination frequency between the two markers of the marker bracket, and:

$$\text{Prob}(0 < r_1 < R) = (\delta_R N_Q)/L_t \quad \{7.50\}$$

with δ_R equal to the length of the marker bracket in map units, again assuming a uniform distribution for the QTL location. $f(r_1)$ is computed as in Equation {7.46} for a single marker.

7.12 Formula for Bayesian estimation and tests of significance of a segregating QTL in a simulated grand-daughter design

In order to derive Bayesian estimates for the QTL parameters, the prior density function is multiplied by the likelihood function. The likelihood function for the daughter design including a polygenic sire effect is given in Equation {6.23} and will be repeated here:

$$L = \prod_{k=1}^{K} \int \left\{ f(g_k - \mu_g, \sigma_g^2) \sum_{v=1}^{4} P_v \prod_{i=1}^{3} \prod_{l=1}^{L_i} \sum_{j=1}^{3} c_{j|i,v}\, f(y_{ikl} - \mu_j - g_k, \sigma_e^2) \right\} dg_k \quad \{7.51\}$$

where K is the number of sires, P_v is the probability of sire QTL genotype v, $c_{j|i,v}$ is the probability of progeny QTL genotype j conditional on the combination of sire QTL genotype v and progeny marker genotype i, L_i is the number of daughters with marker genotype i, x_{ikl} is the trait value for progeny l of sire k, with marker genotype i, $f(g_k - \mu_g, \sigma_g^2)$ represents the normal density function for the sire effects. This function has a mean of μ_g and a variance of σ_g^2, which will be equal to one-quarter of the additive genetic variance not explained by the segregating QTL. $f(y_{ikl} - \mu_j - g_k, \sigma_e^2)$ represents a normal density function with a mean of $\mu_j + g_k$ and a variance of σ_e^2. σ_e^2 includes the residual variance, and three-quarters of the genetic variance not explained by the segregating QTL. The likelihood function is the joint density of the observations, integrated over g_k, the polygenic sire effect, which is assumed to be random.

This will be nearly the same function for the grand-daughter design if the analysis is preformed on DYD with a single record for each son. The only difference is that the residual variances of the DYD are not equal, but are a function of the number of daughters per son, as explained in the previous chapter (Hoeschele and Vanraden, 1993b). The posterior distribution of the QTL parameters given a single marker also consists of discrete part, if the marker is not linked to a segregating QTL; and a continuous part, if a linked QTL is detected. The complete posterior distribution can be described as follows:

$$\text{Posterior}(a, p, r) = \begin{cases} \text{Prob}(r=0.5|y,M) \\ [1 - \text{Prob}(r=0.5|y,M)]*f(a, p, r|y, M) \end{cases} \quad \{7.52\}$$

where y, M represents the phenotypic and marker data. The posterior probability of no linkage is calculated as follows:

$$\text{Prob}(r=0.5|y,M) = \frac{\text{Prob}(r=0.5)E[L(r=0.5)]}{\text{Prob}(r=0.5)E[L(r=0.5)] + [1-\text{Prob}(r=0.5)]E[L(r<0.5)]} \quad \{7.53\}$$

where $E[L(r=0.5)]$ and $E[L(r<0.5)]$ are the expectations of the likelihood function with $r=0.5$, and $r<0.5$, respectively. $E[L(r<0.5)]$ is computed as follows:

$$E[L(r<0.5)] = \int_{0.5}^{0.5}\int_{a_l}^{a_u}\int_{p_l}^{p_u} L(y|M; r, p, a)f(p, a)f(r)dpdadr \quad \{7.54\}$$

where $L(y|M; r, p, a)$ is the likelihood function as computed in Equation {7.51}. Similarly, $E[L(r=0.5)]$ is computed with r fixed at 0.5. That is, the expectation of the likelihood without a segregating QTL linked to the marker, which is a standard polygenic sire model. The posterior density of the QTL parameters is computed as follows:

$$f(r, p, a|y, M) = L(y|M; r, p, a)f(a, p)f(r)/f(y|M) \quad \{7.55\}$$

where $f(y|M)$ is the denominator of {7.53}. Assuming a uniform loss function, the point estimates for r, p, and a are derived by maximizing the statistical density, that is the mode of the distribution. With a quadratic loss function, the parameter estimates are derived by maximizing the mean of the distribution.

Linkage of the genetic marker to a segregating QTL can be tested by comparing the posterior probabilities of $r=0.5$, as given in Equation {7.53} and the posterior probability that $r<0.5$. If both errors are on equal economic value, then the hypothesis of $r=0.5$ will be rejected if the posterior probability is less than half.

7.13 Comparison of ML and Bayesian analyses of a simulated grand-daughter design

A grand-daughter design with six families was simulated. Three grandsires were heterozygous for a QTL with an additive effect of 1.08 genetic standard deviations (0.54 phenotypic standard deviations). In a grand-daughter design the contrast between the two son groups will be half of the QTL substitution effect.

Computed over all families, the ML estimate for the QTL additive effect was 4% greater than the simulated effect. The Bayesian modal estimate, appropriate for a linear loss function, was about 2% greater than the estimate, but was slightly dependent on λ. Decreasing $1/\lambda$ by 40% decreased the estimate of a by less than 1%. The Bayesian estimate with a quadratic loss function was 1.5% less than the simulated value. Estimates of r and p were very similar for all methods.

Bayesian QTL additive effects estimated separately for each family were also smaller than the ML estimates. As expected with Bayes estimators the difference between the ML and Bayes estimates increase with decrease in the number of sons per grandsire. With fewer sons, the assumed value of λ was also more critical. With only 30 sons, the Bayes estimate of the additive effect was 15% less than the ML estimate. However, decreasing $1/\lambda$ by 40% decreased the estimate of the QTL additive effect by an additional 10%.

Although the estimates behaved as predicted, practical application of Bayesian methodology is limited by the fact that there is at present no method to derive a good estimate for the prior distribution of QTL effects. This question of fixed vs. random estimation of QTL effects will be considered again in Section 11.7.

7.14 Markov Chain Monte Carlo algorithms, Gibbs' sampling

Markov Chain Monte Carlo (MCMC) algorithms for parameter estimation are based on Bayesian principles. Thus, a prior distribution must be postulated for the parameters of the distribution. In Gibbs' sampling, a value is generated for each unknown parameter and missing data point from its distribution, conditional on the observed data and on all other sampled values. After many repeat samples empirical posterior distributions of the parameters are derived, which can be used to estimate parameter values and confidence limits. The parameter estimates derived in the early iterations are highly dependent on the initial values.
Therefore these estimates, denoted "burn-in cycles" are discarded. Furthermore, parameter estimates derived from adjacent samples are highly correlated. Thus only widely spaced sample estimates are used to derive the empirical posterior distribution. Therefore, very large samples, in the order of 10,000, are required to obtain results that are independent of the starting values and of each other (Hoeschele, 1994).

Thaller and Hoeschele (1996a) derived equations for Bayesian point estimators for the parameters of the grand-daughter design analysis described in Sections 7.11 through 7.13 via a Gibbs' sampler. They also derived formula for MCMC Bayesian tests of marker-QTL linkage, vs. the null hypothesis of $r=0.5$.
Thaller and Hoeschele (1996b) applied this method to simulated grand-daughter design data. An advantage of this method is that any population structure can be analysed. In their example, a specific relationship structure among the grandsires was assumed. Otherwise the analysis model was the same as given previously in Section 7.11. Analyses were based on a single Gibbs' chain with 5000 burn-in cycles and a length of 750,000 cycles. The effective number of estimates retained was greater than 200 for all parameters. With a simulated population of 20 grandsires, each with 100 sons, they found power greater than 80% to reject the null hypothesis of $r=0.5$ if $a=0.5$ and $r=0.1$. Power reduced dramatically if either the QTL effect was halved, or recombination frequency was doubled.

Although Gibbs' sampling requires much more computing time than any of the methods considered previously, it has the advantage that any population structure can be modeled. Similar to other Bayesian methods, the results obtained are dependent on assumptions used to construct the prior parameter distributions. Gibbs' sampling can also be readily modified to analyse multiple markers and QTL (Uimari and Hoeschele, 1997).

7.15 Summary

In this chapter we considered methods for QTL parameter estimation as random effects. Both the Haseman-Elston sib-pair model, and the Fernando-Grossman gametic model were considered. In the former model only the variance contributed by the QTL and the QTL location were estimated, while in the Fernando-Grossman model, QTL additive effects were also estimated. For both models we considered the situations of a QTL linked to a single marker, and a QTL bracketed between two markers. Multiple QTL were also considered for the Fernando-Grossman model. Although both models assume an infinite number of possible QTL alleles, the estimated QTL variances were robust to deviations from this assumption, and good estimates were derived even if only two alleles were simulated.

Methodology to derive Bayesian estimates of QTL parameters in a grand-daughter design, under the assumption of a biallelic QTL was also presented. As expected, the Bayesian estimates of QTL effects were "shrunken" as compared to ML estimates. The Bayesian and ML estimates converge to the same values as the number of observations increases. Application of Bayesian methodology requires rather specific knowledge about the prior distribution of QTL effects, which is generally lacking.

Chapter eight:

Statistical Power to Detect QTL, and Parameter CIs

8.1 Introduction

The type I error, denoted α, is the probability that the null hypothesis will be rejected, even though it is correct. The probability of not rejecting the null hypothesis when the alternative hypothesis is correct is called the type II error, and is denoted by β. Statistical power is defined as the probability to reject the null hypothesis, provided that it is incorrect. Thus power is equal to $1 - \beta$. For QTL detection the null hypothesis is generally defined as no difference between the genotype means for the putative QTL. With a QTL linked to a single marker, the null hypothesis can also be defined as independent distribution of the marker and QTL genotypes (Simpson, 1989).

Statistical power can be computed analytically only for linear models. For the other analysis methods power can be estimated by repeat simulation. Power to detect segregating QTL will be chiefly a function of the number of individuals genotyped for the genetic markers and phenotyped for the quantitative traits, and the effect of the segregating QTL in comparison to the polygenic and residual variances. Statistical power will also depend on the magnitude of the Type I error allowed, the recombination distances between the QTL and the genetic markers, and the specific experimental design employed. Since the number of possible combinations described is quite large, we will present only a few examples from the literature, and describe in general terms the effect of various parameters on the statistical power of the experiment.

A priori, it would seem that the method of statistical analysis should also affect the power of detection, but this is rarely the case. The exceptions will also be considered in this chapter.

In Section 8.2 we will estimate power for crosses between inbred lines. In Section 8.3 we will consider designs that use replicated progeny, and in Section 8.4 will consider power for segregating populations. In Section 8.5 we will consider estimation of power for likelihood ratio tests, and in Section 8.6 we will consider the effect of the analysis method on QTL detection power. In Section 8.7 we will give examples of power estimates for models that assume QTL effects are random. Power estimates for likelihood ratio tests can be derived only by simulation.

CIs for QTL parameter estimates will be considered in Sections 8.8 through 8.10. Parameter CIs are derived from the parameter estimate variances. These variances can be estimated from the matrix of second differentials computed using the maximum likelihood (ML) parameter estimates, as described in Section 2.9, but these estimates are only lower bounds. Several studies have empirically estimated CIs by repeat simulation. These estimates are generally close to the theoretical values for all parameters, except QTL location, which is the most problematic parameter to estimate, and generally has a non-symmetric error variance distribution. Examples will be presented.

8.2 Estimation of power in crosses between inbred lines

Different studies that estimate the power of QTL detection considered the substitution effect of QTL alleles in terms of the phenotypic, the residual, or the genetic standard deviation. However, since residual and genetic variances only are known *a posteriori*, QTL effects will be given in units of the phenotypic standard deviation (SDU). Soller et al. (1976) analytically computed the required number of offspring required to obtain a given power for the BC and F-2 designs, based on a t-test. For the BC design there is only a single contrast that can be evaluated. For the F-2 design the contrast between the homozygote genotypes was considered. The required number of progeny can be computed as follows:

$$n = \frac{2(Z_{\alpha/2} + Z_\beta)^2}{(\delta_n/\sigma)^2} \quad \{8.1\}$$

where: n = number of progeny per marker genotype class, $Z_{\alpha/2}$ and Z_β are the standard normal distribution values for a type I and type II errors of $\alpha/2$ and β, respectively, δ_n = expected contrast between marker groups, and σ is the residual standard deviation. As shown in Table 4.5, the variance due to a segregating codominant QTL in the F-2 design will be $a^2/2$, where a is the additive effect, measured in SDU. Thus for a = 0.141, the variance contributed by the QTL will be 1% of the phenotypic variance. The expectation of the contrasts, and required numbers of progeny for 2a = 0.282σ, α = 0.05, β = 0.1, and r = 0, are given in Table 8.1 for power of 0.9.

The effects of the magnitude of the QTL, and the proportion of recombination between the marker and the QTL on sample size to achieve a given power will be quadratic. That is, for an effect of half the magnitude, it will be necessary to increase the number of individuals scored four-fold to achieve the same power. In either the F-2 or backcross (BC) designs, the magnitude of the effect measured will decrease proportional to 1–2r, as compared to complete linkage. Thus, to achieve power equal to the case of complete linkage, it will be necessary to increase the experiment's size by a factor of $1/(1-2r)^2$. For example, for r=0.1 the sample size must be increased by a factor of 1.5625, that is 1641 individuals instead of 1050.

144 Quantitative Trait Loci Analysis in Animals

Table 8.1 The expectation of the contrasts, and required numbers of progeny to obtain statistical power of 0.9 for the BC and F-2 designs. ($2a = 0.282\sigma$, $\alpha = 0.05$, and $r = 0$)

Cross	Contrast	Sample size	Dominance		
			$d = -a$	$d = 0$	$d = a$
Backcross	$(a-d)(1-2r)$	$2n$	525	2100	
F-2	$2a(1-2r)$	$4n$	1050	1050	1050

For the F-2, power can also be estimated by ANOVA including all three genotypes. The probability for the alternative hypothesis is computed based on the non-central F distribution. Power including the heterozygotes will be greater if the absolute value of d is greater than $a/2$ (Soller et al., 1976).

For QTL bracketed by two markers, the effect measured will not be reduced by recombination, except for double crossovers. The QTL effect can be estimated in a linear model analysis by deleting recombinant progeny. The proportion of recombinants for the F-2 and BC designs will be $(1-R)^2$ and $(1-R)$, respectively, where R is the recombination frequency between the markers. Power with a marker bracket, therefore, will be reduced by this factor relative to complete linkage. The relative power with a marker bracket as compared to a single marker will be a function of r_1/R, where r_1 is the recombination frequency between the QTL and the nearer marker. The optimum case for a marker bracket is: $r_1 = R/2$. In this case power with a marker bracket will be increased by $(1-R)$ for the BC design, and will be equal to a single-marker analysis for the F-2 design (Weller, 1992).

8.3 Replicate progeny in crosses between inbred lines

In Chapter four, analysis of recombinant inbred lines produced by self-breeding of BC or F-2 individuals was briefly considered. All mating among relatives increases inbreeding, and reduces the frequency of heterozygotes. Inbreeding is measured by the probability that an individual will receive the two copies of the same allele both derived from the same ancestor. These two alleles are termed identical by descent.

Soller and Beckmann (1990) considered F-3, and F-4 generations, recombinant inbred lines (RIL), vegetative clones, and double haploid lines (DHL). In the F-3 design each F-2 individual is mated to itself. This is termed "selfing". It is assumed that only the F-2 individuals are genotyped, but quantitative trait records are produced for the F-3 individuals. Similarly, for the F-4 design, the F-3 individuals are selfed, and the F-4 individuals are phenotyped, but not genotyped. Genotype data from the F-2 generation is analysed. In both these designs recombination in the generations after the F-1 generation does not affect the analysis, because only the F-2 individuals are genotyped.

RIL are produced by several generations of selfing, starting with the F-2 individuals. At each generation inbreeding is increased, so that after several generations of selfing the progeny will be almost completely homozygous. At the final generation, several of progeny from each parent are scored for the quantitative trait, but only a single individual is genotyped for the markers. Since each "line" is now nearly completely homozygous and isogenic, it is only necessary to genotype a single individual for the genetic marker, and genetic variance within each RIL will tend to zero. However, because the RIL individuals are genotyped after several generations of inbreeding, the recombination between the markers and the QTL relative to the F-2 is increased. Recombination will affect linkage between the QTL and the genetic marker, only if the parent is heterozygous for both loci. The probability of these individuals in the F-2 population are $½(1 - 2r + r^2)$. Of these $½(1–2r)$ represent non-recombinants, while the frequency of double recombinants is $½r^2$. For either of these groups, the probability of a single event of recombination will be $2r - r^2$, and the fraction of recombinant chromosomes is increased. After several generations, recombination between the marker and the QTL for RIL will tend towards $r_L = 2r/(1+2r)$ (Soller and Beckmann, 1990).

Vegetative clones produced from F-2 individuals are similar to RIL in that genetic variance within each clone is zero, but no additional recombination has occurred. DHL have the same statistical features as RIL when recombination between the marker and the QTL tends to zero, as described below.

The effect of replicate progeny on statistical power for all these designs can be derived by the analysis of the following model:

$$Y_{ijkl} = A_i + B_j + L_{ik} + e_{ijkl} \qquad \{8.2\}$$

where: Y_{ijkl} = record of individual l from "line" k with genotype i with "block" effect j, A_i = effect of genotype i., B_j = effect of the jth "block", L_{ik} = effect of "line" j nested within genotype i, and e_{ijkl} is the random residual. This model differs from the model of Equation {4.1} in the inclusion of a line effect. Significance of a segregating QTL can be tested by an F-test of the ratio of the mean-squares of A and L times the number of inbred lines. This can be computed as follows. The expectation of the mean-squares of L will be $\sigma_G^2 + \sigma_e^2/N_l$, where σ_G^2 = genetic variance between lines, σ_e^2 = residual variance, and N_l = number of individuals per line. The expectation of the mean-squares for A for inbred lines derived from an F-2 population with codominance at the QTL and complete linkage will be: $a^2 + \sigma_G^2/N_g + \sigma_e^2/(N_g N_l)$, where N_g = number of inbred lines. Thus, the ratio of the MS of A and L times m will have a central F distribution under the null hypothesis that $a^2 = 0$. (An F-test of the ratio of the MS of the marker effect to the residual MS as done for the model of Equation {4.1} will give erroneous results.) A similar situation is encountered for the grand-daughter design, and was discussed by Ron *et al.* (1994).

σ_G^2 will be a function of the heritability, dominance, and the specific mating strategy considered. The advantage of inbred lines is greatest when σ_e^2 is large compared to σ_G^2. Following Soller and Beckmann (1990), the between- and within-progeny group variance components and the required numbers of lines relative to the F-2 design, to obtain equal power are given in Table 8.2.

The variance between lines will be h^2 for all the replicate progeny designs considered above, except RIH and DHL, which will have a variance component of $2h^2$. The saving in genotyping can be quite significant. For example, for $h^2=0.2$, and $N_I = 10$, only 0.29 as many genotypes are required by the F-3 design as compared to the F-2. For all designs, except RIL with large N_I the number of lines required will be a direct function of the heritability. For RIL, the power will also be a function of r. As noted above, recombination between the marker and the QTL for RIL will tend towards $r_L = 2r/(1+2r)$. Thus, the power for RIL will be proportional to $1/(1-2r_L)^2$ as compared to $1/(1-2r)^2$ for the F-2 design.

Table 8.2 Between- and within-progeny group variance components, and the required number of lines relative to the F-2 design for equal power, as a function of the heritability (h^2) and the number of individuals per line (N_I)

Progeny type	Variance component		Required number of lines relative to the F-2
	Between lines	Within lines	
F-2	h^2	$(1-h^2)$	1
F-3	h^2	$(1-h^2/2)/N_I$	$h^2+(1-h^2/2)/N_I$
F-4	h^2	$(1-h^2/4)/N_I$	$h^2+(1-h^2/4)/N_I$
Vegetative clones	h^2	$(1-h^2)/N_I$	$h^2+(1-h^2)/N_I$
Recombinant inbred lines	$2h^2$	$(1-h^2)/N_I$	$[h^2+(1-h^2)/N_I][1-2r]^2/[1-4r/(1+2r)]^2$
Double haploid lines	$2h^2$	$(1-h^2)/N_I$	$h^2+(1-h^2/2)/2N_I$

8.4 Estimation of power for segregating populations

Soller and Genizi (1978) estimated power for the daughter design assuming a nested ANOVA analysis. Weller et al. (1990) estimated power for the daughter and grand-daughter design assuming a χ^2 test, first proposed by Neimann-Sorensen and Robertson (1961). The two methods differ in their treatment of the residual variance. The χ^2 method assumes that the estimated residual variance is the true value, while the ANOVA analysis accounts for inaccuracy in estimation of the residual variance. With large samples the two methods give virtually identical results.

Weller *et al.* (1990) assumed that the squared sum of the within-family paternal allele contrasts would have a central χ^2 distribution under the null hypothesis, and a non-central χ^2 distribution under the alternative hypothesis. Their calculations were based on the assumption of two QTL alleles with equal frequency segregating in the population. Thus, half of the sires would be homozygous for the QTL, and expected paternal allele contrasts for these families are zero. They also assumed complete linkage, and considered substitution effects of 0.1, 0.2 and 0.3. With no dominance at the QTL, the substitution effect is equal to a (half the difference between the homozygote means). Results for a type 1 error of 0.01 are given in Table 8.3. For the daughter design, power of 0.7, with a type I error of 0.01, is obtained for a QTL with a substitution effect of 0.2 SDU if 400 daughters of each of 10 sires are analysed for a trait with heritability of 0.2. This entails genotyping 4000 individuals. Power is maximized when the frequency of the two QTL alleles is equal. For a codominant allele the allele frequency effects power only through the expected frequency of heterozygous sires, which will be close to 0.5 over the range of 0.3 to 0.8. Thus, within this range, allele frequency has only a small effect on power for a codominant locus.

The situation with the grand-daughter design is similar to the F-3 design considered above, in that the sons are genotyped, while records from their progeny are analysed. Power for the grand-daughter design for a QTL additive effect of 0.2 residual standard deviations, and a type 1 error of 0.01 are given in Table 8.4 (after Weller *et al.*, 1990).

Similar to the F-3 design, power for the grand-daughter design is increased per individual genotyped, because many phenotypes are analysed for each individual genotyped. Also power is not affected by an additional generation of recombination. Unlike the F-3 design, both the QTL contrast and the common polygenic effect passed to the grandprogeny are halved. As in the case of inbred lines, increasing the number of grand-daughters will reduce the residual variance, but not between-son genetic variance. Thus, the advantage of the grand-daughter design is greatest for low heritability traits. With heritability of 0.2 and a type I error of 0.01, power is 0.74 to detect a segregating QTL with a substitution effect of 0.2 SDU if genetic markers are analysed on 100 sons of each of 10 grandsires, with 50 quantitative trait-recorded grand-daughters per son. Comparing this example to the example above for the daughter design, greater power is obtained to detect an effect of the same magnitude with the grand-daughter design, even though only one-quarter the number of individuals are genotyped (4000 vs. 1000). The following conclusions can be drawn from the daughter and grand-daughter design power tables:

1. For both the daughter and grand-daughter designs with equal number of genotypes, power is greater for a few big families than for many small ones.
2. With heritability of 0.2, power equal to the daughter design can be obtained

by the grand-daughter design with only one-quarter the number of genotypings.
3. For a given substitution effect measured relative to the phenotypic standard deviation, power for the grand-daughter design decreases with increase in heritability.
4. Similar to replicate progeny designs for inbred lines, increasing number of grand-daughters per son above 50 increases power only marginally.

Table 8.3 Power of the daughter design to detect a segregating QTL as a function of the number of sires, daughters per sire, and gene effect, with a type I error of 0.01

	Number of		Power with QTL effects of:*		
Sires	Daughters per sire	Assays	0.1	0.2	0.3
5	200	1000	0.03	0.18	0.50
	400	2000	0.07	0.44	0.80
	600	3000	0.12	0.64	0.90
	800	4000	0.18	0.76	0.94
	1000	5000	0.25	0.83	0.96
	2000	10,000	0.55	0.95	0.97
10	200	2000	0.05	0.31	0.76
	400	4000	0.11	0.70	0.96
	600	6000	0.21	0.88	0.99
	800	8000	0.32	0.95	0.99
	1000	10,000	0.43	0.97	0.99
	2000	20,000	0.81	0.99	0.99
20	200	4000	0.07	0.56	0.95
	400	8000	0.20	0.93	0.96
	600	12,000	0.38	0.99	0.99
	800	16,000	0.56	0.99	0.99
	1000	20,000	0.70	0.99	0.99
	2000	40,000	0.97	0.99	0.99

* Gene effect = a/SD, where a = half the difference between the mean trait values for the two homozygotes, and SD = the residual standard deviation.

Chapter eight: Statistical Power to Detect QTL

Table 8.4 Power of the grand-daughter design to detect a segregating QTL as a function of the number of sires, daughters per sire, with a gene additive effect of 0.2 residual standard deviations, and a type I error of 0.01

	Number of		Power with heritability of:		
Grandsires	Sons per grandsire*	Grand-daughters per son	0.1	0.2	0.5
5	40 (200)	10	0.05	0.05	0.04
		50	0.26	0.15	0.06
		100	0.38	0.19	0.07
	100 (500)	10	0.20	0.16	0.10
		50	0.67	0.48	0.21
		100	0.79	0.58	0.23
	200 (1000)	10	0.47	0.41	0.28
		50	0.89	0.79	0.49
		100	0.93	0.85	0.53
10	40 (400)	10	0.09	0.07	0.05
		50	0.45	0.26	0.10
		100	0.62	0.34	0.10
	100 (1000)	10	0.35	0.29	0.18
		50	0.90	0.74	0.37
		100	0.96	0.83	0.41
	200 (2000)	10	0.73	0.66	0.48
		50	0.99	0.96	0.75
		100	0.99	0.98	0.79
20	40 (800)	10	0.15	0.12	0.08
		50	0.72	0.47	0.16
		100	0.88	0.59	0.19
	100 (2000)	10	0.59	0.50	0.33
		50	0.99	0.95	0.62
		100	0.99	0.98	0.68
	200 (4000)	10	0.94	0.90	0.76
		50	0.99	0.96	0.95
		100	0.99	0.98	0.97

* Number of assays are given in parentheses.

Power for replicate progeny designs decrease with increase in heritability, if the QTL effect is measured relative to the phenotypic standard deviation. Although it is the phenotypic standard deviation that is economically relevant, it is the genetic variance that must be explained by segregating QTL. With the QTL measured relative to the genetic standard deviation, there is virtually no relationship between heritability and power, if the number of grand-daughters is large.

8.5 Power estimates for likelihood ratio tests - general considerations

As first noted in Section 2.9, the log likelihood ratio times 2 will have a central χ^2 distribution under the null hypothesis. Under the alternative hypothesis, the log likelihood ratio will have a non-central χ^2 distribution with non-central parameter equal to twice the expectation of the log likelihood ratio. In most cases of interest this expectation cannot be computed analytically. We have already noted in Equation 5.29 that for the simple case of a backcross design with complete linkage, the expectation of the log likelihood ratio will be: $0.5 N \log(1 + \sigma_v^2/\sigma_e^2)$. Using the values given above in Table 8.1 for a QTL additive effect of 0.141 standard deviations and a sample size of 2100, $\sigma_v^2 = a^2/4 = 0.005$, and the expectation of the log likelihood ratio is 5.237. Thus, under the alternative hypothesis, the test statistic should have a χ^2 distribution with one degree of freedom, and a non-central parameter of 10.474. Using these values and a type I error of 0.05, power of 0.9 is obtained, which is exactly the same as for a normal test.

Several studies, beginning with Simpson (1989), have attempted to approximately estimate power of likelihood ratio tests for more complicated models by repeated simulation of populations generated under the null and alternative hypotheses. Since hundreds of simulations must be generated to obtain approximate distributions of both the null and alternative hypotheses, power can be estimated only for a few, selected, situations.

8.6 The effect of statistical methodology on the power of QTL detection

Although intuitively it would seem that statistical methodologies that are able to provide more accurate parameter estimates should also increase power of detection, this is generally not the case. Maximum likelihood, which utilizes all information in the data, should apparently be more powerful than ANOVA, which utilizes only the mean and variance of the distributions. Simulation results to this effect were in fact obtained for ML with individual markers by Simpson (1989), but later retracted (Simpson, 1992).

Darvasi *et al.* (1993) compared power for a single marker t-test to power obtained by a likelihood ratio test with marker brackets. Maximum difference in power was obtained with wide marker brackets, and the QTL located in the middle of the bracket. Even with a distance of 50 cM between markers, the difference in power between the two methods was at most 8%. Haley and Knott (1992) found similar results. These results differ from the linear model results presented in Section 8.2, because in the ML analysis the recombinant individuals for the genetic markers are included in the analysis.

For the sib-pair design, Fulker and Cardon (1994) found a greater difference in power between single marker analysis and marker brackets. With marker brackets of 20 cM, and a QTL in the middle of the bracket, the same power could be obtained with interval mapping, by genotyping only 64% as many individuals. Xu and Atchley (1995) found that power was slightly greater with a likelihood ratio test, assuming a random QTL effect, as opposed to a fixed regression model of Fulker and Cardon (1994). The number of different QTL alleles simulated did not affect this conclusion.

Significant differences in power between ML and linear model analysis can be obtained in situations where the linear model analysis cannot utilize all of the data (Knott *et al.*, 1996). In the case of daughter or grand-daughter design, where only sires and their progeny are genotyped, progeny will be informative for a specific marker only if their sires are heterozygous for the marker, and their genotypes are different from their sires. Thus a particular progeny will be informative for only some of the markers. In this case, an ML or non-linear regressions analysis that utilizes data from all linked markers will have greater power than an analysis based on evaluation of the effects of individual markers, or specific marker brackets.

Knott *et al.* (1996) used simulations to compare power by ML and non-linear regression for daughter and grand-daughter designs. They found that power of the two methods were very similar, although the assumptions employed were somewhat different. The ML analysis assumed that only two QTL alleles were segregating, and that the family mean was estimated without error.

8.7 Estimation of power with random QTL models

In the previous chapter we considered models for segregating populations that assume random QTL effects. In segregating populations the number of QTL alleles is not known, and there will be a non-random distribution of polygenic effects. Power cannot be estimated analytically for these models, and has therefore been estimated by simulation. Results will be presented for the Haseman and Elston (1972) full-sib model.

As mentioned in Chapter four, very large samples will be required in the sib-pair design of Haseman and Elston to obtain reasonable power to detect QTL of the magnitude considered above. Most of the calculations for the full-sib design have assumed QTL of much larger magnitude than the examples presented in the previous sections (Sribney and Swift, 1992; Xu and Atchley, 1995). Xu and Atchley (1995) compared power to detect a QTL explaining either 0.25 or 0.5 of the phenotypic variance by a regression model, as described in Section 5.4, and a likelihood ratio test, as described in Section 7.2. In the latter case the QTL effect is assumed to be random. The QTL was located in the middle of a 100 cM chromosome with six equally spaced, fully informative, markers. Models with two and six segregating alleles were simulated, with codominance for all alleles. No polygenic variance was simulated. The number of full-sib families was varied from 250 to 1000, with two sibs in each family. A type I error of 0.05 was assumed.

Similar to results for other experimental designs, power was generally slightly greater for the likelihood ratio test, as compared to the regression model, in which the QTL is a fixed effect. Power was also slightly higher for the six-allele model. For a QTL explaining 0.25 of the variance power approached 0.5 only if 1000 families (2000 individuals) were analysed. Power was greater than 0.9 only if the QTL accounted for 0.5 of the variance and 1000 families were analysed. Tens of thousands of individuals will be required to obtain power greater than 0.5 for loci with substitution effects in the range of 0.2.

8.8 Confidence intervals for QTL parameters – analytical methods

As shown in Equation {2.24}, for maximum likelihood estimation (MLE) the estimation error variance-covariance matrix can be estimated from the inverse of the ML matrix of second differentials. This is also the case for linear model estimation. The prediction error variance estimates can then be used to derive CIs (CI) for all the parameters. This is not an option for interval mapping by the non-linear regression method. Even for MLE this method of deriving CI has limitations. First, in some cases, the likelihood function cannot be readily differentiated twice for all parameters, especially if multiple markers and QTL are included in the analysis. Second, estimation of CI by a linear function of the square roots of the prediction error variances assumes that the distributions of the parameter estimates are symmetric. This will of course not be the case for variances, which can only be positive, but will also not be the case for recombination parameters, especially if the putative QTL location is close to a marker or the end of the chromosome. Alternative methods to estimate CI, especially for QTL location have also been proposed.

Lander and Botstein (1989) proposed estimating "support intervals" for QTL location, based on the likelihood ratio test. As explained previously, in a likelihood ratio test, the likelihood maximized over all parameters is compared with the ML obtained with some of the parameters fixed. If the null hypothesis is correct, the log of the ratio of the two likelihoods times 2 should have a χ^2 distribution with degrees of freedom equal to the number of parameters fixed in the null hypothesis that are allowed to float in the alternative hypothesis. Similarly, the lower bound of the CI of $1-\alpha$ probability for any of the parameter estimates can be constructed based of the following statistic:

$$\chi^2_{(1-\alpha/2)} = 2 \ln [L_{max}/ L_{(\theta=\theta_0)}] \qquad \{8.3\}$$

where $\chi^2_{(1-\alpha/2)}$ is the χ^2 value for $1-\alpha/2$ with one degree of freedom, L_{max} is the likelihood value with the likelihood maximized over all parameters, and $L_{(\theta=\theta_0)}$ is the likelihood maximized over all parameters with θ fixed at θ_0, which is a value for the parameter θ less than the ML value, but closest to its ML value that gives the appropriate χ^2 value. Similarly the upper bound of the CI is determined by the same statistic with θ_0 computed as a value of θ greater than the ML value that satisfies equation $\{8.3\}$.

Mangin et al. (1994) showed that for QTL location, the support interval as given is Equation $\{8.3\}$ underestimated the actual CI, especially for small QTL effects. They were able to derive a rather complicated test statistic that accurately estimates the CI for small QTL effects, but the distribution of this test statistic must be computed empirically.

Furthermore, this method does not account for the possibility that the QTL is outside the marker bracket. In this case there is still likely to be a maximum for QTL location within the marker bracket (Martinez and Curnow, 1992). It does account for the possibility that the CI is asymmetric, which will generally be the case, especially if the QTL is located near an end of the chromosome.

Mackinnon and Weller (1995) proposed estimating CIs and standard error (SE) by computing the expectation of the likelihood function as a function of each parameter with the other parameters held constant. The expectation of the likelihood is computed as follows:

$$E(L_{(\theta=\theta_0)}) = \int (L_{(\theta=\theta_0)})dx \qquad \{8.4\}$$

where x is the trait value, and $L_{(\theta=\theta_0)}$ is as defined above. This integral can be estimated by summation. As noted previously, the difference of the log ML to the log likelihood with one parameter fixed has a $\frac{1}{2}\chi^2$ distribution with one degree of freedom. Based on the expectation of the likelihood function and the χ^2 distribution, the 95% CI for each parameter can be determined. Although this method behaved well for a QTL linked to a single marker, it is difficult to compute, and has not been applied to interval mapping.

8.9 Simulation studies of confidence intervals

To obtain accurate estimates of the CI by simulation, it is necessary to generate a large number of samples. For example, if 1000 samples are generated, the 95% confidence limits are obtained by determining the 25 lowest and 25 highest estimates for each parameter. Thus the effective number of samples can be considered to be 50. In much smaller samples, the estimated confidence limits will vary widely.

Darvasi *et al.* (1993) estimated QTL parameter estimation error variances based on Equation {2.24}, and by repeat simulation for the BC design with marker brackets. The 95% CI was then estimated as ±2 estimation SE for each parameter. They also directly estimated the 95% CI for each parameter by repeat simulation. All methods were very accurate for estimation of QTL effect variances. Estimates based on the second differential matrix tended to slightly overestimate SE for QTL means relative to the empirical estimates, especially for large spacing between markers. Neither the QTL effect nor marker spacing had any appreciable effect on CI for QTL means. The effect of sample size was quadratic, as expected. That is, doubling the sample decreased the CI by a factor of about the square root of two.

For QTL map location, the estimates based on the empirical 95% CI, and estimates based on four times the empirical SE were generally similar. However, estimates based on the second differential matrix tended to underestimate the CI for small marker intervals, and overestimate the CI for large marker intervals. Differences were in some cases were more than two-fold. Clearly, for this parameter the asymptotic properties of the second differential matrix do not hold. For the BC design and a single marker, the matrix of second differentials tended to overestimate error variance for all parameters, even though by theory the opposite should occur. It should be noted though, that even for very large samples the error variance estimated by the matrix of second differentials is correct only at the point of ML. The likelihood function can behave marked differently for other parameter values.

Mackinnon and Weller (1995) estimated parameter SE both empirically and by the matrix of second differentials for the daughter design for a single marker, and also analytically computed the 95% CI, as described above. In addition to QTL means, r, and the residual variance, they also estimated the QTL allele frequencies. CI estimates based on assuming that all other parameters were fixed tended to underestimate the SE derived by either repeat simulation or the matrix of second differentials. As for the BC design with a single marker, the matrix of second differentials tended to overestimate the SE, even though the opposite was expected. Discrepancies increased with decrease in sample size. CI were largest for recombination rate. The standard error for r with a substitution effect of 0.5 was about 0.1 with 2000 individuals. For the BC design and a marker bracket of 50 cM, a similar SE was obtained with only 1000 individuals, although, in both cases the number of QTL genotypes performed was the same.

8.10 Empirical methods to estimate confidence intervals, parametric and non-parametric bootstrap and jackknife methods

In the "parametric bootstrap" method parameter estimates are first derived by any of the methods considered. In the second step a large number of sample distributions of equal size to the actual data sample are then derived from the assumed theoretical distribution, assuming that that the original parameter estimates are the parameter values. Parameter estimates are then derived for each sample. The CI for each parameter is then derived from the empirical distributions of the parameter estimates from the samples generated.

The weakness of the parametric bootstrap method is that it assumes that both the theoretical distribution and the original parameter estimates are correct. If either of these assumptions is incorrect, then estimated CI can differ widely for the true values.

Efron and Tibshirani (1993) proposed empirical "bootstrap" methods to estimated CI in situations where analytical methods cannot be applied. In "non-parametric bootstrapping", a large number of repeat samples of size equal to the actual data are generated by sampling *with repeats* from the original data. Thus, in a particular sample some of the actual records will appear more than once, while other observations will be missing. If the actual data consists of at least several hundred points, it will be possible to draw a virtually unlimited number of different samples in this method. The parameter estimates are then derived for each sample, and as in parametric bootstrapping, the distribution of these estimates is used to derive empirical CI limits. This method is not strictly "non-parametric," because assumptions about the distribution are still employed to derive parameter estimates for each sample. This method is more robust to violations of assumptions used to derive parameter estimates.

"Jackknife" samples are derived from the original data sample by generating new samples consisting of the original data, with one observation deleted. Thus, unlike the empirical bootstrap, the number of jackknife samples that can be derived is only equal to the sample size. Bootstrap and jackknife sampling can be combined to analyse complex problems.

Visscher *et al.* (1996b) applied the non-parametric bootstrap method to estimate CI for QTL location in a BC design with multiple markers and a single QTL segregating on the chromosome. Accuracy of the CI estimate was determined by the proportion of CI that actually contained the QTL. They found that this method was able to estimate accurately the CI for QTL location, provided that the CI was less than two-thirds of the entire chromosome. If the CI estimate was larger than two-thirds of the chromosome, it tended to overestimate the actual CI. This is inevitable as the QTL effect and sample size become smaller. The estimated CI for QTL location approaches the entire chromosome, and assuming the model is correct, the QTL must lie somewhere on the chromosome.

As noted previously by Mangin *et al.* (1994), the support interval or "LOD drop-off" method of Lander and Botstein (1989) consistently underestimated the CI. Similar to the results of Darvasi *et al.* (1993) decreasing the marker spacing from 20 to 10 cM had virtually no effect on the estimated CI. The bootstrap method was also able to derive accurate CI for the other QTL parameters, such as QTL effect, but these were shown by Darvasi *et al.* (1993) to be "well-behaved". It is not clear how bootstrapping will behave if there is more than a single QTL segregating on the chromosome.

8.11 Summary

Numerous misconceptions with respect to the power of QTL detection and experiment design optimization are prevalent. In most cases power to detect a segregating QTL explaining only a few percent of the phenotypic variance will require genotyping at least 500 individuals, and often many more. It is unlikely that a QTL of a magnitude much greater than this will be segregating in the population for moderately heritable trait. Most experiments have been too small to find effects of the magnitude that could be reasonably expected.

Analytical formulas that compute estimation error variances for QTL ML parameter estimates are accurate for means and variances, but not for recombination parameters. CI for QTL location can be significantly larger than estimated by interval mapping support intervals. Increasing marker density above a certain level has only a minor effect on the CI for QTL location. As the marker density increases the number of events of recombination in the sample becomes the limiting factor in estimating QTL location.

Chapter nine:

Optimization of Experimental Designs

9.1 Introduction

Optimization of experimental designs will be defined as obtaining maximum statistical power per unit cost. The major cost elements of QTL detection are producing the individuals for analysis, scoring the quantitative traits, genotyping for the genetic markers, and data analysis. Optimization of experimental designs to obtain maximum power per unit cost will depend on the relative costs of these factors.

Generally the cost of data analysis will be negligible with respect to the other costs. Genotyping individuals for the genetic markers is often the most expensive part of the experiment. Furthermore, if the analysis is based on existing records, marker genotyping is the only significant expense. We will consider the whole range of possibilities, from the dairy cattle situation, in which records are available for analysis at virtually no cost, to human diseases, in which the data set is of limited size, and additional records cannot be obtained regardless of cost.

In Section 9.2 we will first consider the economically optimum spacing of genetic markers for a preliminary genome scan. Replicate progeny, which was considered in the previous chapter, will be considered in Section 9.3 within the framework of optimization of the experimental design. Several other techniques have been proposed to increase statistical power to detect segregating QTL as a function of the number of genotype assays performed: selective genotyping, sample pooling, and sequential sampling. These techniques will be considered in Sections 9.4 to 9.8. Replicate progeny, selective genotyping and sample pooling require increasing the number of individuals produced and scored for quantitative traits, as compared to designs in which all individuals scored for the quantitative traits are also genotyped. Unlike replicate progeny, these other techniques are trait specific.

9.2 Economic optimization of marker spacing when the number of individuals genotyped is non-limiting

With microsatellites it is now possible to develop virtually unlimited numbers of markers. For a complete genome search, the total number of genotypes will be the number of individuals genotyped times the number of markers genotyped for individual. Darvasi and Soller (1994a) considered a number of experimental designs and cost ratios of genotyping to phenotyping. They assumed the Haldane

(1919) mapping function. If both the numbers of individuals and markers available for genotyping are unlimited, and costs of phenotyping are low relative to genotyping costs, then marker spacing of close to 80 cM between will give maximum statistical power per unit cost for crosses between inbred lines or half-sib families. This is equivalent to recombination between markers of R = 0.4 for the Haldane mapping function. For recombinant inbred lines (RIL), optimum spacing will be about 50 cM. With RIL the optimum marker spacing is smaller, because recombination frequency is greater, as explained in Section 8.3. Even if the cost of obtaining trait records, including producing the recorded individuals where necessary, is 100-fold the cost of each marker genotype, optimum marker spacing is still 30 cM for designs other than RIL. In any event, over the range of sample sizes tested, decreasing marker spacing below 20 cM has virtually no effect on power (Darvasi et al., 1993).

9.3 Economic optimization with replicate progeny

The effect of replicate progeny on statistical power was considered in detail in the previous chapter. With replicate progeny, power per individual genotyped is increased if multiple individuals from each line are phenotyped for the quantitative trait. The economically optimum economic design in terms of the number of individuals phenotyped from each line, N_l, will be a function of the relative costs of genotyping and phenotyping a single individual. Economic optimization will be considered under the assumption that a single individual is genotyped from each line, and that N_l individuals are phenotyped from each line.

As show in Table 8.2, statistical power will be a function of N_g/F, where N_g is the number of individuals genotyped (the number of lines), and F is the term in the last column in Table 8.2. Thus, for the case of vegetative clones, power will be a function of :

$$N_g / [h^2 + (1 - h^2)/ N_l] \qquad \{9.1\}$$

The optimum experimental design in terms of N_g is computed by maximizing this function with fixed cost. Total costs of the experiment, T_C, will be defined as:

$$T_C = C_g N_g + C_p N_g N_l \qquad \{9.2\}$$

Where C_g is the cost of genotyping a single individual, and C_p is the cost of phenotyping a single individual. Total costs of the experiment per cost of individual phenotyped, T_C', will be defined as:

$$T_C' = CN_g + N_g N_l \qquad \{9.3\}$$

where C is the ratio of the cost of genotyping each individual to the cost of phenotyping each individual, and the other terms are as described previously. Solving for N_g in equation {9.3} and substituting into expression {9.1} gives:

$$\frac{T_C'}{[C + N_1][h^2+(1-h^2)/ N_1]} \qquad \{9.4\}$$

The optimum experimental design in terms of N_1 can then be computed by setting the differential of this function with respect to N_1 equal to zero and solving. Note that T_C' is a multiplicative constant, and will not affect the optimum value of N_1, which will be a function of C and h^2. This derivative will not be a linear function of N_1. We therefore iteratively solved for the optimum value of N_1 for a range of values of C, and three value of h^2, 0.1, 0.2, and 0.5. Results are given in Figure 9.1. C is plotted on a $\log_{10}$ scale. As heritability increases, N_1 decreases as a function of C. This was explained in the previous chapter, and can also be seen by inspecting Expression {9.4}. The advantage of multiple phenotypes is greater for low heritability traits. Even with log C = 3 (C = 1000), and h^2 = 0.1, the optimum number of individuals per line is still less than 100. Similar calculations can be made for the other progeny group types given in Table 8.2.

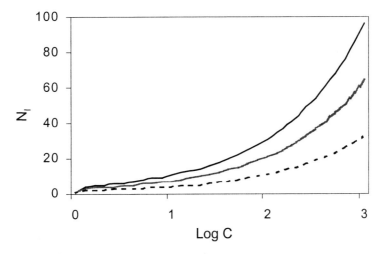

Figure 9.1 Optimum number of individuals phenotyped from each line, N_1, as a function of the ratio between the cost of genotyping and phenotyping each individual, C, for three values of heritability. h^2 = 0.1, heavy solid line; h^2 = 0.2, light solid line; h^2 = 0.5, dotted line. C is given on a $\log_{10}$ scale

9.4 Selective genotyping

Selective genotyping was first proposed by Lebowitz et al. (1987), and elaborated by Lander and Botstein (1989), and Darvasi and Soller (1992). An example for a backcross population is shown in Figure 9.2. The effect of gene substitution in this example is one residual standard deviation. It can be seen from this figure that the distributions of the two genotypes are quite similar close to the means, but very different in the tails of the distributions. Thus, most of the information with respect to QTL detection for any given trait is derived from the individuals with the extreme phenotypic values. If the sample of individuals recorded for the quantitative trait is large, power per individual genotyped can be increased by selectively genotyping those individuals with the highest and lowest trait values.

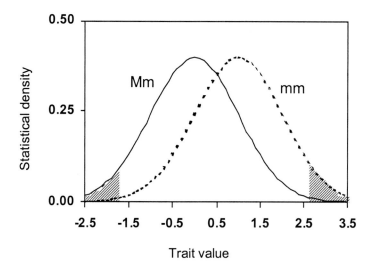

Figure 9.2 Demonstration of selective genotyping in a backcross population. The two genotypes differ by a single standard deviation. All individuals are phenotyped, but only the individuals in the distribution tails are genotyped

Darvasi and Soller (1992) derived equations to estimate the number of individuals that must be genotyped and phenotyped with selective genotyping to obtain the same power with random genotyping. For selective genotyping they assumed that only individuals with the most extreme phenotypes were selected for genotyping and that equal numbers of individuals from each tail of the distribution were genotyped. If N_z individuals are scored for the quantitative trait, but only N_g individuals are genotyped, then the statistical power can be derived from the following equation:

$$Z_\beta = \frac{N_g^{1/2} D_t}{2\sigma_t} - Z_{\alpha/2} \quad \{9.5\}$$

where $Z_{\alpha/2}$ and Z_β are the standard normal distribution values for a type I and type II errors of $\alpha/2$ and β, respectively; D_t is the difference between the mean of the tail samples for the quantitative trait; and σ_t is the within-marker genotype standard deviations for the tail samples. D_t/σ_t is approximately equal to: $\delta_n(1 + Z_p i_p)^{1/2}$, where δ_n is the expected contrast between the two marker genotypes with random genotyping, Z_p is the standard normal distribution value with a probability of p in the upper tail, p is the probability of each tail selected for genotyping and is equal to $N_g/(2N_z)$, and i_p is the mean value of the upper tail of a standard normal distribution with a frequency of p. In quantitative genetics, "i_p" is termed the selection intensity, and is equal to φ/p, where φ is the ordinate, or density, of the standard normal distribution at the point of truncation (Falconer, 1981).

Power equal to that obtained when N randomly selected individuals are both genotyped and phenotyped will be obtained with selective genotyping if:

$$N_z = N/[2p + 2Z_p \varphi_p] \quad \{9.6\}$$

where φ_p is the density of the distribution at Z_p. $N_g = 2pN_z$, and the relative reduction in the number of individuals genotype compared to random genotyping is N_g/N. N_z/N and N_g/N are plotted in Figure 9.3 as functions of p.

As shown in Figure 9.3, N_g/N is nearly a linear function of p over the range of p=0.01 to p=0.25. With selective genotyping it is possible to obtain the same statistical power by genotyping only one-fourth as many individuals, as compared to a random sample, for p = 0.06. In this case $N_z/N = 2.1$. Thus, if N = 1000, equal power can be obtained by phenotyping 2100, individuals, but genotyping only the 252 individuals with the most extreme phenotypes. Note that even for p=0.25, half the individuals are genotyped, $N_g/N = 0.55$, and there is still a very significant saving in the number of individuals genotyped. In this case N_z/N is only slightly greater than one. In other words, the 50% of individuals in the middle of the distribution contribute virtually no information with respect to QTL detection.

Darvasi and Soller (1992) considered a situation in which there are no absolute limitations on the numbers of individuals genotyped and phenotyped. In this case, the optimum experimental design will be a function of the relative costs of phenotyping and genotyping each individual. If genotyping and phenotyping costs are approximately equal, then optimum power per unit cost is obtained when about half of the individuals phenotyped are selected for genotyping. If genotyping costs are 100-fold phenotyping costs, then the experiment is optimized by genotyping less than 5% of the individuals phenotyped. Even if the cost of genotyping an individual is insignificant relative to the cost of obtaining the phenotype, it is economically optimal to genotype 90% of the individuals phenotyped. The disadvantages of this method are:

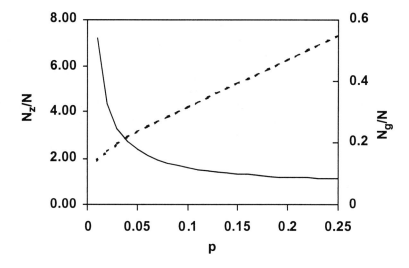

Figure 9.3 Relative number of individuals that must be phenotyped (N_z) and genotyped (N_g) with selective genotyping to obtain power equal to genotyping N individuals selected at random, as a function of p, the fraction of individuals selected for genotyping from each tail. N_z/N, solid line; N_g/N, broken line

1. A much larger sample of individuals must be scored for the quantitative trait.
2. If there are several quantitative traits of interest, it will be necessary to genotype a different sample for each trait. Selective genotyping with multiple traits will be considered in more detail in the following chapter. In general, though, this technique is only useful if the number of traits of interest is low.
3. D_t is a biased estimate of the QTL effect. An approximately unbiased estimate can be derived from the following equation (Darvasi and Soller, 1992) as follows:

$$\delta_n = D_t/(1 + Z_p i_p) \qquad \{9.7\}$$

with all the terms as defined above.

Unbiased estimates can also be derived by maximum likelihood (ML), if all phenotyped individuals are included in the likelihood function (Ronin et al., 1998). The QTL genotype probabilities for the individuals that are not genotyped are the population genotype probabilities.

In Section 6.2 we considered QTL genotype effects on the residual variance. ML can be used to detect QTL variance effects. Power to detect QTL variance effects is reduced with selective genotyping, unless a group of individuals with intermediate trait values are also genotyped (Weller and Wyler, 1992).

9.5 Sample pooling - general considerations

Michelmore *et al.* (1991) proposed that major genes causing diseases could be identified by "bulk segregant analysis". In this technique samples from different groups of individuals displaying a common phenotype are pooled. For example in the case of a disease gene, individuals with the disease are included in one pool, and healthy individuals are included in the second pool. The pooled samples are then genotyped for a series of genetic markers. If there is a significant difference in band intensity between any of the genetic markers tested, it can be deduced that this marker is linked to a gene affecting the trait of interest.

Several studies have shown that this technique, also termed "sample pooling" can also be applied to detection of QTL (Plotsky *et al.*, 1993, Khatib *et al.*, 1994; Lipkin *et a*l., 1998). As will be explained below, the number of genotypings can be reduced by up to two orders of magnitude relative to random genotyping by application of this technique without a reduction in power. For sample pooling to be effective, it must be possible to determine accurately the number of individuals of each genotype in each pool from the band intensity.

Sample pooling must be applied together with selective genotyping. Thus, this method is most useful if the number of quantitative traits of interest is relatively low. There will be some degradation of information with sample pooling relative to selective genotyping due to two factors:

1. Inaccuracy in determination of allele frequency from the band intensity.
2. Lack of knowledge of the specific phenotypic values for individuals of each genotype.

Therefore, more individuals must be scored for the quantitative trait, as compared to individual selective genotyping to obtain the same statistical power. Both selective genotyping and sample pooling are most useful in situations in which many individuals have already been scored for the traits of interest. In this case phenotyping costs can be considered negligible. This situation is common for commercial dairy cattle populations.

Darvasi and Soller (1994b) derived methods to estimate and optimize statistical power as a function of the proportion selected for inclusion in the pools, the QTL effect, and the "technical error" for several experimental designs. The technical error is a measure of the inaccuracy in estimation of the allele frequency from the band intensity. The backcross (BC) design will be considered in detail.

9.6 Estimation of power with sample pooling

As first explained in Chapter four, and shown in Figure 9.2, the progeny will have either Mm or mm genotype for the genetic marker. If the genetic marker is linked to a QTL affecting the quantitative trait, then, as noted above, one genotype will have a higher frequency in the high tail, and the other genotype will have a higher frequency in the low tail. If a single pool from the "high" tail and a single pool from the "low" tail are analysed, then the data consist of four observations, the density of the "M" and "m" allele bands in each pool. The estimates of the two allelic frequencies in each pool are of course correlated. In the BC or F-2 design the correlation will be complete. With no technical error, the frequency of the Mm genotype in a tail will be one minus the frequency of the mm genotype. In the daughter design, these two estimates will be only partially correlated, because the dams will also contribute paternal alleles. If the null hypothesis is correct, the allelic frequencies in the two different pools should be uncorrelated. Therefore, Darvasi and Soller (1994b) proposed a test for the BC design based on the mean of the estimates of the Mm genotype in the high pool, and the mm genotype in the low pool. These estimates are derived by first estimating the relative frequency of the two alleles in each pool.

Under the null hypothesis of no linkage to a segregating QTL, the estimated genotype frequencies in both pools should be equal to 0.5, and the two estimates should be statistically independent. Under the alternative hypothesis, the frequency of Mm should be higher in one tail, and lower in the other. Assuming normality, the null hypothesis will be rejected with a type I error of α if:

$$\hat{\pi}_f - 0.5 > [\text{Var}(\hat{\pi}_f)]^{1/2} Z_{\alpha/2} \qquad \{9.8\}$$

where $\hat{\pi}_f$ is the estimate of π_f, the mean of the genotype frequencies of Mm in the high tail and mm in the low tail, $\text{Var}(\hat{\pi}_f)$ is the variance of $\hat{\pi}_f$, and $Z_{\alpha/2}$ is as defined above. $\text{Var}(\hat{\pi}_f)$, which is the mean of two estimated frequencies, will consist of two components, one due to binomial sampling of genotypes in each tail, and the other due to the technical error in estimating the genotype frequencies from the band intensities, as described above. Assuming that these two components are statistically independent, under the null hypothesis, $\text{Var}(\hat{\pi}_f)$ is computed as follows:

$$\text{Var}(\hat{\pi}_f) = 0.25/(2pN_p) + V_\pi/2 \qquad \{9.9\}$$

where p is the frequency of the individuals selected for inclusion in each pool, N_p is the total number of individuals phenotyped for the quantitative trait, and V_π is the experimental error variance. V_π is a simple function of the technical error variance. This variance can be estimated by analysing pools constructed from individuals with known genotypes. A potential problem in this method is that the technical error variance may be different for different genetic markers. Furthermore, V_π will probably increase as the number of samples included in the pool increases.

For the BC and F-2 designs, the estimated genotype frequencies are derived by doubling the estimated allelic frequencies in each tail, because each diploid individual will contribute two alleles. For example, the frequency of the M allele in a pooled sample is only half of the frequency of the Mm genotype. Thus V_π is equal to four times V_t, the technical error variance of the estimate of marker allele frequency. For the daughter design, V_π can range from V_t to $5V_t$, depending on the frequency of the sire alleles in dam population. If the frequencies of the two sire alleles are close to zero in the dam population, then the frequencies of the two sire alleles in the pooled samples will be equal to the frequencies of the sire haplotypes in the daughter population. In this "best" case $V_\pi = V_t$. Equation {9.9} is based on the assumption that the technical error will be independent of the number of individuals sampled in each pool.

Power of the test was determined for an expected contrast of δ_n between the means of the two marker genotypes in the complete sample of individuals phenotyped. As noted in Chapter four with incomplete linkage and a single marker, the expectation of the contrast between the two marker genotypes in a BC design in terms of the QTL additive and dominance effects will be $(a+d)(1-2r)$. The expected genotype frequencies under the alternative hypothesis, π_f, are:

$$\pi_f = \Phi(Z_{p/2} + \delta_n/2)/2p \qquad \{9.10\}$$

where $\Phi(.)$ is the cumulative normal distribution function. The statistical power can then be derived as follows:

$$Z_\beta = (0.5 - \pi_f)/[\text{Var}(\hat{\pi}_f)]^{1/2} - Z_{\alpha/2} \qquad \{9.11\}$$

with all terms as defined previously. Substituting equations {9.9} and {9.10} into equation {9.11} gives:

$$Z_\beta = \frac{0.5 - \Phi(Z_p + \delta_n/2)/(2p)}{[0.25/(2pN_p) + V_\pi/2]^{1/2}} - Z_{\alpha/2} \qquad \{9.12\}$$

Thus power will be a function of δ_n, p, N_p, and V_π. This equation can be compared to Equation {9.5}, the comparable equation for selective genotyping. For any given set of values for δ_n, N_p, and V_π, the value of p that maximizes power can be found by setting the derivative of Equation {9.12} with respect to p equal to zero. Although it is not possible to solve analytically for p, Darvasi and Soller (1994b) numerically solved for the optimum p value over a range of values for the other parameters. The optimum value for p is a function of δ and the product, NV_π. The value of δ over the range of values from 0.5 to 0.125 phenotypic standard deviations had only a minor effect on the optimum p value, which was slightly higher for smaller QTL effects. The optimum p value approached 0.25 as $N_p V_\pi$ approached zero, but was less than 0.05 for $N_p V_\pi > 10$.

If the technical error is large relative to pN_p, power can be increased by replication of the pools. Replicating each pool n times decreases V_π by a factor of n. Even with several replicates of the pools, the total number of samples analysed will be much less that with individual selective genotyping.

9.7 Comparison of power and sample sizes with random genotyping, selective genotyping, and sample pooling

As noted above, power with sample pooling will be less than with selective genotyping for an equal number of individuals phenotyped. Equal power can be obtained by both methods, if the number of individuals phenotyped is greater with sample pooling. Required sample sizes for random and selective genotyping and sample pooling were compared based on the values used in Table 8.1 for the BC design: type I error, $\alpha = 0.05$; power, $1-\beta = 0.9$; $a = 0.141\sigma$; and complete dominance, $d = -a$. Thus $\delta_n = 0.282\sigma$. With random genotyping, 525 individuals must be phenotyped and genotyped, as given in Table 8.1. For both selective genotyping and sample pooling we will assume $p = 0.05$, which is close to the optimum for both methods for a wide range of situations. With selective genotyping, Equation {9.6} can be used to derive that 1196 individuals must be phenotyped, but only 120 individuals must be genotyped to obtain power of 0.9. Similarly, for sample pooling, N_p, the required number of individuals phenotyped, can be derived from Equation {9.12}. N_p and the number of pools genotyped to obtain equal power are given in Table 9.1 for several combinations of V_π with varying numbers of repeat pool samples.

With no technical error, 1570 individuals must be phenotyped. Since $p = 0.05$, 78 samples are included in each pool. In the second row, following Darvasi and Soller (1994b), $V_\pi = 0.0016$. The square root of V_π is 0.04. Under the null hypothesis, $\pi = 0.5$, and the standard error for the estimate of genotype frequency will be 8% of the mean. In this case the number of individuals that must be phenotyped is nearly doubled, and 156 samples are included in each pool. Still only two pools must be analysed, as compared to 120 genotypes with selective genotyping. With pools of this size, the experimental error variance is nearly equal to the binomial sampling variance.

With four repeats of each pool, the number of individuals that must be phenotyped is only slightly larger than with zero technical error, or about 35% greater than with selective genotyping. Still, only eight pools are analysed, as compared to 120 genotypes with selective genotyping. Without pool repeats, more than 4000 individuals must be phenotyped if the technical error is increased four-fold. Even in this case, the sample phenotyped can be reduced to 1620, if each pool is repeated 16 times. This still requires assaying only one-fourth the number of samples that must be genotyped with selective genotyping, although more labor will be involved in assaying a pool, as compared to genotype determination for a single individual.

Table 9.1 The numbers of individuals that must be phenotyped and included in each pool with different experimental error variances to obtain statistical power of 0.9 for the BC design. ($\delta_n = 0.282\sigma$, $\alpha = 0.05$, and $p = 0.05$). The last two rows give the sample sizes required to obtain the same power with individual selective and random genotyping

Experimental design	Experimental error variance	Number of:			
		Pool repeats	Phenotypes	Samples/pool	Genotypes
Sample pooling	0	1	1570	78	2
	0.0016	1	3120	156	2
		4	1620	82	8
	0.0064	1	4010	205	2
		4	3120	156	8
		16	1620	82	32
Selective genotyping	0	–	1196	1	120
Random genotyping	0	–	525	1	525

9.8 Sequential sampling

Finally, Motro and Soller (1993) suggested sequential sampling as a further tool to reduce the number of individuals genotyped. This method can best be applied to whole genome scans, considered in Chapter eleven. Rather than genotyping a sample large enough to obtain the desired statistical power for all markers, a smaller sample is genotyped in the preliminary step. Further genotyping is not done for those markers that either clearly show no significant effect, or that show a significant effect. Additional individuals will be genotyped only for those markers that display "borderline" significance. By this method it is possible to reduce the total number of genotypings required by nearly half for a single trait.

Unlike the methods described above, sequential sampling requires no increase in phenotyping above the sample size for random genotyping. Furthermore, this method can be used in conjunction with either replicate progeny or selective genotyping. Similar to selective genotyping and sample pooling, sequential sampling is useful only if the number of traits under consideration is small. If several uncorrelated traits are analysed, most chromosomal regions will have borderline significance for at least one quantitative trait, and it will be necessary to genotype the complete sample for nearly all markers.

9.9 Summary

Unless the phenotyping costs are very high relative to genotyping costs, experimental designs with very wide marker spacing are optimum, and decreasing marker intervals below 20 cM will have virtually no effect for most experimental designs. Replicate progeny, selective genotyping, and sample pooling can dramatically increase power per individual genotyped. These three techniques require increasing the number of individuals phenotyped, and are therefore useful only if phenotyping costs are much less than genotyping costs. Sequential sampling does not require an increase in phenotyping costs, but its ability to reduce genotyping costs is rather limited. The effects of sequential sampling and the other techniques are cumulative. Except for replicate progeny, these other techniques are trait specific, and are therefore most appropriate for experiments that consider only a few traits.

Chapter ten:

Fine Mapping of QTL

10.1 Introduction

Smith and Smith (1993) noted the need for close linkage between genetic markers and QTL for application of marker-assisted selection (MAS). Furthermore, MAS becomes much simpler if the actual QTL are determined, as will be seen in the final chapters. In the previous chapter and in the first chapter we noted that relative to the spacing of individual genes, linkage mapping of QTL is a rather crude tool. On average, a 10 cM chromosomal segment will have about 200 genes, and 10^7 base pairs. Although it would seem that increasing the density of markers genotyped should increase the resolution of QTL location, this is true only up to a point. For most practical situations reducing marker spacing below 20 cM does not increase QTL resolution, as noted in Chapter eight (Darvasi *et al.*, 1993).

Even for relatively large QTL effects and sample sizes, minimal confidence interval (CI) for QTL location will still be quite large if the objective is to find the actual gene affecting the trait. In Section 10.2 we will explain the relationship between sample size and the critical interval for the location of a Mendelian gene with complete heritability assuming a saturated genetic map. This can be considered a "best case" relative to QTL mapping. In Section 10.3 we will present methods to compute the minimum CI for QTL location with a saturated genetic map. Darvasi (1998) summarized various strategies that can be applied to further reduce the QTL location CI for crosses between inbred lines. These include advanced intercross lines, selective phenotyping, recombinant progeny testing, interval-specific congenic straits, and recombinant inbred segregation test. These methods will be discussed in detail in Sections 10.4 to 10.8. Methods have also been developed for fine mapping of QTL in segregating populations, and these will be considered in Section 10.9.

10.2 Determination of the genetic map critical interval for a marker locus with a saturated genetic marker map

Before estimating the CI for QTL location, we will first consider determination of genetic map location for a Mendelian factor with complete heritability and "saturated" genetic map. By "saturated" we mean that sufficient markers are genotyped so that marker spacing in no longer a limiting factor with respect to mapping resolution. As noted above, this can be considered a "best case" relative

170 *Quantitative Trait Loci Analysis in Animals*

to QTL mapping.

For a genetic marker it will be possible to determine unequivocally that the gene lies within a specific interval bounded by the closest flanking crossovers (Kruglyak and Lander, 1995c). This interval will be termed the "critical interval", and opposed to a CI, whose boundaries represent only a probability of containing the true location. For a QTL with heritability less than unity there will be a non-zero probability that the gene could be located anywhere in the genome. Therefore, for QTL it is possible to determine only a CI for the gene location.

With a saturated genetic map, the limiting factor in determination of the critical interval is the number of events of recombination, not the number of markers (VanRaden and Weller, 1994). That is, if several closely linked markers are genotyped, but there are no events of recombination between these markers in the sample analysed, then no additional information is obtained as compared to genotyping only those markers closest to the point of recombination.

As first explained in Section 1.6 in the Haldane mapping function (Haldane, 1919), events of recombination are assumed to be distributed randomly with respect to the genetic map, with a frequency of one event of recombination per Morgan per meiosis. In N meioses the expectation is N events of recombination per Morgan. Thus the expected genetic distance between a genetic marker and the nearest event of recombination will be 1/N Morgans, and the expected length of the minimal map interval containing the genetic marker will be 2/N, assuming that the marker is not located near the end of a chromosome. For example, the expectation is that 200 meioses are required to localize a genetic marker to an interval of 1 cM, again assuming a saturated genetic map, and that the genetic marker genotype can be determined without error.

The distribution of the length of critical interval as a function of the number of individuals genotyped is computed as follows. The distance between the genetic marker under analysis and the closest flanking marker on either side will have an exponential distribution, as given in Equation {7.43} with a parameter value of N. Again assuming that the gene is not located near the end of a chromosome, the length of the critical interval will thus be the sum of two exponential distributions. The Gamma distribution with parameters k and λ is defined as the sum of k independent exponentially distributed variables, each with a parameter value of λ. The length of the critical interval will have a Gamma distribution with parameters 2 and N (Kruglyak and Lander, 1995c). The probability density function of a variable x with a Gamma distribution is as follows:

$$f(M) = \frac{\lambda^k M^{k-1}}{(k-1)!} e^{-\lambda M} \qquad \{10.1\}$$

In our case M is the length of the critical interval in Morgans, and the density function of M is: $(N^2 M e^{-NM})/2$. This density is plotted in Figure 10.1 for N = 200 informative meioses. Although the expectation is 1 cM, the statistical density is greater than one-quarter of the maximum density between 0.1 and 1.6 cM.

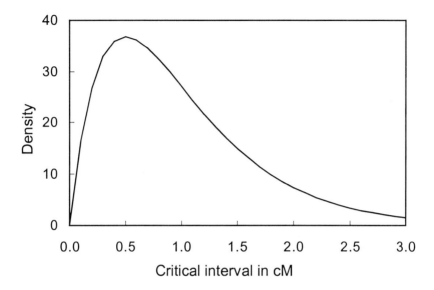

Figure 10.1 The distribution of the critical interval length for a sample of 200 informative meioses

10.3 Confidence interval for QTL location with a saturated genetic marker map

Similar to genetic markers, for a given QTL effect and sample size, there is a minimum CI for QTL location that can be obtained with a saturated genetic marker map. The CI for a QTL will always be greater than the critical interval for a genetic marker. Furthermore, without information on further generations, as described below, there will always be a positive probability that the QTL could be anywhere in the genome.

Kruglyak and Lander (1995c) developed analytical methods to determine the LOD score thresholds for the CI for a QTL affecting a disease trait for the method of allele-sharing described in Section 6.17. (As noted in Section 6.18, LOD scores are the base 10 logarithm of the likelihood ratio of the alternative and null hypotheses.) They were not able to derive a complete analytical formula for the length of the CI, but were able to show that the length of the CI does have a Gamma distribution, as described in the previous section.

Darvasi and Soller (1997) found by simulation that the 95% CI of QTL location in cM with a saturated genetic map could be estimated as follows for many of the common experimental designs:

$$CI = 3000/(mN\delta_g^2) \quad \{10.2\}$$

where m = number of informative meioses per individual [for the backcross (BC) design m = 1, and for the F-2 design m = 2]; N = number of individuals genotyped; and δ_g = substitution effect in units of the residual standard deviation of the design. Thus, the CI is an inverse function of the sample size, and an inverse squared function of the QTL effect. For example, for a QTL with a substitution effect of 0.5 standard deviations, CI = 12 cM if 1000 BC progeny are genotyped. Similar to previous methods that estimate the CI for QTL location, this approximation is effective only if the CI does not include either end of the chromosome.

Results of Darvari et al. (1993) demonstrate that the CI will be only marginally larger if the interval between markers is no more than half the CI obtained with a saturated map. This information can then be used to plan the optimal marker spacing for QTL mapping once a QTL has been detected. Considering the example given above, if the substitution effect has been estimated as 0.5 SD, and 1000 individuals will be genotyped in a BC, optimum marker spacing will be about 6 cM, or half of the CI that can be obtained with a saturated genetic map.

Using the F-2 example in Table 8.1, power will be 0.9 if 1050 individuals are genotyped for a QTL with a substitution effect of 0.141 standard deviations, assuming complete linkage between the genetic marker and the QTL. With a saturated genetic map, CI = $3000/[(2)1050(0.141)^2]$ = 71 cM. Thus, as concluded above, it is possible with a sample size of 1050 to detect a QTL with a substitution effect of 0.141 residual standard deviations, but the CI will be very wide, even with a saturated genetic map.

10.4 Fine mapping of QTL via advanced intercross lines

Darvasi and Soller (1995) proposed that mapping resolution could be increased by production of advanced intercross lines (AIL). AIL are produced by repeated random crossing of progeny resulting from an F-2 or BC. This is different from production of F-3 individuals or recombinant inbred lines (RIL) considered in Section 8.3 in which the progeny of each generation are produced by selfing. Similar to RIL, the events of recombination that occur in future generations affect the phase of QTL and marker alleles. The effect will be greater for AIL, because new heterozygotes are generated at each generation. This has the effect of "stretching" the genome. Again, similar to RIL, for mapping purposes it is only necessary to genotype and phenotype the final generation produced. Recombination frequency for AIL in generation t between two linked loci, r_t can computed as follows:

$$r_t = r_{t-1} + 0.5r(1-r_{t-1})^2 - 0.5r(r_{t-1})^2 = 0.5r + r_{t-1}(1-r) \qquad \{10.3\}$$

where r_{t-1} is the frequency of recombinants in generation t–1. This formula can be explained as follows. If the parent in generation t–1 is already a single recombinant, recombination will not affect the frequency of recombinant gametes. However, the non-recombinant heterozygous parents, with frequency $0.5(1-r_{t-1})^2$ have a probability of r to produce a recombinant gamete. Likewise, the double recombinant heterozygous parents, with frequency of $0.5(r_{t-1})^2$, also have a probabilty of r for recombination, but these gametes will be "non-recombinant" gametes, as compared to the original phase relationship. r_t can be derived from Equation {10.3} as function of the initial recombination rate, r, and t as follows:

$$r_t = [1 - (1-r)^{t-2}(1-2r)]/2 \qquad \{10.4\}$$

For small values of r, r_t can be approximated using a first order Taylor's expansion as follows:

$$r_t = rt/2 \qquad \{10.5\}$$

Thus if the CI for QTL location measured in recombination frequency is C_i, the CI at intercross generation t will be $2C_i/t$. Using the Haldane mapping function, which assumes zero interference, the percent recombination tends toward the distance in cM for short intervals. Thus the CI will decline linearly as a function of t/2. Using the example given above, if the CI is 12 cM, after four intercross generations it can be reduced to about 6 cM. Results obtained from simulation studies approximated the theoretical predictions, provided that the breeding population in each intercross generation was sufficiently large, generally at least 100 individuals. Of course this method is only applicable for species with relative short generation intervals.

10.5 Selective phenotyping

Selective phenotyping is based on the rational that once a QTL is mapped to a given interval only recombinant individuals within that interval contribute to further mapping accuracy. Thus, the total number of phenotypes determined can be reduced by only phenotyping progeny with recombinations within the CI. Selective phenotyping can also be done sequentially. Once an interval is determined to contain the QTL, only recombinant individuals within this interval are phenotyped. Subsequently the length of the interval can be reduced as the QTL location CI is reduced. Potentially this can results in a 10-fold decrease in the number of individuals phenotyped (Darvasi, 1998). Of course this does not reduce the total number of individuals that must be produced and genotyped.

10.6 Recombinant progeny testing

In recombinant progeny testing it is again assumed that a QTL has been localized to a given CI by using either a BC or F-2 design. BC or F-2 individuals carrying a distinguishable recombinant chromosome in the region of interest are selected, as shown in Figure 10.2. Optimally these will be individuals with two closely linked markers, only one of which displays recombination. The event of recombination can then be localized to the chromosomal segment between the two markers. The recombinant individual is then crossed back to one of the parental straits. Depending on where the QTL is located relative to the recombination point, progeny of this cross will either be heterozygous or homozygous for the QTL. By analysis of the progeny of this cross it should be possible to determine unequivocally the QTL location relative to the point of recombination.

In the example given in Figure 10.2, recombination occurred in one individual between markers B and C, and in the other individual between markers D and E. If these two individuals are then mated back to parental strain 1, the QTL will be segregating in the progeny of the cross with recombinant chromosome 1, but not in the progeny of the cross with recombinant chromosome 2. Thus is can be deduced that the segregating QTL is between markers B and E. By analysis of crosses to additional recombinant individuals it should be possible to localize the QTL to a progressively shorter chromosomal segment.

10.7 Interval specific congenic strains

The recombinant individuals analysed by recombinant progeny testing will be segregating at numerous other loci, which may also affect the trait of interest. Therefore, determining whether the QTL is still segregating with recombinant progeny testing will require generating a large progeny sample for each recombinant individual tested. As an alternative strategy, Darvasi (1998) suggested production of interval specific congenic strains. Prior to analysis, several generations of backcrossing to the parental strain are first performed. At each generation only individuals containing the recombinant chromosome are selected for mating to the parental strain. After several generations, the progeny will be nearly homozygous for the entire genome, except for the recombinant chromosomal segment.

By selection of parental individuals, the length of the recombinant segment can also be reduced. Optimally it should be possible to produce a series of recombinant strains, each one homozygous for the entire genome of the first parental strain, except for a small heterozygous segment derived from the second paternal strain. In the final BC generation, these lines are analysed for the presence of a segregating QTL in the recombinant chromosomal segment. If these segments span the original CI for QTL location, it should be possible to localize the QTL to a much small interval than the original CI. It should be possible to localize a QTL with a substitution effect of 0.25 SD to an interval of 1 cM by genotyping only 380 individuals in the final generation (Darvasi, 1998).

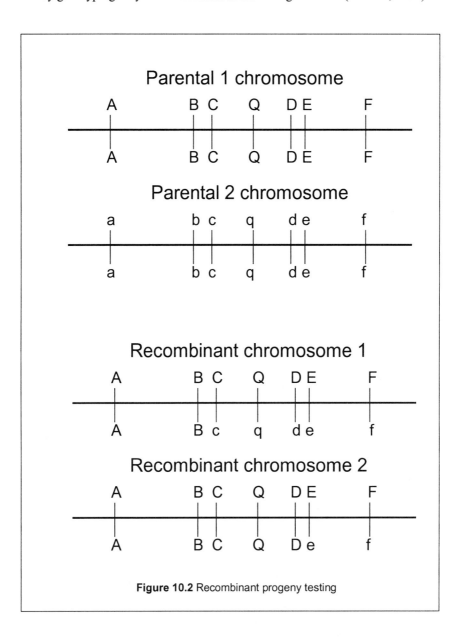

Figure 10.2 Recombinant progeny testing

10.8 Recombinant inbred segregation test

In Chapter eight we considered RIL produced by selfing progeny of an F-2 or a BC. Each RIL will be homozygous throughout the genome, but will contain chromosomal segments derived from either one or the other original parental strains. It is assumed that a number of these strains can be retrieved with recombination points within the original CI for QTL location. These RIL are then mated back to both parental strains, and then are either selfed to produce an F-2 or mated back to the parental strains to produce backcrosses. Each chromosomal segment defined by recombination points in the RIL can now be analysed separately. Both the parental strains and the RIL will be homozygous for the QTL. However, the chromosomal segment containing the QTL will display a segregating QTL in the cross to one parental strait, but not in the other. All chromosomal segments not containing the QTL will give the same results in crosses to both parental strains.

With this design it is possible for a QTL with an effect of 0.25 SD to obtain a CI for QTL location of 1 cM by producing less than 500 individuals in the final generation. This does not consider the number of individuals that must be produced to construct the RIL and the F-1 populations.

10.9 Fine mapping of QTL in outcrossing populations by identity by descent

All the methods considered above, except AIL, are directly applicable only for inbred populations. Furthermore, most of the designs require constructing populations over several generations for the specific objective of fine mapping. As first noted in Chapter four, constructing of specific test populations for QTL analysis is not a feasible alternative for most farm animals, trees, and of course humans.

Riquet *et al.* (1999) proposed that fine mapping in dairy cattle could be accomplished by utilizing historical recombinants. The basic assumption of this method is that a relatively rare QTL allele is due to a single mutation and can be traced back to the original mutant ancestor. The example given in this study is based on a QTL affecting fat concentration, which was found to be segregating in the US, Dutch, and Israeli Holstein dairy cattle populations analysed by daughter and grand-daughter designs. This QTL was found to be located near the centromeric end of bovine chromosome 14.

Riquet *et al.* (1999) analysed 29 Dutch Holstein families by a grand-daughter design. The QTL was segregating in seven of the families analysed. The chromosomal segment containing the QTL was physically mapped based on single nucleotide polymorphisms (SNP, Section 1.5). The seven chromosomal segments with a positive effect on fat percent (the "+" allele), and the seven chromosomal segments with a negative effect on fat percent (the "–" allele) were compared. If many polymorphic markers are genotyped, the probability that all chromosomes with either the + or the – allele would contain the same haplotype in the region of the QTL by chance would be very low. However, if either the + or the – allele was identical by descent in all seven families, then it should be possible to determine a haplotype common to all seven sires. Furthermore, this haplotype must include the segregating QTL.

The chromosomes with the + allele contained a common haplotype, while the chromosomes with the – allele did not. Thus, it can be concluded that all the + alleles are IBD in all of the seven sires analysed. The length of the haplotype common to all seven sires flanked by the closest non-IBD markers was 10.5 cM. Riquet *et al.* (1999) propose that the length of the QTL location CI can be further halved by genotyping for additional markers in the region of interest.

To further strengthen this conclusion, the maternal haplotype was determined for all progeny tested sons and progeny tested grandsons from all the 29 families. The effect of maternal haplotype corresponding to the + allele, vs. all the other maternal haplotypes was compared. The difference was significant, and in the same direction as the original analysis.

10.10 Summary

Even for a Mendelian gene with complete heritability several hundred individuals must be genotyped for many closely spaced markers to determine map location within an interval of a single cM. For a QTL, the CI (CI) will increase as the heritability of the gene decreases. For BC or F-2 designs, CI for QTL location with a saturated genetic map will be an inverse function of the number of individuals genotyped and the square of the QTL effect. Generally CI for QTL will be greater than 10 cM. Various techniques applicable to crosses between inbred lines were presented to decrease CI to the range of from one to a few cM. A CI of this magnitude will still include hundred of genes and millions of DNA base pairs. These methods require large populations and construction of test populations over several generations, and are therefore not applicable to farm animals or human populations. Identical by descent mapping can be applied to outbred population to reduce the CI for QTL location, provided that at least one of the QTL genotypes can be traced to a single common ancestor removed several generations from the current population.

Chapter eleven:

Complete Genome QTL Scans - the Problem of Multiple Comparisons

11.1 Introduction

As we already noted in Chapter one, it is now possible using DNA-level markers to obtain as many polymorphic markers as desired for any species of interest. Thus, it is now possible to conduct complete genome scans for QTL affecting any trait of interest. In Chapters eight and nine we discussed power to detect segregating QTL, based on the assumption that each marker or marker bracket was tested separately. If the number of markers included in the analysis is large, two new problems are encountered.

First, the individual test type I error rate is no longer appropriate. For example, if 100 tests are performed, five should be "significant" at the 5% level purely by chance. The traditional approach to deal with multiple comparisons, which is discussed in Section 11.2, is to control the "family-wise (or experiment-wise) error rate" (FWER), instead of controlling the "nominal" or "comparison-wise error rate" (CWER). The FWER is controlled by setting the rejection threshold sufficiently strict, so that the probability that *any* of the null hypotheses tested are erroneously rejected is below a specified low level, usually 0.05. For uncorrelated hypotheses, the FWER can be readily computed by the "Bonferroni adjustment", which will be explained in Section 11.2. However, linked markers are correlated. Additional methods to deal with the problem of multiple comparisons will be considered in Sections 11.3 to 11.5.

A second level of multiple comparisons in addition to multiple markers is multiple pedigrees. For example in daughter and grand-daughter designs should each family be analysed separately, or should data be analysed jointly over all families, even though the QTL are segregating in only some of the pedigrees? This question will be considered in Section 11.6.

A second problem with multiple marker analyses is that for those effects that are deemed "significant", the estimated effects will be biased upward (Georges *et al.* 1995). The reason for this is that if the true effects are close to the critical value for significance, only those QTL with estimates greater than the true effects will meet the significance criterion. This problem will be considered in the final section of this chapter.

11.2 Multiple markers and whole genome scans

Lander and Botstein (1989) first considered the problem of multiple markers in detail. They presented analytical formula for two specific situations; a "sparse" map, and a "dense" map. Kruglyak and Lander (1995c) also considered the case of intermediate spacing. In the former they assumed that the markers were sufficiently far apart that the individual tests could be considered independent. In this case the FWER can be computed by the "Bonferroni adjustment" (Simes, 1986) as follows:

$$\alpha_f = 1 - (1 - \alpha_c)^m \qquad \{11.1\}$$

where α_f = FWER, α_c = CWER, and m = number of markers. For small α_f, α_c is approximately equal to α_f/m, the formula presented by Lander and Botstein (1989). For example, if 100 tests are performed, and an FWER of 0.05 is desired, the CWER or nominal error rate must be approximately 0.0005. In the dense map case, Lander and Botstein (1989) assumed that the markers are sufficiently close so that all "sites" along the chromosome are being tested for segregating QTL. In this case, the expected number of regions with a standard normal distribution value greater than the critical value for α_c under the null hypothesis of no segregating QTL anywhere in the genome, $\mu(Z)$, can be computed as follows for either the backcross (BC) or F-2 designs (Lander and Kruglyak, 1995):

$$\mu(Z) = [N_c + 2\rho_M M_G Z^2]\alpha_c \qquad \{11.2\}$$

where N_c = number of chromosomes, ρ_M = the expected rate of recombination per Morgan, M_G = genome length in Morgans, and Z = the standard normal distribution value for α_c. For BC and half-sib designs, $\rho_M = 1$, because recombination is followed only for a single chromosome. For the Haseman-Elston full-sib model $\rho_M = 2$, because recombination on either chromosome will affect the estimated QTL effect. In an F-2 design $\rho_M = 1$ if only the additive effect is estimated, and $\rho_M = 1.5$ if both additive and dominance effects are estimated.

For a genomic scan of intermediate density, Equation {11.2} can be modified as follows (Kruglyak and Lander, 1995c):

$$\mu(Z) = [C + 2\rho_M M_G Z^2 v(2Z\sqrt{\Delta})]\alpha_c \qquad \{11.3\}$$

where Δ is the mean map distance between markers in Morgans, and $v(2Z\sqrt{\Delta})$ represents a function of $2Z\sqrt{\Delta}$. For small values of Δ, $v(2Z\sqrt{\Delta})$ is approximately equal to $e^{-1.166Z\sqrt{\Delta}}$. For larger values of Δ, $v(2Z\sqrt{\Delta})$ is approximately equal to $1/(2Z^2\Delta)$. As Δ approached zero, the intermediate density function approaches the dense map function, and as Δ increases, Equation {11.3} approaches $(N_c+m)\alpha_c$, which can be compared to the sparse map function of $\alpha_f = m\alpha_c$, given previously. The discrepancy between these two formulas is due the fact that in Equation {11.3} it is assumed that each chromosomal interval is tested for a QTL, while the sparse map function of Equation {11.1} assumes that each marker is tested. Assuming that each chromosome has at least one marker, the number of chromosomal intervals, including the chromosomal ends will be one more than the number of markers on each chromosome, or N_c+m.

For small values of $\mu(Z)$, $\mu(Z)$ tends to α. This is because with low $\mu(Z)$ it is very unlikely that more than a single region can have a Z-value greater than the critical value. Lander and Botstein (1989) present a similar formula for likelihood ratio tests. For a dense map scan of the bovine genome by the daughter design, (C=30, and G=30) a CWER of approximately 5×10^{-5}, comparable to a Z-value of 3.9, is required to obtain an FWER of 0.05. Requirement of such a stringent type I error results in a corresponding increase in the type II error. That is, many true effects will be missed.

To deal with the problem of appropriate thresholds for declaration of significance, Lander and Kruglyak (1995) propose the following criteria:

1. Suggestive linkage - obtaining a test statistic with the CWER corresponding to $\mu(T) = 1$, or the expectation that a test statistic of this magnitude should occur no more that once by chance in a complete genome scan. For the bovine genome, this requires a nominal probability of 0.0019.
2. Significant linkage - obtaining a test statistic with a CWER required for $\mu(T) < 0.05$.
3. Highly significant linkage - obtaining $\mu(T) < 0.001$.
4. Confirmed linkage - significant linkage confirmed by obtaining p<0.01 on a second, independent study.

Lander and Kruglyak (1995) also propose that, unless there is a reason to focus *a priori* on a specific chromosomal region, type I errors should be based on complete genome scans, even if the number of markers actually analysed was limited. They maintain that even if the original marker spacing is quite wide, additional markers will be genotyped for those regions that display marginal significance. Thus, the whole genome is potentially under observation.

The problem of multiple comparisons is somewhat alleviated if those effects deemed "significant" are repeated on a second, independent, analysis. Since only these effects are considered in the second analysis, the number of comparisons is drastically reduced. However, this is not a viable option in many cases. For analysis of disease traits, and generally for analysis of data on large animals, a second independent data set is not available. Contrary to the assumption of many researchers, adding additional markers in chromosomal regions with marginal significance cannot be considered verification of significant effects, even if they type I error is decreased. The "new" analysis based on the added markers will be highly correlated to the original analyses. Two other methods that provide alternative solutions to this problem will now be considered.

11.3 QTL detection by permutation tests

Churchill and Doerge (1994) proposed a method to empirically estimate FWER rejection thresholds that can be applied to a very wide range of experimental designs. Many different samples are generated from the actual data by "shuffling" the trait values with respect to the marker genotypes. Each individual genotyped is randomly assigned one of the trait values from the sample. Since the trait values for all individuals are now random with respect to marker genotypes, the null hypothesis of no linkage between the genetic markers and QTL is correct by definition. The test statistics computed from these "permutation samples" are then used to construct the empirical distribution of the test statistic under the null hypothesis. The appropriate rejection threshold for any desired comparison-wise or experiment-wise type I error can then be derived from the empirical distribution of the test statistic. This method has the advantage that no assumptions are required with respect to distributional properties of either the quantitative traits or the genetic markers. Rejection thresholds are computed based on the actual number and genomic distribution of markers genotyped. A disadvantage of this method is that thresholds must be computed anew by permutation for each data set analysed.

Churchill and Doerge (1994) computed CWER and FWER based on permutation tests for simulated data. This method can also be applied to the problem of multiple traits, considered in detail in Chapter twelve. The fact that no assumptions are made with respect to the distribution of the test statistic under the null hypothesis is especially important for computation of the FWER. As demonstrated above, to obtain a reasonable FWER for a complete genome scan, a very small CWER is required. At these very low probabilities it is likely that minuscule divergence of the actual data distribution from the theoretical distribution may result in a significant divergence of the analytically computed probability from the actual probability for the specific data set analysed. An example will be given in the following section.

11.4 QTL detection based on the false discovery rate

Benjamini and Hochberg (1995) proposed controlling the "false discovery rate" (FDR) as an alternative to controlling the FWER for the general problem of multiple testing. They defined the FDR as: "The expected proportion of true null hypotheses within the class of rejected null hypotheses". Derivation of rejection thresholds based on controlling the FDR, and important properties of this method will be described. We will then present examples based on actual data.

Assume that m multiple comparisons are tested. For each null hypothesis H_1, H_2, ..., H_m, a test statistic and the corresponding p-values, P_1, P_2, ..., P_m, are computed. Let $P_{(1)}$, $P_{(2)}$, ..., $P_{(m)}$ be the ordered P values, and denote by $H_{(i)}$ the null hypothesis corresponding to $P_{(i)}$. If all null hypotheses are true, but K hypotheses, $H_{(1)}$ to $H_{(K)}$, are rejected, then the expectation of the number of hypotheses rejected should be approximately equal to the actual number of hypotheses rejected for any value of K. If in fact, some of the null hypotheses are false (that is actual effects are detected), then the expectation of the number of hypothesis rejected should be less than K. The expectation of the number of hypotheses rejected assuming that all null hypotheses are true is $mP_{(K)}$. Defining q = $mP_{(i)}/i$, Benjamini and Hochberg (1995) prove that the FDR can be controlled at some level q*, by determining the largest i for which: $q^* < mP_{(i)}/i$. That is, out of K hypothesis rejected, it is expected that the proportion of erroneously rejected hypotheses is no greater than q*. Illustrative examples and important properties of the FDR will now be considered.

Weller et al. (1998) applied the FDR to the QTL detection. Comparison of FDR and FWER will be illustrated using the example of Weller et al. (1998) for a grand-daughter design analysis of the US Holstein population. A total of 1555 sons of 18 US grandsires were genotyped for 128 microsatellites. Daughter yield deviations (DYD) were analysed by the following linear model for seven economic traits:

$$Y_{ijk} = GS_i + M_{ij} + e_{ijkl} \qquad \{11.4\}$$

where Y_{ijk} is the DYD (VanRaden and Wiggans, 1991) for k^{th} son of the ith grandsire with paternal allele j, GS_i is the effect of the ith grandsire, M_{ij} is the effect of the jth marker allele, progeny of the ith grandsire. For each marker-trait combination an F statistic was computed for the paternal marker allele effect nested within grandsire. Thus, 896 comparisons were tested.

The comparisons with the 10 smallest p-values are given in Table 11.1. Assuming uncorrelated tests, only two F-values have a FWER less than 0.05. Using Lander and Kruglyak's (1995) criterion of "suggestive linkage" (FWER <0.5 for a complete genome scan) only four null hypotheses would be rejected. If all 10 hypotheses are rejected, q, and thus, FDR are still <0.25, even though FWER=0.811. Thus, seven or eight marker-trait combinations should represent "true" effects, and can be expected to repeat on a second population sample. Unlike FWER, $q = mP_{(i)}/i$ is not monotonic. For example, as *i* increases from 5 to 6, and from 9 to 10, q *decreases*. A decrease in q occurs when the increase in successive probabilities is low.

Results for q, FWER, and CWER, computed as the individual F probabilities, up to *i*=30 are plotted in Figure 11.1. For i>10, q and FWER are very close, with both close to unity. For i=10, p is still <0.05. Thus in this case, the criteria of controlling the FDR at 0.5 and a CWER of 0.05 give similar results.

These results were compared to the p-values computed from a typical permutation of the same genotype data against the trait data. The permutation results are plotted in Figure 11.2. Since the relationship between the markers and traits after permutation is random by definition, no null hypotheses should be rejected, and FDR and FWER would be similar. For the lowest F probability,

Table 11.1 Estimation of FDR for grand-daughter design results

I	Trait	Chrom.	Marker	F-value	p-value	Exp*	FWER	q
1	Fat %	14	15	11.157	10^{-8}	10^{-5}	10^{-5}	10^{-5}
2	Fat %	3	1	5.295	0.00003	0.025	0.024	0.012
3	Fat yield	14	15	4.146	0.00009	0.077	0.074	0.026
4	Protein %	2	4	5.279	0.00042	0.378	0.315	0.094
5	Protein %	3	8	4.246	0.00091	0.818	0.559	0.163
6	SCS†	22	1	3.819	0.00101	0.907	0.596	0.151
7	SCS	22	2	4.590	0.00124	1.112	0.671	0.159
8	Fat %	3	8	3.880	0.00194	1.734	0.823	0.217
9	Milk	7	3	3.466	0.00231	2.068	0.874	0.230
10	SCS	23	1	4.218	0.00242	2.166	0.885	0.217

* Expectation for the number of hypothesis rejected under the null hypothesis.
† Somatic cell score.

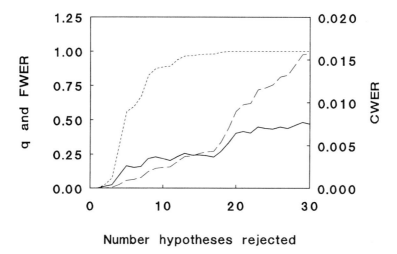

Figure 11.1 The q value (—), FWER (- - -) and comparison-wise type I error rate (CWER) (⋯) for analysis of the GD data

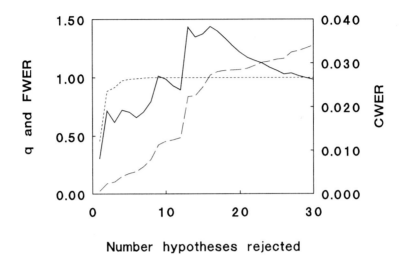

Figure 11.2 The q value (—), FWER (- - -) and comparison-wise type I error rate (CWER) (⋯) for the permuted grand-daughter design data

FWER was 0.45, and q was 0.31. Thus, one hypothesis would be rejected with FWER controlled at 0.5, but not with FDR controlled at any reasonable level. For i values >5, the FWER is nearly equal to unity. By theory, the expectation of q is unity for all values of i, but this criterion is affected much more by random fluctuation than FWER. q is nearly equal to unity for $i = 9$, but then rises to nearly 1.5 before settling down to close to unity by $i = 30$. With $i = 9$, CWER is still 0.01, which is almost exactly the expectation by chance (0.01 × 896 comparisons). Thus, by the criterion of CWER < 0.01, nine hypotheses would be rejected, as compared to 17 for the actual data (Figure 11.1). This illustrates the unreliability of the CWER criterion. The examples presented demonstrate the following important properties of the FDR.

1. If all null hypotheses are true, controlling FDR is equivalent to controlling FWER.
2. If some of the null hypotheses are false, then the FDR is smaller than the FWER. The difference between the two criteria increases with increase in the number of "false" null hypotheses (that is actual effects). Thus, any procedure that controls the FDR at a given level will also control the FWER at this level.
3. Unlike methods for controlling FWER, it is not necessary to assume that relationships among the test statistics are known. As demonstrated, the FDR can be readily controlled both for multiple linked markers and linked traits.
4. Even though $P_{(i)}$ increases monotonically with i, q does not. Thus, it may be

necessary sometimes to *increase* i to control the FDR at the desired level.
5. Although the true FDR is less than q; as i increases, the FDR approaches q. This will be true even if the hypotheses are correlated.
6. By controlling the FDR, the number of hypotheses rejected, i. e. QTL detected, is a function of the actual number of segregating QTL in the population; this is not true if either the FWER or CWER are controlled.
7. The dilemma of the appropriate rejection criterion for a partial genome scan is solved. The FDR can be controlled at the same level whether the complete genome or only part of the genome has been analysed.
8. Additional levels of contrasts, such as multiple traits or multiple populations can be handled without the necessity of a proportional increase in the critical test value.

Controlling the FDR is recommended primarily for a preliminary genomic scan. A second, independent, experiment will be required to determine which hypotheses tentatively rejected by the first analyses represent actual segregating QTL. A further advantage of the FDR is that an accurate prediction can be made of the proportion of hypotheses rejected in the first analyses that represent true effects. A weakness of the FDR is that it tends to fluctuate widely for low i if the total number of hypotheses tested is very large.

11.5 *A priori* determination of the proportion of false positives

Controlling the false discovery rate can only be applied after the experimental results are obtained. Thus it cannot be used to determine *a priori* the power of a planned experiment. Southey and Fernando (1998) proposed estimating the expected proportion of false positive tests based on the assumed prior probabilities of true and false null hypotheses. For a single test, the expected proportion of false positives, $E(q)$, can be computed as follows:

$$E(q) = \frac{\alpha P(H_o)}{\alpha P(H_o) + P(H_\alpha)(1-\beta)} \qquad \{11.5\}$$

where α is the nominal significance level (the type I error), $P(H_o)$ is the prior probability of the null hypothesis, $P(H_\alpha)$ is the prior probability of the alternative hypothesis, and $(1-\beta)$ is the power of the test. If multiple tests are performed, then Equation {11.5} becomes:

$$E(q) = \frac{\sum \alpha_i P(H_{oi})}{\sum [\alpha_i P(H_{oi}) + P(H_{\alpha i})(1-\beta_i)]} \qquad \{11.6\}$$

where α_i is the significance level for test i, $P(H_{oi})$ is the prior probability for the null hypothesis for test i, $P(H_{\alpha i})$ is the prior probability for alternative hypothesis i and $(1-\beta_i)$ is the power to reject this null hypothesis. If these probabilities are the same for all tests, then this equation reduces to:

$$E(q) = \frac{m\alpha P(H_o)}{m[\alpha P(H_o) + P(H_\alpha)(1-\beta)]} \qquad \{11.7\}$$

where m is the total number of tests. The problem with applying this method is that generally good estimates are not available for the prior probabilities. To compute these probabilities, Southey and Fernando (1998) assumed that the population was genotyped for N_k intervals of equal lengths and that N_Q QTL of equal size were scattered throughout the genome. They further assumed that there was no more than one QTL per interval. Thus the prior probability of the alternative hypotheses is N_Q/N_k, and the prior probability of null hypotheses is $1 - N_Q/N_k$. They further assumed that these QTL explained all the genetic variance. With 10 QTL and heritability of 0.25, the probability of false positives was 0.3 with a significance level of 0.001 if 1000 individuals were genotyped in a BC design. This can be compared to the value of 5×10^{-5} required to obtain a FWER of 0.05 for a whole genome scan (Lander and Kruglyak, 1995).

Similar to the FDR, but unlike computation of the FWER, the method of Southey and Fernando (1998) is affected by the frequency of detectable QTL segregating in the population. Furthermore, this method can used to plan an experiment in advance, and answer the question: is power sufficient to detect segregating QTL, provided they are present. However, in practice prior knowledge about the number, distribution and effects of QTL is very vague. Similar to the Bayesian analysis of Hoeschele and VanRaden (1993b) presented in Chapter seven, the assumptions made with respect to prior knowledge will affect the conclusions of the analysis.

11.6 Analysis of multiple pedigrees

With daughter and grand-daughter designs the question arises whether the different families should be analysed jointly or separately. This question was considered previously in Section 6.10. For the full-sib design with many small families, separate analysis of each family is generally not a viable option, because not enough data is available in single families to obtain reasonable power. A joint analysis over all families has the advantage that the number of tests is reduced, and thus a less restrictive CWER is required to obtain the desired FWER. However, if a QTL is segregating in only a small fraction of the families, then power may be reduced as compared to a separate analysis of each family.

Analysis models must also be more complicated if several families are analysed jointly. Georges *et al.* (1995) used a maximum likelihood (ML) algorithm to estimate QTL parameters including chromosomal location for a grand-daughter design, but analysed each grandsire family separately.

Knott *et al.* (1994, 1996) proposed a regression method in which information from all families is used to determine the QTL's map location, but a separate effect is estimated for each family. Thus, each sire included in the analysis is considered heterozygous. Analysis by this method or a simple ANOVA analysis on the individual markers are similar to the FDR and that even if significance is found over all families, it is not known which families actually have segregating QTL.

Bovenhuis and Weller (1994), Mackinnon and Weller (1995), and Song and Weller (1998) analysed all families jointly, but assumed that only two QTL alleles were segregating in the population. With a two-allele model, at least half of the families should be homozygous for a segregating QTL. Grignola *et al.* (1996a) assumed that the QTL effect was random. Similar to Knott *et al.* (1996), they assumed that two different QTL alleles were segregating in each family. Rather than estimate the substitution effect for each family, they estimated the variance due to the QTL effect based on the model of Fernando and Grossman (1989), as modified by Goddard (1992) to include marker brackets.

For most populations of interest, the number of alleles segregating for a particular locus will be very low. If all alleles have equal fitness, then the effective number of alleles, k_M, at equilibrium can be estimated as a function of the effective population size, N_e, and the mutation rate, η, as follows (Spiess, 1977):

$$k_M = 4 N_e \eta + 1 \quad \quad \{11.8\}$$

For example, with $N_e = 10^4$ and $\mu = 10^{-5}$, $k_M = 1.4$. The effective number of alleles is defined as the number of alleles required to obtain a given level of heterozygosity in the population, assuming all the alleles are of equal frequency. Thus, assuming that this mutation rate is more-or-less representative of mutations that are selectively neutral, but have a measurable effect on some trait of interest, it is unlikely that more than two alleles with frequencies greater than 0.1 will be segregating in populations of this size. Selection will further reduce the number of allele maintained in the population. Thus, mathematical models that assume many different QTL alleles in a population cannot be justified biologically.

Although some commercial animal populations consist of millions of individuals, effective population sizes will still be quite small due to the extensive use of a very few sires via artificial insemination (AI). The US Holstein cattle population of about 10 million cows has an effective population size of only about 100 (Riquet *et al.* 1999). If this is the case, then according to Equation {11.8} there should be virtually no polymorphism in these populations.

This apparent discrepancy can be explained by considering the number of generations that has elapsed since the widespread use of AI. Maruyama and Fuerst (1985) found that approximately $2N_e$ generations are required to approach equilibrium after a major reduction in the effective population size. Assuming a mean generation interval of 5 years, fewer than 10 generations have elapsed since the widespread use of AI with frozen semen. Maruymna and Fuerst (1985) also found that the rate of decrease in allelic number differs from the rate of decrease in heterozygosity. The rate of decrease in allele number is dependent on $4N_o\eta$, where N_o is the original effective population size, while the decrease in heterozygosity is proportional to $1/N_e$, but independent of N_o. Thus, if $4N_o\eta$ is initially large, several generations after the reduction in population size there will be a surplus of heterozygotes in the population, as compared to the frequency expected for a population at equilibrium. The discrepancy is greatest approximately $0.2N_e$ generations after the bottleneck. Thus it is likely that there are currently more heterozygotes for QTL than expected based on Hardy-Weinberg equilibrium. This may explain the relatively large numbers of bulls found to be heterozygous for QTL in many studies.

11.7 Biases with estimation of multiple QTL

Smith and Simpson (1986) first noted that if multiple QTL are estimated as fixed effects, the estimated effects of those QTL that meet the "significance" criterion will be biased upward. This has been documented by simulation studies (Beavis, 1994; Georges et al., 1995), and is supported by results of an actual experiment (Eshed and Zamir, 1996)

Georges et al. (1995) simulated a half-sib design, but considered each family separately, so that the results are comparable to a BC design. The number of progeny in each family was varied from 50 to 200, and the QTL effects were varied from 0.25 to 1 phenotypic standard deviation. In all cases the QTL was bracketed by two markers 20 cM distant. The simulated QTL position was 5 cM from one of the markers. ML interval mapping was used to estimate QTL effect and location, and significance was determined by a likelihood ratio test. As simulated QTL effect or sample size decreased, the fraction of QTL determined as "significant" (LOD score $\geq$ 3) decreased, and bias of the estimated effect increased. Bias was under 10% of the simulated effect only if more than 90% of the simulated effects were "detected".

Beavis (1994) found an approximately linear relationship between the ratio of estimated to simulated QTL effect, and the power of detection. If power of detection was only 10%, then the estimated effect was approximately four-fold the simulated effect. Furthermore, even if the simulated QTL were of equal size, the distribution of "significant" effects was positively skewed if power of detection was low.

Further support for these simulation studies come from the results of Eshed and Zamir (1996), summarized in Section 6.3. They analysed the complete tomato genome for QTL affecting five quantitative traits using chromosomal segment substitution lines. The background parent was *Lycopersicon esculentum* (common tomato), and the donor parent was *L. pennellii*. Fifty substitution lines, each containing a single chromosomal segment from *L. pennellii* on the background of the *L. esculentum* genome, were analysed. Of 250 line-by-trait combinations, 81 were significantly different from the control isogenic line ($p<0.05$). The different substitution lines were then crossed to produce lines differing from the control each in two chromosomal segments. For those cases in which both *L. pennellii* chromosomal segments gave significant effects in the same direction, the effect estimates for the double substitution lines were consistently less than the sum of the effect estimates in the single chromosomal segment substitution lines. As noted in Section 6.3, Eshed and Zamir (1996) proposed that these results were due to epistasis. However, this result is expected even without epistasis, if the "significant" effect estimates in the single segment substitution lines were overestimated. The effects should not be overestimated in the double segment analysis, because these effects are no longer a selected sample.

It should be possible to obtain unbiased estimates of a selected sample of effects if the QTL are estimated as random effects, or if Baysian estimation methods are used, as described in Chapter seven. Zhang and Smith (1993) simulated a whole genome scan with 100 segregating QTL. The 20 greatest estimated effects were then used in a marker-assisted selection programme. Selection response was more than double if the QTL effects were estimated as random, as compared to least-squares estimation.

In order to estimate QTL as random effects, it is necessary to know, or at least estimate, the variance of the distribution of effects. Good information on this distribution is nearly always lacking. Methods to derive reasonable estimates for these parameters were considered by Hoeschele and VanRaden (1993a), and are summarized in Chapter seven.

11.8 Summary

With multiple markers, and the possibility of complete genome scans, comparison-wise type I error rates for individual tests are virtually meaningless. Furthermore, estimates of QTL effects deemed "significant" would be biased. Four methods were presented to deal with the problem of multiple comparisons; computation of error rates for complete genome scans, permutation tests, controlling the false discovery rate, and a Bayesian analysis based on prior information on the distribution of segregating QTL in the population. None of these methods completely solve the problem of multiple comparisons. Various solutions have been presented to analyse multiple pedigrees, covering the range from a separate analysis of each family, to a joint analysis with the same allele segregating in all families, but again there is no uniformly "best" solution.

Chapter twelve:

Multiple Trait QTL Analysis

12.1 Introduction

A third level of complexity, in addition to multiple markers and multiple pedigrees, is multiple traits. Although the vast majority of QTL studies have considered multiple traits, nearly all studies have analysed each trait separately. Only a few studies have considered the theoretical aspects of multiple-trait QTL analysis (Jiang and Zeng, 1995; Korol *et al.*, 1987, 1995; Weller *et al.*, 1996). In Section 12.2, we will consider the specific theoretical problems related to multiple trait analysis. In the following sections the methods that have been proposed to deal with multiple trait analysis will be described

Two main methods have been proposed for multiple trait QTL analysis that alleviate some of the problems considered above. Jiang and Zeng (1995) and Korol *et al.* (1995) proposed a maximum likelihood (ML) multivariate analysis. This method will be described in Section 12.3. Both studies applied this method to simulated data sets. Only the bivariate situation was considered in depth, and normal distributions of the residual variance was assumed for both traits. In Section 12.4 power of single and multitrait analyses will be compared. It will be shown that in most cases, multiple trait analyses are more powerful than single trait analyses, even if the QTL affects only one of traits analysed. If QTL effects are found on two correlated traits in the same chromosomal region, this may be due to a single gene affecting both traits, or two linked loci. The question of pleiotropy vs. linkage will be considered in Section 12.5.

Weller *et al.* (1996) proposed a canonical transformation of the original traits in order to derive an uncorrelated set of variables, and this method will be described in Section 12.6. The advantages and disadvantages of both methods will be considered. Determination of statistical significance with multiple traits will be considered in Section 12.7. Finally, in Section 12.8 we will consider selective genotyping with multiple traits.

12.2 Problems and solutions for multiple trait QTL analyses

The main problems with multiple trait QTL analysis were summarized by Weller *et al.* (1996), and will be reviewed here with some additions.

Chapter twelve: Multiple Trait QTL Analysis 191

1. Most studies have determined statistical significance based on each marker-trait combination. As noted above, increasing the number of tests performed increases the probability that some markers will display statistical significance "by chance". This problem becomes more severe as the number of markers and traits increase.
2. If a significant effect is found associated with more than one trait, it is not clear whether several different QTL, each affecting a single trait, or a single locus with correlated effects on several traits has been detected. This will be especially acute if some of the traits are highly correlated.
3. Several techniques have been suggested to increase statistical power per individual genotyped at the expense of individual phenotyped (Darvasi and Soller, 1992, 1994a; Lander and Botstein, 1989; Lebowitz *et al.*, 1987). As noted in the previous chapter, some of these techniques are trait specific, for example selective genotyping and sample pooling. How will these techniques be affected, and what is the optimum strategy in a multiple trait analysis?

12.3 Multivariate estimation of QTL parameters for correlated traits

We will consider in detail the simple case of analysis of a single QTL flanked by two markers in backcross (BC) between two inbred lines. Two traits, x and y with residual variances of σ_x^2 and σ_y^2 and a residual covariance σ_{xy} of will be considered. In the basic case it will be assumed that the QTL can affect the means of either trait, but will not affect the residual variances or covariances. The likelihood function for the BC design with two flanking markers was described in Equation {5.20} as follows:

$$L = \prod^{n_{M1N1}} f_{M1N1} \prod^{n_{M1N2}} f_{M1N2} \prod^{n_{M2N1}} f_{M2N1} \prod^{n_{M2N2}} f_{M2N2} \quad \{12.1\}$$

where n_{M1N1}, n_{M1N2}, n_{M2N1}, n_{M2N2} are the number of individuals with genotypes M_1N_1/M_2N_2, M_1N_2/M_2N_2, M_2N_1/M_2N_2, and M_2N_2/M_2N_2, respectively, and f_{M1N1}, f_{M1N2}, f_{M2N1}, and f_{M2N2} are the density functions for the four possible marker genotypes. The density functions for the possible marker genotypes are computed then as follows:

$$f_{M1N1} = (1-a)f(Q_1) + af(Q_2) \quad \{12.2\}$$

$$f_{M1N2} = (1-b)f(Q_1) + bf(Q_2) \quad \{12.3\}$$

$$f_{M2N1} = (1-b)f(Q_2) + bf(Q_1) \quad \{12.4\}$$

$$f_{M2N2} = (1-a)f(Q_2) + af(Q_1) \qquad \{12.5\}$$

where $a = r_1r_2/(1-R)$, $b = r_1(1-r_2)/R$. In the bivariate model, $f(Q_1)$ and $f(Q_2)$ are the bivariate normal density functions for each observation. The bivariate normal distribution was given in Equations {3.14} and {3.15} and will be repeated here:

$$f(Q_1) = [2\pi\sigma_x^2\sigma_y^2(1-\rho^2)]^{-1/2} e^{\phi_1} \qquad \{12.6\}$$

$$f(Q_2) = [2\pi\sigma_x^2\sigma_y^2(1-\rho^2)]^{-1/2} e^{\phi_2} \qquad \{12.7\}$$

where $\phi 1$ and $\phi 2$ are computed as follows:

$$\phi_1 = -\frac{1}{2(1-\rho^2)}\left[\frac{(x-\mu_{x1})^2}{\sigma_x^2} - 2\rho\frac{(x-\mu_{x1})(y-\mu_{y1})}{\sigma_x^2\sigma_y^2} + \frac{(y-\mu_{y1})^2}{\sigma_y^2}\right] \qquad \{12.8\}$$

$$\phi_2 = -\frac{1}{2(1-\rho^2)}\left[\frac{(x-\mu_{x2})^2}{\sigma_x^2} - 2\rho\frac{(x-\mu_{x2})(y-\mu_{y2})}{\sigma_x^2\sigma_y^2} + \frac{(y-\mu_{y2})^2}{\sigma_y^2}\right] \qquad \{12.9\}$$

where μ_{x1} and μ_{x1} are the means of the two genotypes for trait x, μ_{y1} and μ_{y2} are the means of the two genotypes for trait y, σ_x^2 and σ_y^2 are the residual variances for x and y, and $\rho = \sigma_{xy}/\sigma_x\sigma_y$ is the residual correlation. Thus, it is necessary to maximize the likelihood in Equation {12.1} for at least eight parameters: the means of x and y for each genotype, μ_{x1}, μ_{x2}, μ_{y1}, and μ_{y2}; the residual variances of x and y, σ_x^2 and σ_y^2; the residual correlation, ρ; and recombination frequency between one of the markers and the QTL, r_1. If different residual variances are assumed for each genotype, then the number of parameters increases to 12.

Presence of a segregating QTL within the marker interval can be tested by a likelihood ratio test. The null hypothesis will be a standard bivariate normal distribution, which has five parameters: the means and variances for x and y, and the correlation. Therefore under the null hypothesis of no segregating QTL, the χ^2-statistic will have three degrees of freedom. Similarly, it is possible to test a hypothesis that the QTL effects only one of the two traits, say x. In this case, the null hypothesis will differ from the alternative hypothesis in that μ_{y1} and μ_{y2} will be set equal. In this case the χ^2 statistic will have only one degree of freedom.

As noted first in Section 5.11, the distribution of the likelihood ratio test statistic for interval mapping under the null hypothesis is between the χ^2 distributions with one and two degrees of freedom (Jansen, 1994). Apparently this is due to the correlation between the estimated QTL location and estimated QTL effect. The distribution of the likelihood ratio test statistic for a bivariate analysis will be considered in the next section.

12.4 Comparison of power for single and multitrait QTL analyses

A priori it could be assumed that power to detect a segregating QTL should be less with a multivariate analysis, because it is necessary to estimate more parameters. However, this is often not the case. For a QTL affecting two correlated traits, three basic situations exist. These are illustrated in Figures 12.1, 12.2, and 12.3. In all cases it will be assumed that the two traits have a positive residual correlation. For a two-dimensional distribution, the density function will be a surface, and a three-dimensional figure is required. In these figures, the situation is simplified by showing only the density peaks and the density at half of the maximum.

Figure 12.1, the simplest case, shows a QTL affecting only trait x, but not trait y. Figure 12.2 represents a case in which the QTL affects both traits, and the direction of the effects is in the same direction as the residual correlation. That is, the allele with the higher mean for trait x also has the higher mean for trait y. Note that the distance between the means in the two-dimensional trait space is greater than the projection in either individual trait. In Figure 12.3 the direction of the QTL effects is in opposite direction to the residual correlation, that is, the allele with a positive effect on trait x has a negative effect on trait y, even though the residual correlation is positive.

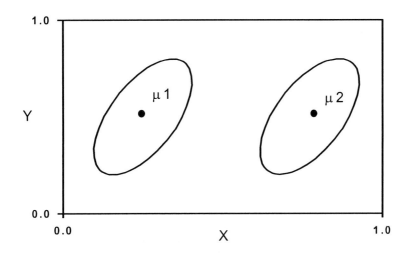

Figure 12.1 Bivariate density plot of a QTL affecting trait x, but not trait y. The distribution peaks, μ_1 and μ_2, and the density at one-half of the maximum density are shown. The two traits are positively correlated

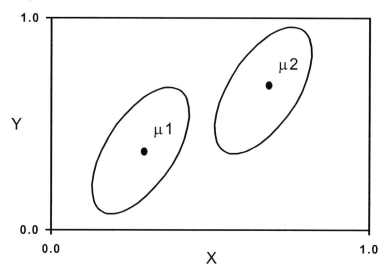

Figure 12.2 Bivariate density plot of a QTL affecting traits x and y in the same direction. The distribution peaks, $\mu1$ and $\mu2$, and the density at one-half of the maximum density are shown. The two traits are positively correlated

Korol et al. (1995) compared expected power between the bivariate and univariate analyses in terms of expected LOD scores. (As noted in Section 6.18, LOD scores are the base 10 logarithm of the likelihood ratio of the alternative and null hypotheses.) For the situation of complete linkage between a QTL and a genetic marker for a single trait, the expectation of the log of the likelihood ratio, ELOD, was given in Equation {5.29}, and will be repeated here:

$$\text{ELOD} = 0.5N\log(1 + \sigma_v^2/\sigma_e^2) = -0.5N\log(1 - H^2) \qquad \{12.10\}$$

where σ_v^2 is the variance due to the QTL, σ_e^2 is the residual variance, and H^2 is the "heritability" of the QTL, that is the fraction of the total variance due to the QTL, which is $\sigma_v^2/(\sigma_v^2+\sigma_e^2)$. As noted in Chapter four, for the BC design, $\sigma_v^2 = a^2/4$. For a bivariate analysis, Korol et al. (1995) showed that with complete linkage between the QTL and a genetic marker:

$$\text{ELOD} = -0.5N\log(1 - H_{xy}^2) \qquad \{12.11\}$$

where H_{xy}^2 is the two-dimensional analog of H^2, and is computed as follows:

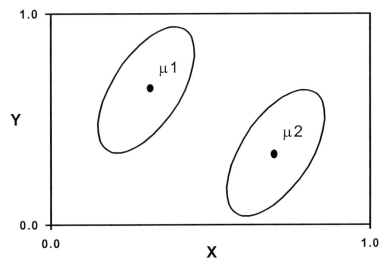

Figure 12.3 Bivariate density plot of a QTL affecting trait x and y in opposite directions. The distribution peaks, μ_1 and μ_2, and the density at one-half of the maximum density are shown. The two traits are positively correlated

$$H_{xy}^2 = 1 - \frac{\sigma_x^2 \sigma_y^2 (1-\rho^2)}{(\sigma_x^2 + a_x^2/4)(\sigma_y^2 + a_y^2/4) - \sigma_x^2 \sigma_y^2 [\rho + a_x a_y/(4\sigma_x \sigma_y)]^2} \quad \{12.12\}$$

where a_x and a_y are the QTL substitution effects on x and y, and the other terms are as defined for equations {12.7} through {12.9}. The proof of Equation {12.12} is rather complicated and is given in Korol et al. (1995). Unlike single trait QTL analysis, in multivariate analysis the signs of a_x and a_y are critical. That is, if $a_x a_y > 0$, then the effects of the QTL on both traits are in the same direction.

It can readily be shown that Equation {12.12} reduces to Equation {12.10} if $\rho = 0$ and $a_y = 0$. Thus, if there is no residual correlation between the two traits, and the QTL affects only one of the two traits, there is no increase in power by a bivariate analysis. Further analysis of this equation is aided if it is assumed that the QTL effects are measured in units of the residual standard deviations. Equation {12.12} then becomes:

$$H_{xy}^2 = 1 - \frac{(1-\rho^2)}{(1+a_x^2/4)(1+a_y^2/4) - [\rho + a_x a_y/4]^2} \quad \{12.13\}$$

For a given set of values for a_x and a_y, H_{xy}^2 will be maximum when $\rho = -a_x a_y/4$.

This implies that the genetic correlation is in opposite direction to the effect of the QTL on the two traits, as shown in Figure 12.3. Power for the bivariate analysis will always be greater if ρ and $a_x a_y$ are of opposite sign, but could be less if ρ and $a_x a_y$ are of the same sign. Similar results were found by Mangin et al. (1998).

From Equation {12.13} it can also be seen that if the QTL affects only a single trait, $H_{xy}^2 > H^2$ for trait x, if $\rho \neq 0$. However, this does not necessarily mean that power is greater with the bivariate analysis, because more parameters must be estimated. Mangin et al. (1998) found that power for the bivariate analysis would be greater than the single trait analyses, provided that the correlation is not close to zero. For example, with an effect of $a_x = 0.6$, power for the bivariate analysis will be greater if the correlation is >0.4 or <–0.4. As a_x increases, a smaller absolute value for the correlation is required to obtain greater power for the bivariate analysis.

In simulation studies using the model of Equations {12.1} through {12.9} Korol et al. (1995) found that the empirical critical value for the likelihood ratio statistic under the null hypothesis of no segregating QTL was very close to the theoretical value with three degrees of freedom. For the null hypothesis, which assumes no segregating QTL in the marker interval, five parameters must be estimated; two means, two variances, and the correlation. However, they did not present the data, so it is not clear if this result in fact contradicts the results of Jansen (1994) for single trait interval mapping. Theoretical χ^2 distributions with three and four degrees of freedom are not that different. If the QTL affected only a single trait, power was increased in the bivariate analysis if the two traits were correlated, as predicted by Equation {12.13}.

12.5 Pleiotropy vs. linkage

As noted at the beginning of this chapter, if significant effects are found for two correlated traits in the same chromosomal region by single trait analyses, it is of interest to determine whether the two effects are pleiotrophic effects of the same locus, or the effects of two linked QTL. This question is important, because linkage relationships will be broken in future generations, while pleiotrophic effects will continue unaltered.

If single trait analyses are performed, the only information that can be used to distinguish between these alternatives will be the estimated location of the QTL. As noted previously, unless the sample size is huge, the confidence interval for QTL location will be rather broad. Thus if the effects are due to two different QTL separated by as much as 20 cM, it will not be possible to reject the single locus hypothesis.

This question was investigated in detail by Jiang and Zeng (1995). A multivariate analysis assuming two QTL is required. The complete model will include at least 13 parameters, eight parameters for the means of the two QTL genotypes on each trait for the two loci, the two residual variances, the residual correlation and two map location parameters. This "complete" model assumes that each QTL has an effect on each trait. The reduced models that can be tested against the complete model are a model with a single QTL affecting both traits, or a model with two QTL each affecting only one of the two traits. It is not possible to test the latter two hypotheses against each other by a likelihood ratio test, because these hypotheses are not "nested". As explained in Section 2.9, a likelihood ratio test is valid only if the null hypothesis is "nested" within the alternative hypothesis. That is, all parameter values fixed in the null hypothesis are allowed to "float" in the alternative hypothesis. However, in the case of one QTL with effects on both traits vs. two QTL each with effects on a single trait, different parameters are fixed in each hypothesis.

Jiang and Zeng (1995) therefore proposed the following test model. In the complete model, two QTL are assumed, one affecting trait x, by not y, and the other affecting trait y, but not x. A different location is estimated for each QTL. In the reduced model, it is assumed that the QTL location is the same for both QTL. In this case, the alternative hypothesis can be tested against the null hypothesis, since the only difference between the two models is the QTL location parameters, which are fixed to be equal in the null hypothesis, but allowed to float in the alternative hypothesis.

It is not clear if this really solves the problem of nesting, since the hypothesis of two QTL each affecting only a single trait, but with identical location, is equivalent to the hypothesis of a single QTL affecting both traits. This question of pleiotropy vs. linkage will be considered again below.

12.6 Estimation of QTL parameters for correlated traits by canonical transformation

As noted in the previous sections, with two traits and a single segregating QTL in a backcross population it is necessary to estimate at least eight parameters (a recombination frequency, two means for each trait, a variance for each trait, and a correlation coefficient). For the F-2 situation, at least 10 parameters, including six means, must be estimated. As the number of traits increases, the number of parameters that must be estimated increases exponentially.

Weller *et al.* (1996) proposed a canonical transformation of the original traits in order to derive an uncorrelated set of variables. The canonical variables are a set of linear functions of the original traits. In a canonical transformation, the vector of trait values for each individual is multiplied by the matrix of eigenvectors derived from the variance matrix. (For computation of eigenvectors and eigenvalues, see Searle, 1982.) The QTL analyses are then performed on the canonical variables, which are uncorrelated by definition. QTL effects on the actual traits can then be derived by reverse transformation. In addition to the eigenvectors, the eigenvalues are generally computed. The values of eigenvalues, relative to the total of all eigenvalues indicate how much of the total variance is determined by each canonical variable. The advantages of this method are as follows:

1. Any number of traits can be readily analysed, since only a single trait analysis is performed for each variable. Thus, analysis is relatively simple.
2. Since the canonical variables are by definition uncorrelated, it is possible to compute the FWER by the Bonferroni correction, as described in Section 11.2.
3. It may also be possible to reduce the total number of traits analysed, and thus increase the power of detection, by deleting canonical variables with very low eigenvalues.
4. By analysis of the canonical variables it should be possible to directly determine whether the observed effect is due to pleiotropic effects of a single loci, or two linked QTL. Since the canonical variables are uncorrelated, a QTL with correlated effects on two traits should affect only a single canonical variable, while two separate effects should be observed for linked QTL.

The disadvantages of this method are:

1. If the model includes only a single random effect, an infinite number of canonical transformations is possible. Significant effects found for one transformation may not be significant by another transformation. This problem can be alleviated by computing the matrix of eigenvectors from the correlation matrix, as opposed to the variance-covariance matrix, which is dependent on the trait units. In this case all traits are given equal value.
2. A canonical transformation can be applied only if all traits are recorded on all individuals, although methods have been developed to solve the problem of missing data (Weller et al., 1996).
3. It is generally more useful to determine effects on the biological scale of interest, rather than some arbitrary scale of the canonical variables. As noted above, the effects on the actual traits can be determined by reverse transformation, but these will not be equal to the effects estimated directly on the actual traits, especially if some of the canonical traits are deleted from the analysis.

Technically, the canonical variables should be computed from the matrix of residual correlations, rather than phenotypic corrections, which include the QTL effect, in order to obtain a set of variables with uncorrelated residuals. However, as noted in previous chapters, for nearly all cases of interest the variance due to the QTL will be small relative to the phenotypic variance. Thus, if the canonical variables are derived from the phenotypic variance matrix, the residual variance matrix will also be nearly uncorrelated.

This problem can be solved by an iterative procedure in which the canonical variables are first computed based on the phenotypic variance matrix. QTL effects are then estimated, and residual variances and covariances are computed. A new set of canonical variables is then computed based on the residual variance matrix. The QTL effects are again estimated, and a new residual variance-covariance matrix is computed. Iteration is continued until convergence to a residual variance matrix with zero covariances.

A canonical transformation was applied to daughter design data for milk, fat, and protein production of Israeli Holsteins (Weller *et al.*, 1996). A significant QTL effect was found associated with milk and protein production, but not fat. Milk and protein production are highly correlated. By a canonical transformation, it was possible to reduce the number of variables from three to two. A significant effect was found associated only with one of the two remaining variables, which was highly correlated with both milk and protein production. Thus, it was concluded that a single QTL was affecting both traits.

12.7 Determination of statistical significance for multitrait analyses

Both methods described above provide partial answers to the problem of determination of statistical significance in the multitrait situation. For a multivariate analysis it is possible to maximize the likelihood for the complete model and for a "restricted model" with equal means for all QTL genotypes for all traits. Significance of an effect can then be tested by a likelihood ratio test of the two hypotheses. Similarly it is possible to test the hypothesis that the QTL affects only one of the two traits. With the canonical transformation, each trait is analysed separately, and a p-value is computed for each trait. The family-wise error rate (FWER) can then be computed as described above.

Mangin *et al.* (1998) proposed the following test statistic, T, for the analysis of m canonical variables with interval mapping:

$$T = \sum_{v=1}^{m} T^v(r_1) \quad \{12.14\}$$

where $T^v(r_1)$ is the likelihood ratio statistic for a QTL with recombination frequency r_1 from the first marker of the interval for canonical variable v. They proved that under the null hypothesis of no segregating QTL this test is asymptotically equivalent to the multivariate likelihood ratio test given above. Furthermore, under the null hypothesis, T will have an asymptotic central χ^2 distribution with m degrees of freedom. This test is similar to the false discovery rate (FDR) and an ANOVA analysis across families in that even if overall significance is found, it is not known which of the QTL effects on the individual variables were in fact significant.

Although power will generally be greater for the multivariate analysis, it will in some cases be greater for single trait analyses. Even if the individual traits are analysed separately on the original, correlated scale, a FWER can still be computed empirically by a permutation test, as suggested by Churchill and Doerge (1994) for multiple linked loci. For multiple traits, the vector of trait values for each individual is permuted against the genotypes numerous times. For each permutation, a test statistic and its p-value under the null hypothesis are computed for each trait. The lowest p-value at each permutation is then selected, and these are ranked over all the permutations. The nominal probability for the 5% lowest p-value over all traits is then an approximate 5% FWER. For correlated traits, this method should result in a higher p-value than computation of FWER assuming an equal number of uncorrelated traits.

This method was applied to a single marker and seven correlated traits for grand-daughter design data considered in the previous chapter. The genotype data were permuted against the vector of daughter yield deviations (VanRaden and Wiggans, 1991) for the seven traits. F-values were computed for the seven traits at each permutation. The correlation matrix of the traits is given in Table 12.1, and the results of the permutation analysis are in Figure 12.4. The empirical comparison-wise type I error computed by ranking all 7000 F-values computed is compared to the empirical FWER computed by ranking on the highest F-value of the seven traits at each permutation. The expected comparison-wise probabilities assuming six or seven independent traits are also plotted.

The correlations among milk, fat, and protein were all >0.5, as was the correlation between fat and protein percentage. It therefore seems reasonable to assume that the empirical FWER for these seven traits would be considerably smaller than the theoretical FWER assuming seven uncorrelated traits. However, the empirical FWER was generally between the theoretical FWER computed for six or seven uncorrelated traits, and at some points even higher. The relatively low gain in reducing the number of traits can be explained by the fact that the empirical distributions for the individual traits are not exactly the same, and are not equal to the theoretical F-distribution. Even slight discrepancies from the theoretical distribution may become important at very low p-values.

12.8 Selective genotyping with multiple traits

As considered in Section 9.4, power to detect segregating QTL can be increased per individual genotyped by selectively genotyping those individuals with extreme values for the quantitative traits (Darvasi and Soller, 1992; Lebowitz *et al.*, 1987; Lander and Botstein, 1989). If only the highest and lowest 5% of individuals are genotyped, it is possible to obtain equal power as compared to random genotyping with only one-fourth as many genotypes. Although power is increased per individual genotyped, it is reduced per individual phenotyped. Since selective genotyping is trait specific, the question arises as to the effect of selective genotyping for one trait on correlated traits.

Table 12.1 Correlations among daughter yield deviations for the seven traits analysed in the US Holstein population

	Milk	Fat	Protein	Fat %	Protein %	Herdlife	SCS[1]
Milk	1.	0.512	0.821	-0.456	-0.419	0.304	0.020
Fat		1.	0.633	0.537	0.122	0.214	-0.066
Protein			1.	-0.155	0.174	0.309	0.010
Fat %				1.	0.539	-0.075	-0.087
Protein %					1.	-0.028	-0.017
Herdlife						1.	-0.270
SCS							1.

[1] Somatic cell score.

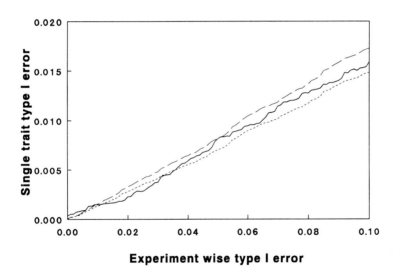

Figure 12.4 Nominal single-trait type I error as a function of the empirical experiment-wise type I error (——), the experiment-wise type I error assuming six independent traits (-- --), and the experiment-wise type I error assuming seven independent traits (····)

Darvasi and Soller (1992) demonstrated that the estimates of the QTL effect are biased if only individuals genotyped are used to estimate the effect. They also derived a method to estimate the actual QTL effect as a function of observed effect and the proportion selected for genotyping. Results on simulated data from the study of Ronin et al. (1998) are presented in Table 12.2 for single trait ML. All individuals with phenotypes are included in the analysis. For individuals with phenotypes, but without genotypes, the population genotype probabilities are assumed. For example, in a BC, it is assumed that each of these individuals has a one-half probability of each genotype. Estimates of the QTL parameters for the trait under selection are unbiased.

Table 12.2 ML single trait estimates of QTL parameters with selective genotyping*

Simulated effect	a_x	a_y	σ_x	σ_y	L_x	L_y	Power for $x^\dagger$	Power for y
X	0.261	0.260	0.999	0.988	412.11	54.16	0.89	0.48
	(0.005)	(0.010)	(0.001)	(0.001)	(1.11)	(1.98)		
Y	-0.005	0.168	0.998	1.001	60.86	56.55	0.11	0.22
	(0.009)	(0.012)	(0.001)	(0.001)	(2.89)	(2.40)		

*Results are the mean and standard deviations (in parentheses) of 200 simulated data sets for each set of parameters. For each data set 2000 individuals from a BC population were simulated, with a QTL effect of a = 0.25 on either trait x or y at position 50 cM on the chromosome. The marked chromosome had a length of 120 cM, with markers spaced at 20 cM intervals. In both cases the 200 highest and lowest individuals for x were selected for genotyping. The correlation between x and y was 0.5, and the residual standard deviations were $\sigma_x=\sigma_y=1$. Parameter estimates for a_x, a_y, σ_x, σ_y, and QTL location (L_x and L_y) were derived by single ML interval mapping, including individuals with unknown genotypes.
$\dagger$ Empirical power to detect a segregating QTL by a likelihood ratio test with a type-1 error of 0.05.

If, however, selective genotyping is applied to a single trait, but other correlated traits are also analysed by single trait ML, then QTL effects associated with the correlated traits will be biased, even if all individuals with phenotypes are included in the analysis. In the example in Table 12.2, selective genotyping was performed relative to trait x, and the QTL was associated with this trait, but not the correlated trait, y. Although single trait ML was able to estimate accurately the effect on trait x and the QTL location, a "ghost" effect of nearly the same magnitude, and a power of nearly 0.5, was found associated with trait y. In the second row of Table 12.2, the segregating QTL was simulated for y, but not x, and selective genotyping was still relative to x. Although no effect was found associated with x, the effect associated with y was underestimated, and the power was only 0.22.

Results of the multivariate analyses for both situations are presented in Table 12.3 (Ronin et al., 1998). Unbiased estimates were obtained for the effects on both traits, whether an effect was simulated for trait x or y. Power of detection for an effect on x was similar for both analyses, but much greater for a true effect on y. Moreover, power of detection is increased as compared to random sampling, whether the QTL is associated with the trait under selection, or with the correlated trait. Thus, wiht selective genotyping it is possible by multivariate ML to derive accurate estimates of QTL effects for both traits under selection and correlated traits. For correlated traits with selective genotyping, power is increased relative to single trait ML with either selective genotyping or random sampling.

Table 12.3 ML multiple trait estimates of QTL parameters with selective genotyping[1]

Simulated effect	a_x	a_y	σ_x	σ_y	Location	Power[2]
X	0.256	0.011	0.999	0.996	412.96	0.87
	(0.006)	(0.012)	(0.001)	(0.001)	(1.33)	
Y	-0.004	0.264	0.999	0.994	55.81	0.45
	(0.007)	(0.012)	(0.001)	(0.001)	(2.19)	

[1] Data sets were simulated as described for Table 12.2. Parameter estimates for a_x, a_y, σ_x, σ_y, and QTL location were derived by multitrait ML interval mapping, including individuals with unknown genotypes.
[2] Empirical power to detect a segregating QTL for the trait with the true effect by a likelihood ratio test with a type1 error of 0.05.

12.9 Summary

Analysis of multiple traits presents additional problems that can be solved by either a multitrait analysis, which is computationally demanding, or by a canonical transformation, which is not. The advantages of the multitrait analysis are that effects are estimated on the scale of the actual traits, and power of detection is generally increased, even if the QTL affects only a single trait. By a multitrait analysis it is also possible to obtain unbiased estimates of QTL parameters even with selective genotyping for one of the correlated traits. The multitrait analysis becomes extremely demanding computationally if the number of traits included in the analysis is greater than two. This is not a problem for canonical transformation, which can readily handle any number of traits. By canonical transformation an answer is obtained immediately as to the number of different QTL affecting the traits analysed, since the canonical variables are by definition uncorrelated. The main disadvantage of this method is that effects are computed on the scale of the canonical variables, which do not of themselves have economical value. If individuals are selected for genotyping based on their phenotypic values for a specific trait, but additional correlated traits are included in the analysis, biased parameter estimates are obtained for the correlated traits.

Chapter thirteen:

Principles of Selection Index and Traditional Breeding Programmes

13.1 Introduction

Currently nearly all breeding programmes, especially for farm animals, are based on the principles of selection index. No information on the individual genes affecting the economic traits is utilized. In those situations in which traditional selection index works well, little is gained by identification of the individual loci affecting quantitative traits. However, many practical breeding situations are encountered in which trait-based selection index is very inefficient or impractical. In these instances marker-based selection can make a very significant gain.

In Section 13.2 we will review the principles of single trait selection index, and in the following section we will estimate the changes in QTL allelic frequency due to traditional selection. In Section 13.4 we will consider multitrait selection index and in Section 13.5 we will describe methods to estimate the cumulative long-term economic value of genetic gain, which is much higher than generally thought. We will then consider in detail the main traditional breeding schemes for dairy cattle, and estimate the genetic gains that can be obtained. In the final section we will consider nucleus breeding schemes, based on extensive use of multiple ovulation and embryo transplant.

In the next two chapters we will consider the potential gain that can be obtained by marker-assisted selection in conjunction with trait-based selection, and in the final chapter we will consider marker-assisted introgression.

13.2 Selection index for a single trait

Lush and Hazel (Hazel, 1943; Hazel and Lush, 1942; Lush, 1935) formulated the principles of economic selection index. Although they did not phrase the derivation of selection index in matrix terms, we will do so because it greatly facilitates explanation. For selection on a single trait based only on trait records and relationships among animals, the expected gain is maximized by selecting individuals based on their estimated genetic values, u, which can be computed as follows:

$$u = E(u) + \mathbf{C}\mathbf{V}^{-1}[\mathbf{y} - E(\mathbf{y})] \qquad \{13.1\}$$

where E(.) denotes an expectation, **y** is a vector of trait records, **C** is the covariance matrix between u and **y**, and **V** is the variance matrix of **y**. For the case of a single record per individual and no relationships, $\mathbf{CV}^{-1}$ is equal to the heritability of the trait. The expected gain due to one generation of selection, ϕ, based on u is computed as follows.

$$\phi = i_p \rho_a (\sigma_A) \quad \{13.2\}$$

where i_p is the selection intensity, ρ_a is the accuracy of the evaluation, and σ_A is the additive genetic standard deviation. As defined in Section 9.4, the selection intensity is the difference between the mean of the selected group and the population prior to selection in units of the trait standard deviation. As noted previously, i_p can be computed as follows:

$$i_p = \varphi_p / p \quad \{13.3\}$$

where φ_p is the ordinate of the normal curve, and p is the proportion of individuals selected.

The accuracy of the evaluation is the correlation between the estimated and actual breeding values. The accuracy squared is termed the "reliability" of the genetic evaluation. For genetic evaluations computed by selection index, or the mixed model described in Chapter three, reliabilities of evaluations can be computed as pev($\hat{u}$)/var (u), where pev($\hat{u}$) is the prediction error variance of the estimated breeding value, and var (u) is the variance of u. The prediction error variances can be computed as described in Section 3.4. For selection based on a single record per individual and no relationships, ρ_a is the square root of the heritability.

Genetic gain per year, ΔG, is computed as follows:

$$\Delta G = i_p \rho (\sigma_A) / L_G \quad \{13.4\}$$

where L_G = generation length in years. In most animal breeding programs, selection intensities, accuracies of genetic evaluations and generation intervals are different along the four paths of inheritance: sires to sons (SS), sires to daughters (SD), dams to sons (DS), and dams to daughters (DD). In this case, mean annual genetic gain for the population, ΔG, is computed as follows (Rendel and Robertson, 1950):

$$\Delta G = \frac{\phi_{SS} + \phi_{SD} + \phi_{DS} + \phi_{DD}}{L_{SS} + L_{SD} + L_{DS} + L_{DD}} \quad \{13.5\}$$

where: ϕ_x = genetic gain per generation for path x (SS, SD, DS, or DD), and L_x = generation interval for path x.

Equation {13.2} is based on the assumption that candidates for selection have equal genetic mean and accuracy. However, in most commercial animal breeding programs this is not the case. In practice, selection will be among individuals of differing ages. As animals age, the accuracy of their evaluations generally increase, due to additional expressions of the economic traits and the accumulation of information on relatives. However, in an ongoing breeding programme, younger animals will have a higher mean genetic value than older animals. In this case, truncation selection based on the estimated genetic values of all candidates for selection will still result in optimum genetic gain, but Equation {13.2} is no longer correct. The expected genetic gain will be a function of the fraction of individuals in each age group, their mean accuracies, and the rate of genetic gain in the population. Ducrocq and Quaas (1988) derived iterative methods to estimate the optimum truncation point and expected annual genetic gain with overlapping generations. Typical breeding programmes will be considered in detail in Section 13.5.

13.3 Changes in QTL allelic frequencies due to selection

Genetic gain in a population under selection is achieved by increasing the frequencies of alleles with a positive effect on the trait under selection. Under the simple case of phenotypic selection for a relatively large population, the change in allele frequency, Δp, for a codominant QTL with two alleles can be approximately computed as follows (Falconer, 1981):

$$\Delta p = i_p a p (1-p) / \sigma \qquad \{13.6\}$$

where p is the allele frequency before selection, a is the additive effect, and σ is the phenotypic standard deviation. For example with $i_p=2$, a=0.5 phenotypic standard deviations, and p=0.5, the change in allele frequency will be approximately 0.25. A selection intensity of 2 is achieved if the top 5% of the population are selected as parents. With a high selection intensity it does not take many generations to bring a "favourable" rare allele to near fixation in the population for a QTL of moderate size. This is illustrated in Figure 13.1 for the case of $i_p a = 1$. As can be seen in this figure, it takes only nine generations for allelic frequency of a favourable allele to increase from 0.01 to 0.99. For selection other than phenotypic selection on a single record, σ should be replaced with the standard deviation of the selection criterion, which will generally be smaller than σ.

Selection index is remarkably efficient under the optimum conditions: high heritability, high selection intensity (this requires a high fertility rate), and the possibility to score the quantitative trait on all individuals prior to breeding. However, very few actual situations correspond to these ideal conditions. Although it would seem that if the individual genes affecting the trait were known, it should be possible to devise a more efficient selection strategy than mass selection on the phenotype, this is apparently not the case (Weller and Soller, 1981).

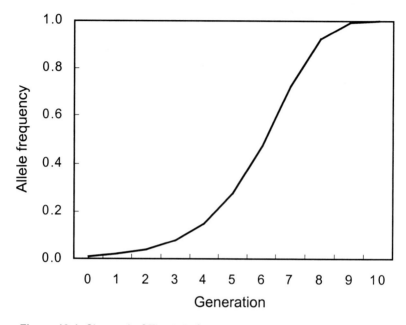

Figure 13.1 Change in QTL allelic frequency due to mass selection. a*i = 1, initial allelic frequency = 0.01

13.4 Multitrait selection index

We will now consider selection index for a multitrait breeding objective. Assume that for each individual there is a vector **u**, of length m, consisting of the individual's breeding values for traits of economic importance and a vector **y** of n measured traits to be included in the selection index. Although **u** and **y** may include the same traits, this does not have to be the case. Assume further that the economic values associated with **u** are linear functions of the trait values. We can then define a vector **v**, also of length m, consisting of the economic values of the traits in **u**. The aggregate economic breeding value, H, can then be computed as **v'u**. H, the optimum selection index, is a scalar in monetary units. For a given selection intensity, the response to selection will be greatest, in monetary units, if candidates for selection are ranked by H. Since the elements of **u** are generally unknown, the goal is to derive the linear index, I_s, of **y**, that maximizes the correlation between I_s and H. Specifically, **b** is defined as a vector of index coefficients, $I_s = $ **b'y**. In scalar notation:

$$I_s = b_1y_1 + b_2y_2 + ... + b_ny_n \qquad \{13.7\}$$

where b_i is the index coefficient for trait i. The objective is to solve for the vector **b** that maximizes the correlation between **b'y** and **v'u**. Defining $\mathbf{V_p}$ as the n × n phenotypic variance matrix of the traits in **y**, and **C** as the n × m genetic covariance matrix between the measured traits in **y** and the breeding values in **u**; the selection index coefficients are then derived by the following equation:

$$\mathbf{b} = \mathbf{V_p^{-1}Cv} \qquad \{13.8\}$$

For single trait selection, $\mathbf{V_p^{-1}C}$ is equal to the heritability. Brascamp (1984) presents several methods to derive this equation, and summarizes the important properties of the selection index. If all traits included in the selection index are also included in the breeding index, then **C** is equal to the genetic variance matrix.

If economic values are linear functions of the biological trait values, and if no information other than trait values and relationships are known, then selection of parents based on I_s is the most efficient method to increase the mean economic value of the population. The response of the vector of individual traits, ϕ, to one generation of selection on I_s is computed as follows:

$$\phi = i_p\mathbf{C'b}/\sigma_{Is} \qquad \{13.9\}$$

where σ_{Is} is the standard deviation of the selection index, which can be computed from the variance of the selection index, which is equal to $\mathbf{b'V_pb}$. The right-hand side of Equation {13.9} reduces to $ih(\sigma_A)$ for phenotypic selection on a single trait, which is the same as Equation {13.2}. The economic value of response to selection on the index, $\mathbf{v'}\phi$, is computed as follows:

$$\mathbf{v'}\phi = i_p(\mathbf{v'C'\ V_p^{-1}Cv})/(\mathbf{v'C'\ V_p^{-1}Cv})^{0.5} = i_p(\mathbf{v'C'V_p^{-1}Cv})^{0.5} = i_p\sigma_{Is} \qquad \{13.10\}$$

13.5 The value of genetic gain

As already noted, many of the studies that have considered marker-assisted selection (MAS) are quite pessimistic. In certain breeding programmes gains obtained by information on specific genes will be minuscule. Like any other investment, genotyping must be considered in terms of potential gains vs. costs. Two basic methods have been considered in the literature to evaluate genetic gain: the gain accrued to the national economy, and the gain that will be obtained by a specific breeding enterprise in competition with other breeding companies (Dekkers and Shook, 1990). In the latter case the economic value is determined in terms of increased returns due to increase in market share and increased profit per unit product. We will now consider the first alternative in detail.

The annual rate of genetic gain in most domestic species is from about 1 to 5% of the mean (Lande and Thompson, 1990; Weller and Fernando, 1991). Although these numbers seem small, they in fact represent huge increases in economic value, as will be demonstrated. Genetic gain is unlike all other investments, in that gains due to genetic improvement are eternal and cumulative. Unlike investment in new machinery, genetic gain never is "used up" and never has to be replaced. Unlike introduction of a new treatment or process, which must be continually applied, once genetic gain is obtained no further investment is required to maintain this gain.

The calculations that follow are based on Weller (1994) for the calculation of the value of gains from breeding to the national economy. Consider an ongoing breeding programme with a constant rate genetic gain per year. The annual rate of genetic gain will have a nominal value of V. The *cumulative* discounted returns to year T, R_v, will be a function of the nominal annual returns, the discount rate, d, the profit horizon T, and the number of years from the beginning of the programme until first returns are realized τ. R is computed as follows (Hill, 1971):

$$R_v = V \left[\frac{r_d^\tau - r_d^{T+1}}{(1 - r_d)^2} - \frac{(T - \tau + 1)r_d^{T+1}}{1 - r_d} \right] \quad \{13.11\}$$

where $r_d = 1/(1+d)$, and the other terms are as defined previously. For example, with d = 0.08, T = 20 years, and t = 5 years, R_v = 32.58V. That is, the cumulative returns are equal to nearly 33 times the nominal annual returns. For an infinite profit horizon, Equation {13.11} reduces to:

$$R_v = \frac{V r_d^\tau}{(1 - r_d)^2} = \frac{V}{d^2(1 + d)^{\tau - 2}} = 124.04V \quad \{13.12\}$$

We will now compare the value of nominal annual genetic gain to annual costs of a breeding programme, assuming a fixed nominal cost per year. Costs, unlike genetic gain, only have an effect in the year they occur. We will assume that annual costs are equal during the length of the breeding programme, and that first costs occur in the year after the base year. C_T, the net present value of the total costs of the breeding programme, is computed as follows:

$$C_T = \frac{C_c r_d (1 - r_d^T)}{1 - r_d} \quad \{13.13\}$$

where C_c = annual costs of the breeding programme. Using the same values for T, and d, C_T = 9.82C_c. Thus, with a profit horizon of 20 years, cumulative profit is positive if V > 0.31C_c. For an infinite profit horizon, C_T = 12.5C_c, and profit will be positive if V > 0.1C_c.

Therefore, a breeding programme can be profitable even if the nominal annual costs are several times the value of the nominal additional annual genetic gain. For example, we will consider the US dairy cattle population, which consists of about 10,000,000 cows. Annual genetic gain is about 100 kg milk/year. The value of a 1 kg gain in milk production has been estimated at $0.1 (Weller, 1994). Thus, the annual value of a 10% increase in the rate of genetic gain (10 kg/year) is:

$$V = (10 \text{ kg/cow/year})(\$0.1/\text{kg})(10,000,000 \text{ cows}) = \$10,000,000/\text{year} \quad \{13.14\}$$

The cumulative value with a profit horizon of 20 year and an 8% discount rate would be $326 million, and break-even annual costs are $32,000,000/year. Thus, it would be profitable to spend quite a lot for a relatively small gain.

The value of genetic gain to a specific breeding enterprise will generally be less than the gain to general economy. This is because most of the gains obtained by breeding will be passed on to the consumers. Brascamp et al. (1993) considered the economic value of MAS based on changes in returns from semen sales for a breeding organization operating in a competitive market. In this case a breeding firm that adopts a MAS program can increase its returns either by increasing its market share or increasing the mean price of a semen dose. Although the value of genetic gain will be less, relatively small changes in genetic merit can result in large changes in market share.

13.6 Dairy cattle breeding programmes, half-sib and progeny tests

A number of studies have investigated in depth how MAS can be applied to dairy cattle breeding programmes. The studies will be considered in detail in the next chapter. In this section we will describe the specific problems related to dairy cattle breeding, and the major breeding schemes that have been applied or proposed. Dairy cattle are unique in that:

1. Males have nearly unlimited fertility via artificial insemination (AI), while females have very limited fertility.
2. Nearly all of the traits of interest are expressed only in females. Thus most genetic gains are obtained by selection of males. However, the males can only be genetically evaluated based on the production records of their female relatives.

Recently, it has become possible to increase fertility of females by multiple ovulation and embryo transplant, although these techniques are still relatively expensive.

Considering these limitations, commercial dairy cattle programmes have traditionally been based on either half-sib or progeny test designs. Bulls reach sexual maturity of the age of 1 year. The male generation intervals in commercial breeding programmes are usually much longer than the biological minimum. A typical half-sib breeding programme is described in Figure 13.2, and a typical progeny test breeding programme is described in Figure 13.3.

Both designs as described assume a total cow population of 100,000 cows, but this is not a critical element of either design. Both designs can be applied to much larger populations. In the half-sib design, bull sires are selected based on the records of their daughters. These elite bulls are then mated to elite cows based on pedigree and their own production records. Of the 20 bull calves produced each year, about 10 are used for servicing the general cow population, once they reach sexual maturity at the age of 1 year. Thus the bulls used for general service are selected based on the production records of the daughters of their sires', which are the half-sibs of the bulls used for general service. In this design the maximum accuracy of sire evaluations is 0.5, assuming that no information is available on the dam of the sire. With information on the dam, the accuracy can be slightly higher, but will not account for the "Mendelian sampling" of the two parental genotypes by the son.

Most advanced dairy cattle breeding programmes are based on a progeny test of young sires based on a relative small sample of daughters. Sires with superior evaluations based on the first crop of daughters are returned to service. However, by the time daughter milk production records are available these sires are 5 years old. As will be shown, theoretical studies demonstrate that the gain in accuracy obtained by the progeny test outweighs the loss incurred by increasing the generation interval.

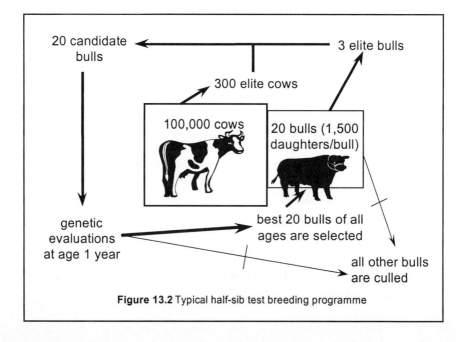

Figure 13.2 Typical half-sib test breeding programme

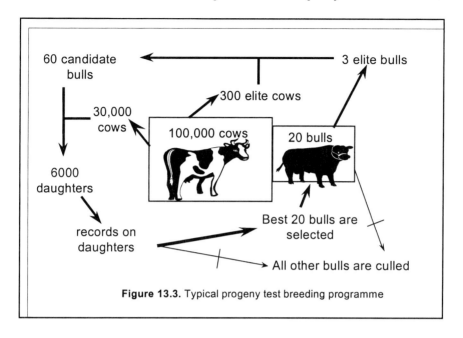

Figure 13.3. Typical progeny test breeding programme

In the progeny test design described in Figure 13.3, sires for general service are selected based on the production records of a sample of 50 to 100 daughters. Since the daughters completely reflect the additive genotype of the sire, it is possible with this design to approach an accuracy of unity for sire evaluations. With about 100 daughters the accuracy of sire evaluations will be about 0.9. Thus the accuracy of the sire evaluations is nearly double by the progeny test scheme. Sires are used in general service only after their daughters complete their first lactation. As noted above, by that time the sires are at least 5 years old.

The expected genetic gains in units of the genetic standard deviation by these two breeding schemes are summarized in Table 13.1, assuming that the breeding objective has a heritability of 0.25. Both schemes assume equal selection along the dam-to-cow path. As noted above, selection intensity is low, because most female calves produced must be used as replacement cows. Although there is no selection along the sire-to-cow path in the half-sib design, the expected annual genetic gain by this scheme is nearly equal to the genetic gain obtained by the progeny test design, because the mean generation interval is decreased.

Table 13.1 Expected annual genetic gains in units of the genetic standard deviation for the half-sib (HS) and progeny test (PT) designs for a trait with a heritability of 0.25

Design	Path	Generation interval	Proportion selected	Selection intensity	Accuracy	Genetic gain*
HS	Sire-to-bull	4.8	0.05	2.0	0.8	1.6
	Sire-to-cow	2.5	1.00	0	0.6	0
	Dam-to-bull	4.8	0.0017	3.2	0.7	2.24
	Dam-to-cow	4.0	0.85	0.3	0.7	0.21
	Total	16.1				4.05
	Annual					0.2516
PT	Sire-to-bull	7.4	0.02	2.4	0.95	2.28
	Sire-to-cow (young)†	2.0	1.00	0	0.6	0
	Sire-to-cow (proven)	7.4	0.11	1.7	0.95	1.614
	Dam-to-bull	4.8	0.005	2.9	0.7	2.03
	Dam-to-cow	4.0	0.85	0.3	0.7	0.21
	Total	22.5				5.796
	Annual					0.2576

* Computed as selection intensity multiplied by accuracy for each path.
† 21% of the cows are mated to young sires, and the remaining 79% are mated to proven sires.

13.7 Nucleus breeding schemes

We will now briefly consider breeding schemes that utilize multiple ovulation and embryo transplant (MOET). Nearly all advanced commercial breeding programs already use MOET to produce bull calves from elite cows. This slightly increases the selection intensity along the dam-to-bull path, but selection intensity is already very high along this path, 2.9 in the example given in Table 13.1. This is based on the assumption that 300 bull dams are selected from a potential cow population of 60,000 live cows with production records. The further reduction in the number of bull dams required by application of MOET has only a small effect on the selection intensity. The can be seen by comparing the increase in selection intensity obtained in the half-sib design in which the number of bull dams is reduced to 100.

Theoretically, genetic gain would be maximized if all cows were progeny of a small sample of selected cows. This would require applying MOET to the entire cow population. However, at current costs the potential increase in genetic gain cannot be justified economically. Therefore, several studies have suggested nucleus breeding programs based on a population of several hundred cows (Nicholas and Smith, 1983).

In the nucleus population, MOET is applied to the 5 to 10% of cows with the highest genetic evaluations, and all replacement cows are daughters of these cows. Since the total nucleus population size is relatively small, the total costs, including MOET, are not excessive. It is not possible in a population of this size to progeny test young sires. Therefore, the other elements of the nucleus breeding programme resemble the half-sib scheme. Rates of genetic gain up to 20% greater can be obtained by a nucleus breeding scheme (Nicholas and Smith, 1983). Bulls produced in the breeding nucleus are then used as sires in the general population. In this way the genetic gain obtained in the nucleus is transferred to the general population.

Even without markers, genetic gains were greater for nucleus schemes than traditional progeny testing schemes, although several studies have disputed these claims. All the theoretical studies that have considered MOET schemes have assumed that selection of all animals was based on a single trait with moderate heritability. In practice this is not the case, and secondary traits are also considered, especially in the selection of bull dams. On the positive side, it should be possible to obtain more accurate and unbiased trait and pedigree records from a small population maintained specifically for breeding purposes. In most commercial breeding programmes large sums are paid to farmers for bull calves from elite cows. Thus there is a tendency among many farmers to provide preferential treatment to superior cows, in order to inflate their genetic evaluations. These undesirable tendencies can be controlled in a breeding nucleus kept under a single management.

A potential problem in nucleus breeding programmes is the rapid buildup of inbreeding, because of the small effective population size. This problem is somewhat alleviated if animals with superior genetic merit in the general population are incorporated in the breeding nucleus. Breeding programs in which genetic material flows in both directions are called "open nucleus" schemes, as opposed to "closed nucleus" schemes in which genetic material only flows in one direction: from the nucleus to the general population. As yet, no national breeding programmes are based on nucleus breeding schemes.

13.8 Summary

Traditional selection index based on phenotypic records and information on relationships is very efficient, provided that it is possible to obtain high selection intensities, the selection criterion has a relative high heritability, and the selection criterion can be measured on all candidates for selection. However, many situations exist in which these conditions are not met. In many important mammalian species, such as cattle, the rate of genetic gain that can be obtained by traditional selection index methodology is limited, because the economic traits are expressed only in females, which have low fertility rates. Breeding schemes based on genetic evaluations of males by their female relatives have been developed. It is in these situations that MAS can have a significant impact. A small increase in the rate of genetic gain can have a huge economic value, measured in terms of its contribution to the national economy. Thus, relatively large costs in genotyping can be justified to increase rates of genetic gain by only a few percent. Economic values measured in terms of the gain to a specific breeding enterprise in competition with other firms are lower.

Chapter fourteen:

Marker-Assisted Selection - Theory

14.1 Introduction

Much more has been written with respect to methods for detection and analysis of individual quantitative trait loci as compared to application of these genes in breeding programs. Many of the reviews that were published on this topic were quite pessimistic (Smith and Simpson, 1986; Stam, 1986). As noted in the previous chapter, in those situations in which traditional selection index works well, little is gained by identification of the individual loci affecting quantitative traits. However, many practical breeding situations are encountered in which trait-based selection index is very inefficient or impractical. In these instances marker-based selection can make a very significant gain.

In this chapter we will first review the situations in which selection index is inefficient, and in Section 14.3 we will present the general consideration for marker-assisted selection (MAS) within a breed, and in the following section we will consider the specific problems of MAS in segregating populations. Formula to compute the optimum selection index with phenotypic and marker information, and to compare phenotypic selection and MAS for individual selection will be presented in Section 14.4. MAS with traits expressed only in a single sex, and selection on juveniles will be considered in the next two sections. Optimization of MAS with family selection will be considered in Section 14.7, and the reduction of selection gain with MAS due to sampling will be considered in Section 14.8. Problems of MAS related to segregating problems will be considered in the next two sections, and the final section will briefly consider "Velogenetics" – the synergistic use of MAS and germ-line manipulation

14.2 Situations in which selection index is inefficient

The practical situations in which selection index is not efficient can be listed as follows:

1. Low heritability for trait included in the economic objective.
2. Traits that cannot be scored on all individuals (males, juveniles, live animals, disease challenge).
3. Negative genetic correlations among traits.
4. Non-additive genetic variance (dominance, epistasis).

5. Crossbreeding.
6. "Cryptic" genetic variation.
7. Introgression

We have already mentioned the first two situations above. Many traits of major economic importance have been neglected in breeding programmes because of low heritability. Prime examples are fertility traits and disease resistance. Selection index works best on traits with near normal continuous distributions. Thus, traits such as conception rate, number of progeny, or disease have received less emphasis in breeding programs. Selection index is less efficient when the trait is expressed only in one sex, or only in mature individuals. Certain traits cannot be scored on live animals, such as carcass composition. In this case genetic values can only be estimated though records of relatives.

As shown by Falconer (1981) negative genetic correlations among traits included in the selection objective tend to build up over time. Nearly all commercial breeding programs include traits with negative genetic correlations. The effect of negative genetic correlations among traits included in the selection objective will be considered below in detail.

Clearly, selection index does not utilize non-additive genetic variance, nor does it provide an answer for crossbreeding among straits. The three main goals of crossbreeding are: (1) utilization of heterosis, (2) increased genetic variation, and (3) introgression. The "classical" explanations for heterosis are elimination of inbreeding depression, and overdominance at the level of the individual locus. Even in the absence of these "true" genetic effects, crossbreeding is often more profitable than selection within a single line. Moav (1966) defined five types of "economic" heterosis.

Different breeds are sometimes crossed to produce a population with increased genetic variance. Selection index can then be used to increase the economic value in future generations. However, desirable genes of individuals with overall inferior phenotypes can be lost through trait-based selection. Generally only the economically best breeds will be considered as parental candidates. Again, some breeds with overall inferior phenotypes may carry some desirable genes, which will not be found by trait-based selection. This is especially true of wild progenitors of domestic species. This "cryptic" genetic variation can be utilized via MAS.

14.3 Potential contribution of MAS for selection within a breed - general considerations

Potentially, MAS can increase annual genetic gain by:

1. Increasing the accuracy of evaluation
2. Increasing the selection intensity
3. Decreasing the generation interval.

Most of the studies on MAS have dealt with increasing the accuracy of evaluation. Information on the individual genes affecting the trait of interest does increase the accuracy of the evaluation, but the effect decreases as the heritability increases. Assume that marker information is available for QTL affecting some of the traits included in the breeding objective. We will define m_s as the "net marker score", which is the sum of the additive effects associated with the markers for a given individual. With information on individual loci in addition to phenotypic trait values, selection index methodology can be used to construct an optimum linear selection index of the form: $\mathbf{b_y'y} + b_m m_s$ (Lande and Thompson, 1990), where $\mathbf{b_y}$ represents the index coefficients for the quantitative trait records, $\mathbf{y}$, and b_m represents the index coefficient for m_s. $\mathbf{b_y}$ and $\mathbf{y}$ are vectors, while b_m and m_s are scalars. That is, the marker information can be considered the addition of a single trait to the selection index. The index coefficients can be computed, based on Equation {13.8}, which will be repeated here:

$$\mathbf{b} = \mathbf{V_p^{-1} C v} \quad \{14.1\}$$

In the case of selection on phenotype and marker information, $\mathbf{C = G}$. The marker score has no intrinsic economic value. Therefore, the coefficient of the net marker score in $\mathbf{v}$, the vector of economic values, will be equal to zero. We will now consider in detail several situations of interest.

14. 4 Phenotypic selection vs. MAS for individual selection

In the simplest case we will assume that for trait-based selection, individuals are selected based on a single phenotypic record, and that for MAS individuals are selected based on the phenotypic record, and their own marker information. Information from relatives is not considered. The phenotypic and genetic variance matrices are computed as follows:

$$\mathbf{V_p} = \begin{bmatrix} \sigma_z^2 & \sigma_m^2 \\ \sigma_m^2 & \sigma_m^2 \end{bmatrix} \quad \text{and} \quad \mathbf{G} = \begin{bmatrix} \sigma_A^2 & \sigma_m^2 \\ \sigma_m^2 & \sigma_m^2 \end{bmatrix} \quad \{14.2\}$$

where σ_z^2 and σ_A^2 are phenotypic and genetic variances, and σ_m^2 is the additive genetic variance explained by the genetic markers. In terms of the additive genetic variance these equations become:

$$\mathbf{V_p} = \begin{bmatrix} 1/h^2 & p_m \\ p_m & p_m \end{bmatrix} \quad \text{and} \quad \mathbf{G} = \begin{bmatrix} 1 & p_m \\ p_m & p_m \end{bmatrix} \quad \{14.3\}$$

where h^2 is the heritability, and p_m is the fraction of the additive genetic variance associated with the genetic markers, that is: $p_m = \sigma_m^2/\sigma_A^2$. Inverting $\mathbf{V_p}$ and substituting into Equation {14.1} gives index coefficients of: $(p_m - p_m^2)(p_m/h^2 - p_m^2)$ and $(p_m/h^2 - p_m^2)^2$. The actual b-values will be functions of the trait units. Therefore the ratio of the values has more intrinsic meaning. This ratio is computed as follows:

$$b_m/b_x = (1/h^2 - 1)/(1 - p_m) \qquad \{14.4\}$$

where b_m and b_x are the index coefficients for marker and phenotypic information, respectively. From this equation it can be deduced that as the heritability of the selection objective tends toward unity, b_m tends to zero, regardless of p_m.

The relative selection efficiency, RSE, of two different indices is defined as the ratio of their expected genetic gains (Weller, 1994). The economic value of genetic gain by selection on the index is computed by Equation {13.10}. The economic gain by phenotypic selection will be: $i_p h \sigma_A$. Thus the RSE of a selection index including marker information to a selection index based only on trait values for individual selection will be equal to: $(\mathbf{v'G'V_p^{-1}Gv})^{0.5}/(h\sigma_A)$. The elements of $\mathbf{v}$, $\mathbf{G}$, and $\mathbf{V_p}$ are given above. $\mathbf{V_p}$, a 2 × 2 matrix, can be easily inverted. Inverting this matrix and multiplying the vectors and matricies gives (Lande and Thompson, 1990):

$$\text{RSE} = \left[\frac{p_m}{h^2} + \frac{(1-p_m)^2}{1-h^2 p_m} \right]^{1/2} \qquad \{14.5\}$$

As heritability tends to unity, so does RSE. For $h^2 = 0.25$, and $p_m = 0.5$, RSE = 1.5. Thus, gains for individual selection through MAS can be quite significant. Equation {14.5} gives the added gain due to selection on an index including phenotypic information on the selection objective and marker information. If selection is based only on known QTL without information on the economic trait, then the RSE of MAS to trait-based selection is RSE $(p_m/h^2)^{1/2}$. Thus, selection efficiency on markers alone will be greater than trait-based selection if $p_m > h^2$.

14.5 MAS for sex-limited traits

As noted in Section 14.2, selection index is inefficient in situations in which the selection criteria cannot be scored on all individuals, for example a sex-linked trait. Selection efficiency can be increased by selection among individuals without phenotypic expression of trait. For example, milk production is expressed only in females. Therefore selection among males is based only on information from relatives. With only information on relatives, two full brothers will have the same genetic evaluation. Information on markers could be used to differentiate between them. Furthermore, as shown in the previous chapter, in many animal species, although the traits of interest are expressed only in females, females have a low fertility rate, while males have a very high potential fertility rate. Thus, the selection intensities will also be different in the two sexes. For a trait expressed only in females, the RSE of MAS on both sexes relative to individual phenotypic selection of females will be:

$$\text{RSE} = \left[\frac{p_m}{h^2} + \frac{(1-p_m)^2}{1-h^2 p_m} \right]^{1/2} + \frac{i_\male}{i_\female} \left[\frac{p_m}{h^2} \right]^{1/2} \quad \{14.6\}$$

where $i_\male$ is the selection intensity in males, and $i_\female$ is the selection intensity in females. The first term of this equation is the same as equation {14.5}, and refers to selection of females for which both marker and phenotypic information is available. The second term refers to selection in males, for which only marker information can be used.

In this case RSE can be significantly higher, as compared to situations in which the trait is expressed in both sexes. For example, if $p_m = h^2$, and $i_\male/i_\female = 2$, then RSE is doubled, relative to the situation in Equation {14.4}. As heritability tends toward unity, Equation {14.6} tends to: $1+(i_\male/i_\female)\sqrt{p_m}$. The maximum RSE as p_m tends towards unity for any heritability is: $(1+i_\male/i_\female)/h$.

14.6 Two-stage selection: MAS on juveniles, and phenotypic selection of adults

In many agricultural species, especially fruit trees, it is relatively inexpensive to produce large number of juveniles. Thus selection intensity can potentially be quite high. If these individuals do not express the selection criteria, it is still possible to select these individuals based on their genetic markers. In this case a two-stage procedure has been proposed in which juveniles are selected based on genetic markers, and adults are selected based on phenotype (Smith, 1967). Selection on juveniles reduces the additive genetic variance in the selected sample by a factor $p(1 - \sigma_m^{2*}/\sigma_m^2)$, where σ_m^2 is the variance of the marker score prior to selection, and σ_m^{2*} is the variance of the marker score after selection on juveniles. The RSE of this scheme relative to phenotypic selection on adults is computed as follows:

$$\text{RSE} = \frac{1 - p_m(1 - \sigma_m^{2*}/\sigma_m^2)}{[1-h^2 p_m(1-\sigma_m^{2*}/\sigma_m^2)]^{1/2}} + \frac{i_m}{i_A} \left[\frac{p_m}{h^2} \right]^{1/2} \quad \{14.7\}$$

where i_m and i_A are the selection intensities for immature and adults, respectively.

The second term is parallel to the second term of Equation {14.6}, and the first term accounts for the reduction in selection intensity on adults, due to preselection of juveniles. With very strong selection on juveniles, the term: $1-\sigma_m^{2*}/\sigma_m^2$ tends toward unity, and Equation {14.7} tends towards: $(1-p_m)/(1-h^2p_m)^{\frac{1}{2}} + (i_m/i_A)(p_m/h^2)^{\frac{1}{2}}$. Note that the first term is less than unity. That is, the efficiency of phenotypic selection after preselection of juveniles is reduced. Of course, in practice selection in the second stage will be based on both marker and phenotypic information, but the equations to describe this situation are quite complicated. A somewhat similar scheme has been proposed in dairy cattle with respect to sire selection. Young bulls can first be selected based only on genetic markers, and then the remaining bulls can be reselected based on daughter performance (Kashi et al., 1990). This scheme will be considered in detail in the following chapter.

14.7 MAS including marker and phenotypic information on relatives

With both marker and trait information on both the individual and his relatives, selection index theory can again be used to construct the optimum selection index, which will have the following form:

$$I_s = b_{zf}Z_f + b_{mf}m_f + b_{zw}Z_w + b_{mw}m_w \qquad \{14.8\}$$

where Z_f is the mean family phenotype, m_f is the mean family marker score, Z_w is the phenotypic deviation of the individual from the family mean, m_w is the deviation of the individuals molecular score from the family mean, and the bs are the appropriate index coefficients. As in individual selection it is assumed that the marker scores have no intrinsic economic values. We will further assume that the selection objective is measured in units of its economic value. In this case, the vector of economic weights will be: [1 0 1 0]'.

We will define r_f as the fraction of genes identical by descent among family members (½ for full-sibs, and ¼ for half-sibs), n as the number of individuals in each family, and c^2 as the residual correlation among family members. The values for the index coefficients can be derived based on selection index theory as explained in the previous chapter, and are as follows (Lande and Thompson, 1990):

$$\begin{bmatrix} b_{zf} \\ b_{mf} \\ b_{zw} \\ b_{mw} \end{bmatrix} = \begin{bmatrix} r_n h^2(1-p)/D_f \\ (t_n - r_n h^2)/D_f \\ (1-r_f)h^2(1-p)/D_w \\ [1-t-(1-r_f)h^2]/D_w \end{bmatrix} \qquad \{14.9\}$$

where $r_n = r_f + (1 - r_f)/n$, $t = r_f h^2 + c^2$, $t_n = t + (1 - t)/n$, $D_f = t_n - r_n h^2 p$, and $D_w = 1 - t - (1 - r_n h^2 p)$. The expression for RSE using information on relatives is quite complex, and is given in Lande and Thompson (1990).

14.8 Maximum selection efficiency of MAS with all QTL known, relative to trait-based selection, and the reduction in RSE due to sampling variance

The maximum RSE that can be obtained for various selection schemes with $p = 1$ were also computed by Lande and Thompson (1990) and are given in Table 14.1. Very large families are assumed for the combined individual and family selection schemes. The RSE computed for selection based on half-sib or full-sib records are much less than for individual phenotypic selection. With half-sib selection, the maximum gain possible, as p tends towards unity is: $2[(1- h^2/4)/(1+2h^2)]^{1/2}$. For $h^2 = 0.5$, maximum RSE = 1.32, as compared to a RSE of 2 for individual selection with the same heritability.

Table 14.1 Maximum relative selection efficiency of MAS to phenotypic selection, with all QTL identified and large sample size

Selection scheme	Relative selection efficiency
Individual Index including markers and phenotype (on both sexes)	$1/h$
Index on female-limited trait, markers on males*	$(1+ i_\male/i_\female)/h$
Two stage: strong marker-based selection in immatures, phenotypic selection on adults†	$(i_m/i_A)/h$
Combined individual and family index Paternal half-sibs	$2[(1- h^2/4)/(1+2h^2)]^{1/2}$
Full-sibs, No residual within-family correlation	$(2 - h^2)^{1/2}$
With a residual within-family correlation‡	$(2/h)[t(1 - t)]^{1/2}$

* $i_\male$ and $i_\female$ are selection intensities for males and females, respectively.
† i_m and i_A are selection intensities for juveniles and adults, respectively.
‡ $t = h^2/2 + c^2$, where c^2 is the residual within-family correlation.

224 Quantitative Trait Loci Analysis in Animals

In all of the previous equations, RSE were estimated under the assumption that QTL effects were estimated without error. However, if the sample size is finite, there will be sampling errors in the estimated QTL effects. The loss in selection efficiency for MAS due to sampling error will be approximately equal to the following expression (Lande and Thompson, 1990):

$$\frac{(2h^2 p_m + N_Q/N) p_m (1 - h^2)^2}{N h^2 (1 - p_m h^2)[p_m + h^2(1 - 2p_m)]^2} \quad \{14.10\}$$

where N is the number of individuals analysed, and N_Q is the number of marker loci included in the selection index. The reduction in RSE will be less than 2% if at least a few hundred individuals are analysed, for any combination of p_m and h^2. (Lande and Thompson, 1990).

14.9 Marker information in segregating populations

Even if segregating QTL are detected via linkage to genetic markers, there are two major problems that must be addressed if this information is to be included in actual breeding programs:

1. Linkage phase can be different in different individuals. Thus it will be necessary to determine the QTL alleles and phase for each candidate for selection.
2. Unless the markers are very tightly linked to the QTL, linkage relationships will break down in future generations.

The second problem is less acute if the QTL is located within a marker bracket. However, as noted in Chapter ten, the confidence interval for a QTL will generally be greater than 10 cM, unless the sample size is huge, or other methods described in this chapter are used to reduce the confidence interval. Therefore, the marker bracket must be relatively wide to ensure that the bracket does in fact include the QTL. In this case a significant fraction of the progeny will not receive the marker bracket intact.

To overcome both of these problems, a number of studies have assumed that the actual QTL have been identified, and the effects of the different alleles are known *a priori*. Once the QTL effect is determined, it is necessary only to genotype candidates for selection to determine their QTL genotypes. Although several loci with major effects on economic traits have been identified and even sequenced (e. g. Gootwine *et al.*, 1998) this is not as yet a realistic option for QTL that account for only a few percent of the phenotypic variance. Studies that assume that the actual QTL alleles can be identified are still quite useful in that they give an indication of the upper limit that can be achieved by MAS under different breeding strategies. Breeding programmes based on both marker-assisted selection and identification of actual QTL will be considered below.

14.10 Inclusion of marker information in "animal model" genetic evaluations

Most studies that have evaluated MAS have generally assumed that the genome is first scanned to locate chromosomal regions containing QTL. Using additional markers, the QTL are progressively localized to smaller and smaller chromosomal regions, and finally the actual genes are identified. The identified QTL are then used in selection programmes (Soller, 1994). Following this approach, or even localization of the QTL to a very small chromosomal segment, recombination in future generations is no longer a problem, but there is a significant time lag until QTL are utilized in breeding programmes.

An alternative approach was presented by Fernando and Grossman (1989). Their model, first discussed in Chapter four, estimates breeding values of all individuals in the population, including information from genetic markers, but does not directly estimate the QTL effects. Instead, they modified a standard individual animal model so that in addition to the polygenic effect of each individual, two "gametic effects" are estimated for the two parental marker alleles or haplotypes passed to each individual for each locus. Rather than representing specific QTL alleles, these gametic effects include uncertainty with respect to the QTL allele received. Following the principles of selection index, selection based on the estimated breeding values including marker information should result in maximum genetic gain in the next generation, even though QTL information is incomplete.
As noted in Chapter seven, this model was extended to handle a reduced animal model (Cantet and Smith, 1991), and multiple QTL bracketed by genetic markers (Goddard, 1992).

14.11 Velogenetics - the synergistic use of MAS and germ-line manipulation

In future breeding programs, MAS will probably be combined together with other new technologies affecting reproduction, such as multiple ovulation and embryo transplant (MOET) which was discussed in the previous chapter, sexed semen, and cloning. Georges and Massey (1991) considered the possibility of combination of MAS with germ-line manipulation. Spontaneous oocyte maturation and ovulation do not begin until puberty. For cattle this is at the age of close to 1 year. However, waves of oocyte growth are seen even *in utero*. Activation of primordial follicles starts at 140 days of gestation. Georges and Massey (1991) considered the theoretical possibility to grow, mature and fertilize prepubertal oocytes *in vitro*.

This procedure could possibly reduce the generation interval of cattle to as little as 3 to 6 months, as compared to the normal biological minimum of close to 2 years. By using *in vitro* fertilization of fetal oocytes by selected, progeny-tested sires, annual responses in milk yield could be doubled compared to conventional progeny testing. They term this procedure "velogenetics", and propose the following breeding scheme.

1. Selection of "bull grandams" based on records and genetic markers.
2. Selection of fetal "bull dams" based on genetic markers.
3. *In vitro* fertilization of fetal oocytes with semen of elite sires, selected by breeding values based on records of female relatives and genetic markers.
4. Selection among juvenile male calves based on genetic markers.
5. Selected young sires at the age of 1-2 years are mated to cows of commercial population.

Step 3 of this protocol is not possible at present, but until very recently, it was also considered impossible to clone mature mammals.

14.12 Summary

Although trait-based selection is very efficient in certain situations, in many practical cases, this is not the case, and these situations are summarized in this chapter. Formula were presented that can be used to evaluate the relative efficiency of MAS, as compared to traditional trait-based selection, for a number of situations of interest. In some cases the selection efficiency of MAS can potentially be more than 1.5 times traditional selection. As the situations considered approach reality, the formulas become more complicated, and more parameters must be considered. Most situations of real-world interest cannot be evaluated analytically, and simulation of these scenarios is required. A number of schemes of particular interest will be considered in detail in the final chapter.

Chapter fifteen:

Marker-Assisted Selection - Results of Simulation Studies

15.1 Introduction

In the previous chapter we presented mathematical formulas that can be used to evaluate marker-assisted selection (MAS), as compared to trait-based selection. Although a wide range of situations was considered, these still represent only a small fraction of all possible scenarios. Furthermore, many of the questions of interest cannot as yet be answer analytically. Therefore a number of studies have used stochastic simulations to evaluate MAS. Nearly all of these studies confronted the question of a mathematical model for the additive genetic variance that accounts for a finite number of QTL of sufficient magnitude for detection.

In this chapter we will first review the mathematical models that have been used to describe the polygenic variance, and in Section 15.3 we will present formulas to calculate the effective number of QTL for a trait. In Section 15.4 we will present a general overview of scenarios for application of MAS to dairy cattle, and in the following sections we will consider these scenarios in detail. The long-term consequences of MAS and trait-based selection will be considered in Section 15.8. Multitrait selection will be evaluated in the final two sections.

15.2 Modeling the polygenic variance

As noted in the first chapter, the traditional mathematical model for polygenic variance has been the "infinitesimal model". That is, polygenic variance is assumed to be due to an infinite number of loci, each contributing an infinitesimal fraction of the total genetic variance. This model is mathematically tractable, and apparently works very well, provided that no individual locus accounts for a very large fraction of the total genetic variance. However, the infinitesimal model cannot be applied to MAS simulations, which all postulate individual QTL large enough to be detected by linkage to genetic markers.

Nearly all of the simulation studies considered below, and a number of additional studies, have addressed the question of the appropriate mathematical model for polygenic variance with MAS. A number of studies have assumed a single segregating QTL on the background of the infinitesimal model for the remainder of the genetic variance (Gibson, 1994; Villanueva et al., 1999). These simulations will be considered in detail in Section 15.8.

Most MAS simulation studies have attempted to simulate all the additive genetic variance in terms of a finite number of loci, sampled from a theoretical distribution. Generally these studies have applied a distribution that postulates a few big QTL and many small ones. Zhang and Smith (1992, 1993) simulated a normal distribution of QTL effects but they also considered a gamma distribution of QTL effects. Some studies used a theoretical distribution to directly simulate the variance of each QTL, while other studies first simulated QTL effects, and then either simulated allelic frequencies from a uniform distribution, or assumed equal allelic frequencies. De Koning and Weller (1994) used a χ^2 distribution to simulate the variances of QTL effects. Hoeschele and VanRaden (1993a) postulated an exponential distribution, while Mackinnon and Georges (1998) assumed double exponential distribution of allelic effects at each QTL. As given in Equation 7.43, the exponential distribution has the form:

$$f(a) = \lambda e^{-\lambda a} \qquad \{15.1\}$$

where a is the allelic effect, and λ is the parameter of this distribution. The expectation of the distribution is equal to $1/\lambda$. They assumed that all QTL were biallelic, and simulated allelic frequency from a uniform distribution. The double exponential distribution has the following form:

$$f(a) = \tfrac{1}{2}\lambda e^{-\lambda |a|} \qquad \{15.2\}$$

Mackinnon and Georges (1998) simulated either two or four alleles for each QTL. The allelic frequencies were simulated by sampling from a uniform distribution, and then dividing the sampled values by their sum, so that the sum of the allelic frequencies would equal unity. They assumed a heritability of 0.3, which was generated by simulating 5, 10, or 20 QTL. As the number of QTL increased from 5 to 20, it was necessary to increase λ from 6 to 12 to account for the total heritability of 0.3. With any of these theoretical distributions there is no maximum value for QTL effect, although the probability of sampling a very large QTL becomes progressively smaller.

Lande and Thompson (1990) proposed the following deterministic distribution for the variances of the QTL:

$$\sigma_a^2 (1 - \alpha_a)[1, \alpha_a, \alpha_a^2, \alpha_a^3, \ldots] \qquad \{15.3\}$$

The variances of the QTL generated by this model summed to infinity will equal σ_a^2. The parameter α, which must be between 0 and 1, determines the relative magnitude of the individual loci. Assuming additivity, $\alpha_a = 2p(1-p)a$ for biallelic QTL with a as defined previously, and p = allelic frequency. The first QTL in the series is the largest, and has a variance of α_a. Subsequent QTL are progressively smaller, and the total number of loci is infinite. As α tends towards 0, the biggest

QTL explains a relatively larger effect of the total additive genetic variance. With $\alpha_a=0.5$, a single QTL explains half of the genetic variance. If the 1th locus of series is the smallest QTL likely to be detected, then the maximum proportion of the additive genetic variance that can be detected is $1 - a^1$.

15.3 The effective number of QTL

For the theoretical distributions considered above, the "effective number of loci" can be defined as the total additive genetic variance, divided by the expectation of the individual QTL variance. Thus if QTL variances are generated by an exponential distribution, the effective number of loci will be equal to λ. Lande and Thompson (1990) defined a similar parameter for the distribution given in Equation {15.3}.

$$N_E = \left(\sum_{i=0}^{\infty} \alpha_a^i\right)^2 / \sum_{i=0}^{\infty} \alpha_a^{2i} = (1+\alpha_a)/(1-\alpha_a) \qquad \{15.4\}$$

where N_E is the effective number of loci. Values of α_a equal to 1, 1/3, 2/3, 5/6 and 11/12 correspond to N_E of 1, 2, 5, 11, and 23, respectively. As the effective number of loci increases the fraction of the total additive genetic variance that can be detected, $1 - a^1$, decreases. Consider Equation {8.1}, which will be repeated here:

$$n = \frac{2(Z_{\alpha/2} + Z_\beta)^2}{(\delta/\sigma)^2} \qquad \{15.5\}$$

When $Z_\beta = 0$, the power to detect a QTL is 0.5. In a backcross design, the QTL with the smallest variance that will be detected with a power of 0.5 in terms of the total additive genetic variance is:

$$p_1 = \delta_1^2/\sigma_A^2 = \frac{4(Z_{\alpha/2})^2}{N(\sigma_A/\sigma)^2} = \frac{4(Z_{\alpha/2})^2}{Nh^2} \qquad \{15.6\}$$

where p_1 is the faction of σ_A^2 due to the 1th QTL, and $N = 2n$ is the number of individuals analysed. As will be seen below, genetic progress with MAS will be maximized with a relatively low value for $Z_{\alpha/2}$. With $Z_\beta = 0$, half of the QTL "detected" will be spurious.

15.4 Proposed dairy cattle breeding schemes with MAS - overview

Several different schemes have been proposed to incorporate marker information into commercial dairy cattle programs. Most studies have assumed only minor modifications of the existing programmes. *A priori,* dairy cattle improvement should be nearly an ideal situation for application of MAS, as noted in the previous two chapters, because most economic traits are only expressed in females, which have very limited fertility. The following schemes have been considered:

1. A standard progeny test system, with information from genetic markers used to increase the accuracy of sire evaluations in addition to phenotypic information from daughter records (Meuwissen and van Arendonk, 1992).
2. A multiple ovulation and embryo transfer (MOET) nucleus breeding scheme in which marker information is used to select sires for service in the MOET population, in addition to phenotypic information on half-sisters (Meuwissen and van Arendonk, 1992).
3. Progeny test schemes, in which information on genetic markers is used to preselect young sires for entrance into the progeny test (Kashi *et al.*, 1990; Mackinnon and Georges, 1998).
4. Selection of bull sires without a progeny test, based on half-sib records and genetic markers (Spelman *et al.*, 1999).
5. Selection of sires in a half-sib scheme, based on half-sib records and genetic markers (Spelman *et al.*, 1999).

These designs will be considered in detail in the following sections.

15.5 Inclusion of marker information into standard progeny test and MOET nucleus breeding schemes

Meuwissen and van Arendonk (1992) considered two schemes. The first scheme was a traditional progeny test scheme in which information on markers in addition to records on daughters was used to more accurately evaluate young sires. They also considered both "closed" and "open" nucleus breeding schemes. In all three of these schemes no modifications of the comparable breeding programmes without marker information were required. Thus the only costs involved were the actual genotyping costs. This is not the case in the breeding programmes considered in the following sections.

Results are presented in Table 15.1. As in Chapter thirteen, rates of genetic gain are presented in terms of the genetic standard deviation. A heritability of 0.25 was assumed. The rate of annual genetic gain for the progeny test scheme without MAS is slightly less than the value given in Table 13.1. This difference is due to slight differences in the assumptions with respect to the base breeding program. In this scheme MAS increased the rate of genetic gain only 5% when the markers explained 25% of the genetic variance. This result is not surprising, considering that the accuracy of sire evaluations based on a progeny test of 50 daughters is already quite high, as shown in Table 13.1. The advantage of this scheme is that it requires virtually no change in the existing breeding programme either on the part of artificial insemination (AI) institutes or farmers, and would therefore meet with no opposition.

As explained in Chapter thirteen, in nucleus schemes selection is carried out within a relatively small population, and bulls produced from this population are then used to service the general population. In nucleus breeding schemes, progeny testing of sires is not a viable option, and sires are selected based on records of half-sisters. Thus, the accuracies of sire evaluations are much lower, which gives more scope for improvement via MAS. Results for nucleus breeding schemes are also presented in Table 15.1

Table 15.1 Rates of genetic gain with marker assisted selection in progeny test and open and closed nucleus breeding programmes (Meuwissen and van Arendonk 1992)

Scheme	Fraction of the variance of within-family deviation explained by markers	Genetic gain (σ_a/year)	Percent increase
Progeny test	0	0.240	-
	0.05	0.242	0.8
	0.1	0.245	2.0
	0.25	0.253	5.4
Open nucleus	0	0.284	-
	0.05	0.317	15.6
	0.1	0.343	20.8
	0.25	0.408	43.7
Closed nucleus	0	0.297	-
	0.05	0.325	15.4
	0.1	0.350	17.8
	0.25	0.412	38.7

Meuwissen and van Arendonk (1992) assumed that QTL genotypes of sires would be determined by genotyping from 100 to 1000 daughters, and that grand-progeny would be selected based on an index including genotypic and phenotypic information. The fraction of within-family variance of grand-progeny predicted by marker analysis of both grandsires was at most 13% if markers were closely spaced, and 1000 daughters were genotyped per sire. In this case, increases in the rates of genetic gain were 26% and 22% for open and closed nucleus breeding schemes.

15.6 Progeny test schemes, in which information on genetic markers is used to preselect young sires

Kashi *et al.* (1990) and Mackinnon and Georges (1998) considered a standard progeny-test breeding scheme, but used markers to select among young candidate bulls prior to progeny test, in addition to pedigree information. Since the number of candidate bulls is increased, more cows must be selected as bull dams, or the number of progeny per bull dam must be increased by MOET. As in the nucleus schemes considered above, there is significant scope for improvement, since the accuracy of young sire evaluations based only on pedigree information is low. This method also has the advantage that it requires only minimal changes on the part of the AI institutes, and no changes by the farmers.

Both Kashi *et al.* (1990) and Mackinnon and Georges (1998) assumed that although the young sires are genotyped for the genetic markers, the QTL genotype of each young sire must be determined based on production records of their female relatives. Since linkage phase between QTL and the genetic markers are assumed unknown *a priori*, these must be determined by either a daughter or grand-daughter design analysis, as described in Chapter four. Mackinnon and Georges (1998) compared these two genotyping strategies.

In the "top-down" strategy, QTL genotypes are determined for the elite sires used as bull sires by a grand-daughter design. If a dense marker map is available, it will then be possible to determine which QTL allele is passed to each son. Elite bulls from among these sons are then selected as bull sires for the next generation. If the original sire was heterozygous for a QTL, it can be determined which of his sons received the favourable allele. Sons of these sires are then genotyped and preselected based on whether they received the favourable grand-paternal QTL alleles. It is assumed that the dams of the candidate sires are also genotyped, and that these cows will be progeny of the sires evaluated by a grand-daughter design. Thus, grand-paternal alleles inherited via the candidates' dams can also be traced.

Since QTL evaluation is based on a grand-daughter design, a much larger population than that considered in the previous chapter is assumed. Mackinnon and Georges (1998) assumed that 500 young bulls, sons of 10 elite sires, are progeny tested each year in their scheme. A disadvantage of this scheme is that only the grand-paternal alleles are followed. Some of the sons of the original sires that were evaluated by a grand-daughter design will also received the favorable QTL allele from their dams, but not via the genotyped grandsires. However, young sires will be selected based only on the grand-paternal haplotypes.

In the "bottom-up" scheme, QTL genotypes of elite sires are determined by a daughter design. These sires are then used as bull sires. The candidate bulls are then preselected for those QTL heterozygous in their sires, based on which paternal haplotype they received. Since QTL phase is evaluated on the sires of the bull calves (the candidates for selection), no selection pressure is "wasted" as in the "top-down" scheme. In addition, this design can be applied to a much smaller population, because only several hundred daughters are required to evaluate each bull sire. On the negative side, more daughters than sons must be genotyped to determine QTL genotype, as described in Chapter four.

Mackinnon and Georges (1998) assumed that in either scheme it will not be necessary to increase mean generation interval above that of a traditional progeny test program, although this will probably not be the case. In the "bottom-up" scheme, bulls are not used as bull sires until they have been evaluated for QTL based on daughter records. Mackinnon and Georges (1998) also assumed that the daughter design analysis would be based on either 50 or 100 daughters that were produced in each sire's progeny test. As shown by Weller *et al.* (1990), a daughter design analysis based on only 100 daughters per sire will not be very accurate. In the "top-down" scheme, bulls are not used as bull sires until their sires have been evaluated for QTL based on a grand-daughter design. This requires a large number of progeny tested sons, which will only be produced over several years.

Both Kashi *et al.* (1990) and Mackinnon and Georges (1998) address the problem that QTL determination will be subject to error. Mackinnon and Georges (1998) proposed that evaluated sires should be considered heterozygous for the QTL if the contrast for the selection objective between the two haplotypes is greater than a fixed minimum value denoted c. Of course if this value is set too high, then some heterozygous sires will be considered homozygous, while if the value is set too low, then some homozygous sires will be considered heterozygous. In the first case, segregating QTL will be missed, while in the second case, selection for the positive QTL allele will be applied to no advantage.

Mackinnon and Georges (1998) assumed that only bulls that received the positive QTL alleles for all loci for which their sires were heterozygous would be selected for progeny testing. This requires production and genotyping of many more candidate bulls as compared to the traditional progeny test scheme. For example, in the "bottom-up" design, assume that 50 sons are to progeny tested for each bull sire, and the bull sire is heterozygous for two QTL. In this case, 242 candidates must be produced and genotyped to obtain a 95% probability that there will be 50 sons that received the positive alleles for both loci. As noted previously, increasing the number of young sires produced will require many more bull dams. This will decrease selection intensity along the dam-to-son path. It can be argued that in the future, it may be possible to maintain selection intensity along this path by MOET of elite cows. However, MOET of elite cows to produce bull calves also increases the rate of genetic gain without MAS.

Mackinnon and Georges (1998) assumed a heritability of 0.3, and that the additive genetic variance was due to 10 loci, each with four alleles. The QTL effects were assumed to be sampled from a double exponential distribution, with the QTL with the largest effect accounting for about one-third of the genetic variance.

They found that, generally, decreasing c to 0.1 phenotypic standard deviation increased genetic gain. Most of the QTL selected would not meet the criteria of "suggestive linkage" given in Chapter eleven, or even a nominal type I error of 0.01, recommended by Lande and Thompson (1990). The "bottom-up" design was superior to the "top-down" design. With preselection of young sires based on one, two, or five loci, rates of genetic gain were increased by 8, 14, and 23% in the "bottom-up" design. However, most of the genetic gain is lost if the reduction in the selection intensity of the bull-dams is included in the analysis. In the case of five loci, in which the number of candidates bulls is very large, more than three-quarters of the genetic gain obtain by preselection is lost due to increasing the number of bull dams. Therefore neither scheme can be economically justified without efficient and inexpensive MOET.

Kashi et al. (1990) estimated that rates of genetic gain could be increased up to 30% by a similar scheme. However, Brascamp et al. (1993) noted that Kashi et al. (1990) did not account for the expected differences among estimated breeding values of candidate bulls even without information on individual QTL. Furthermore, Kashi et al. (1990) did not account for the reduction in selection intensity expected along the dam-to-son path, if many more bulls are considered as candidates *a priori*. As shown by Mackinnon and Georges (1998), this reduction is significant.

15.7 Selection of sires based on marker information without a progeny test

Spelman et al. (1999) considered three different breeding schemes by purely determinist simulation:

1. A standard progeny test with the inclusion of QTL data.
2. The same scheme with the change that young bulls without progeny test could also be used as bull sires based on QTL information.
3. A scheme in which young sires could be used as both bull sires and cow sires in the general population, based on QTL information.

They assumed that only bulls were genotyped, but once genotyped, the information on QTL genotype and effect was known without error. It was then possible to do a completely deterministic analysis. They varied the fraction of the genetic variance controlled by known QTL from zero to 100%. Their results are summarized in Table 15.2.

The annual genetic gain without MAS is the same as the progeny test scheme given previously in Table 13.1, even though the base conditions were somewhat different. Spelman et al. (1999) also assumed selection for a single trait with a heritability of 0.25. Even without MAS, a slight gain is obtained by allowing young sires to be used as bull sires, and a genetic gain of 9% is obtained if young sires with superior evaluations are also used directly as both sires of sires and in general service. As noted in Section 15.5, genetic gain with MAS used only to increase the accuracy of young bull evaluations for a standard progeny test scheme is limited, because the accuracy of the bull evaluations are already high. Thus, even if all the genetic variance is accounted for by QTL, the genetic gain is less than 25%. However, if young sires are selected for general service based on known QTL, the rate of genetic progress can be doubled. The maximum rate of genetic gain that can be obtained in the "all bulls" scheme is 2.2 times the rate of genetic gain in a standard progeny test. Theoretically, with half of the genetic variance due to known QTL, the rate of genetic gain obtained is greater than that possible with nucleus breeding schemes, as shown in Table 15.1. As explained in the previous chapter, very large expenditures can be justified to obtain this increase in the rate of genetic gain.

Table 15.2 Rates of genetic gain obtained in dairy breeding programmes with sires genotyped for known QTL (Spelman *et al.*, 1999)

Scheme*	Fraction of marked genetic variance	Genetic gain (σ_A/year)	Percent increase
Progeny test	0	0.258	-
	0.1	0.263	1.8
	0.5	0.283	15.5
	1.0	0.320	24.0
Sires of sires	0	0.260	-
	0.1	0.271	4.5
	0.5	0.326	25.4
	1.0	0.395	52.1
All bulls	0	0.282	-
	0.1	0.301	6.7
	0.5	0.437	55.2
	1.0	0.577	104.7

* The progeny test scheme is described in Figure 13.3. In the "sire of sires" scheme, young sires can also be selected as bull sires. In the "all bulls" scheme, young sires can be selected as both sires of bulls and sires of cows in general service.

15.8 Long-term considerations, MAS vs. selection index

Although most studies have looked at the gain obtained by a single generation of MAS, a few studies have also looked at the expected long-term effects of MAS.

Since the effect of long-term selection cannot be solved analytically, all of these studies are based on simulation, and the model used becomes critical. Even though Lande and Thompson (1990) maintain that new additive genetic variance arises by mutation at a rate on the order of 10^{-3} times the environmental variance per generation, all of these studies have assumed that no new genetic variance is generated during the course of the breeding programme.

Several studies simulated long-term selection for a single trait (de Koning and Weller, 1994; Meuwissen and Goddard, 196; Whittaker *et al.*, 1995; Zhang and Smith, 1992, 1993). Zhang and Smith (1992) and Whittaker *et al.* (1995) assumed that all of the genetic variance was due to 100 QTL with effects sampled from a normal distribution. de Koning and Weller (1994) assumed that all of the genetic variance was due to 10 QTL, with QTL variances sampled from a χ^2 distribution with 10 degrees of freedom. Both studies compared MAS to trait-based selection index. Zhang and Smith (1992) also considered selection only on QTL, and selection on a combined index of selection on phenotypic and marker information. Zhang and Smith (1992) assumed that the population was genotyped for 100 markers covering a genome of 20 Morgans. They assumed that the base population for selection was generated by several generations of crossing between two inbred lines, each homozygous for a different allele of each QTL and marker locus.

Zhang and Smith (1992) used a mixed model to estimate QTL effects, with the QTL considered random. The method of Goddard (1992), explained in Chapter seven, was used to derive the numerator matrix relationship for the QTL effects. Although 100 QTL were simulated, only the 20 greatest effects were used in selection. Zhang and Smith (1993) also considered MAS based on least-squares estimation of QTL effects. A modification of the method of Lande and Thompson (1990) described in Section 14.5 was used to generate the optimum selection index for combined selection on marker and phenotypic data. The phenotypic and genetic variance matrices now related to the estimated breeding values. Optimum selection index weights for the two sources of information were computed using Equation {14.4}, based on the variances of the two sources of information and the covariance between them. As noted in the previous chapter, the marker score has no economic value.

Three heritabilities were simulated: 0.1, 0.2 and 0.5. Selection was continued for 10 generations, but no new genetic variance was generated. Zhang and Smith (1992) found that MAS combined with selection index based on relative information always resulted in greater genetic gain than conventional selection index, or selection only on the marker information. Phenotypic selection was greater than selection based only on the 20 QTL with the greatest effects. The advantage of combined selection relative to phenotypic selection decreased as heritability increased, but the mean genetic level of the population was always greater, even after 10 generations of selection. The genetic mean with combined selection at the eighth generation was approximately equal to the genetic mean at the tenth generation with phenotypic selection.

For marker-based selection, Zhang and Smith (1993) found that rates of genetic gain were less than half if the QTL effects were estimated by least-squares. There are apparently two reasons for this result. In Section 6.7 we noted that estimating QTL as fixed effects and ignoring polygenic variance should result in biased QTL estimates (Kennedy *et al.*, 1992). In addition, as noted in Section 11.7, estimates of a sample of QTL effects selected by truncation on a critical value will be biased if the QTL are estimated as fixed effects.

Whittaker *et al.* (1995) compared three methods of MAS to phenotypic selection over 20 generations. Response in MAS was always greater, although the difference declined in later generations. As predicted by the theory given in the previous chapter, the relative gain with MAS was greater with lower heritability and increased population size.

de Koning and Weller (1994) assumed that genotypes for the 10 QTL were known without error in the MAS scheme. de Koning and Weller (1994) found similar results to Zhang and Smith (1992) for high heritability traits. Results for the relative selection efficiency (RSE) of MAS and trait-based selection are presented in Table 15.3 for three levels of heritability. For low heritability traits the advantage of MAS was greater. The difference between selection index and MAS decreased over time, but even after 10 generations, the relative efficiency of MAS to selection index with heritability of 0.2 was 1.24.

Gibson (1994) employed an infinitesimal model for genetic variance, excluding a single segregating QTL. He found that genetic response was greater via MAS in the early generations, but always greater for traditional selection index in subsequent generations. Traditional selection surpassed MAS at around generation 10. These results contradict the results from the four studies presented previously. All of these studies assumed that all the genetic variance was due to a fixed number of QTL, while Gibson (1994) assumed an infinitesimal model.

The apparent explanation for these contradictory results is that with the infinitesimal model genetic variance with MAS is reduced relative to selection index in the early generations due to inbreeding, which results in less genetic gain in later generations. Although the model of Gibson (1994) assumed an infinite number of loci affecting the quantitative trait, genetic variance is reduced due to inbreeding. Fixation is obtained for the segregating QTL, and no additional genetic variance is generated during the course of selection. A selection plateau is obtained by generation seven with MAS, and by generation 15 with phenotypic selection.

Villanuea *et al.* (1999) simulated a model similar to Gibson (1994), but restricted the increase in the rate of inbreeding. In this case, the rate of genetic gain with selection on a single identified QTL was always greater than trait-based selection.

Table 15.3 The relative efficiency of MAS with all QTL known for a two-trait or single-trait selection objective, relative to trait-based selection. The genetic correlation was –0.4, the environmental correlation was 0, and heritability of the two traits were equal, for the two-trait simulations. Results are the means of 10 replicates

Generation	Two-trait heritability			Single-trait heritability		
	0.05	0.20	0.40	0.05	0.20	0.40
1	-	-	-	-	-	-
2	5.10	2.55	1.95	4.10	2.16	1.55
3	4.50	2.40	1.82	3.84	2.03	1.57
4	4.15	2.08	1.67	3.52	1.98	1.50
5	3.58	1.87	1.46	3.27	1.91	1.47
6	3.14	1.63	1.32	3.08	1.78	1.41
7	2.71	1.45	1.23	2.85	1.62	1.37
8	2.42	1.36	1.18	2.71	1.48	1.30
9	2.21	1.29	1.15	2.50	1.35	1.23
10	2.02	1.25	1.13	2.27	1.24	1.16

15.9 MAS for a multitrait breeding objective with a single identified QTL

Lande and Thompson (1990) first considered MAS with a multiple-trait breeding objective. They derived general equations based on the variance matrix of marker scores for the individual traits, in addition to the phenotypic and genetic variance matrices. They noted that even with individual selection, the index weights for the phenotypic information would change if marker information was included. de Koning and Weller (1994) also considered multitrait selection with MAS. Lande and Thompson (1990) assumed a different index coefficient of the marker information for each trait, while de Koning and Weller (1994) used a single coefficient for the marker information.

de Koning and Weller (1994) considered the effect of a single identified QTL. The selection objective consisted of two traits, with phenotypic variances of σ_{p1}^2 and σ_{p2}^2, genetic variances of σ_{a1}^2 and σ_{a2}^2, a genetic correlation of ρ_a, and a phenotypic correlation of ρ_p. They assumed that there were only two alleles for the QTL segregating in the population, with frequencies of p and 1–p, and that the effect of the QTL on both traits was codominant. Thus, the genetic correlation between the traits on the QTL was either 1 or –1. They further assumed that, prior to selection, mating was random with respect to the QTL. No epistasis between the QTL and other loci was assumed. Therefore the correlation between the QTL and the other loci was zero. The genetic variances of the identified QTL on traits 1 and 2, σ_{Q1}^2 and σ_{Q2}^2, were computed as $p_1(\sigma_{a1}^2)$ and $p_2(\sigma_{a2}^2)$ where p_1 and p_2 are the fractions of the genetic variance for each trait attributed to the identified QTL. The effects of the QTL on trait 1 were a_1, 0, and $-a_1$, and the effects of the QTL on trait 2 were a_2, 0, and $-a_2$.

The phenotypic and genetic parameters of the two traits and the QTL were used to derive the optimum linear selection index, of the form:

$$I = b_{y1}Y_1 + b_{y2}Y_2 + b_Q Q \qquad \{15.7\}$$

where Y_1 and Y_2 are the phenotypic trait values for traits 1 and 2, Q is the "value" for the QTL, and b_{x1}, b_{x2} and b_Q are the index coefficients. Q was set equal to 2, 1, and 0 for locus effects of a_i, 0 and $-a_i$. The vector of optimum index coefficients, $\mathbf{b_I}$ is derived based on Equation {13.8}. Since all traits included in the index are also included in the vector of economic weights, $\mathbf{C} = \mathbf{G}$. The elements of $\mathbf{V_p}$ and $\mathbf{G}$ are given in Table 15.4.

Table 15.4 The genetic and phenotypic variance-covariance matrices for selection on two traits and a single QTL*

Trait	Genetic matrix			Phenotypic matrix		
	Trait 1	Trait 2	QTL	Trait 1	Trait 2	QTL
Trait 1	σ_{a1}^2	$\rho_a \sigma_{a1} \sigma_{a2}$	$2p(1-p)a_1$	σ_{p1}^2	$\rho_p \sigma_{p1} \sigma_{p2}$	$2p(1-p)a_1$
Trait 2	$\rho_a \sigma_{a1} \sigma_{a2}$	σ_{a2}^2	$2p(1-p)a_2$	$\rho_p \sigma_{p1} \sigma_{p2}$	σ_{p2}^2	$2p(1-p)a_2$
QTL	$2p(1-p)a_1$	$2p(1-p)a_2$	$2p(1-p)$	$2p(1-p)a_1$	$2p(1-p)a_2$	$2p(1-p)$

* Explanation of symbols is given in the text.

As noted in the previous chapter, the "heritability" of the QTL is 1. Therefore, the phenotypic variance of the QTL is equal to the genetic variance, and the phenotypic covariances are equal to the genetic covariances. These values differs from the values given in Lande and Thompson (1990), because they measured the standard deviation of the QTL in units of the quantitative trait, while de Koning and Weller (1994) measured the QTL in units of the number of alleles with "positive" effects. Since each quantitative trait is measured in different units, this notation is more appropriate for a multitrait breeding objective. The economic values for the two traits were set equal to unity, and the economic value for the QTL was 0, as in the previous chapter.

The RSE of the index including the QTL information was computed based on the formula of Cunningham (1969). Maximum genetic response will be obtained when all traits with genetic correlations with the traits in the aggregate genotype are included in the index. If one of the traits included in the aggregate genotype is deleted from the index, the variance of the selection index will be reduced by b_i^2/w_i, where b_i is the index coefficient for the trait deleted (in this case the marker score), and w_i is the diagonal element for this trait in $\mathbf{P}^{-1}$. RSE is then computed as follows:

$$RSE = \frac{(\mathbf{b_1'V_p b_1})^{1/2}}{(\mathbf{b_1'Pb_1} - b_i^2/w_i)^{1/2}} \quad \{15.8\}$$

Comparisons of RSE for a single-trait and a two-trait selection objective as a function of heritability are given in Table 15.5. The proportion of the additive genetic variance due to the QTL was set at 0.10 or 0.30. For two-trait selection, the genetic and phenotypic correlations were –0.40, and the heritability of the traits were equal. It was assumed that $p_1 = p_2$. Equal frequencies were assumed for the two QTL alleles, thus: $\sigma_{Qi}^2 = \frac{1}{2} a_i^2$, where a_i^2 is the substitution effects of the QTL for trait i. As shown in the previous chapter, the RSE of MAS increased as a function of the proportion of the additive genetic variance associated with the QTL (Lande and Thompson, 1990). This also occurred with two genetically correlated traits. The increase in selection efficiency was generally two to three times greater for the two-trait selection objective, as compared to the single-trait objective. The relative increase for the two-trait breeding objective compared to the single-trait objective increased with increased heritability.

Table 15.5 Comparison of relative selection efficiencies of MAS and phenotypic selection for a single-trait and a two-trait selection objective, as a function of the heritabilities, when a single QTL was known. The proportion of the additive genetic variance due to the QTL was set at 0.10 or 0.30. For two-trait selection, the genetic and phenotypic correlations were –0.40, and the heritabilities of the traits were equal

Heritability	Proportion = 0.10		Proportion = 0.30	
	Two traits	One trait	Two traits	One trait
0.05	2.668	1.678	4.472	2.549
0.10	1.948	1.348	3.162	1.872
0.20	1.464	1.152	2.236	1.422
0.45	1.124	1.035	1.491	1.110
0.80	1.011	1.003	1.118	1.010

15.10 MAS for a multitrait breeding objective with multiple identified QTL

de Koning and Weller (1994) compared selection on known loci affecting quantitative traits to phenotypic selection index for a single- and a two-trait selection objective. Two situations were simulated: a single known quantitative locus, and 10 identified loci accounting for all the additive genetic variance. RSE of MAS relative to trait-based selection was higher for two-trait selection than for single-trait selection. The advantage of MAS was greater when the traits were negatively correlated. RSE of MAS relative to phenotypic selection for a single locus responsible for 0.1 of the genetic variance was 1.11 with heritabilities of 0.45 and 0.2, and zero genetic and phenotypic correlations between the traits.

Results are presented in Table 15.3 for selection based on 10 loci. RSE of MAS for 10 known loci was greater for multitrait selection with a negative genetic correlation between the traits, as compared to single-trait selection. The difference in RSE between multitrait and single-trait selection decreased in later generations. Allele fixation for MAS was obtained for all loci after 10 generations. Response to trait-based selection continued through generation 15, and approached the response obtained with MAS after 10 generations. The cumulative genetic response by MAS was only 80% of the economically optimum genotype, because the less favorable allele reached fixation for some loci, generally those with effects in opposite directions on the two traits. By the tenth generation, more than 90% of the loci reached fixation with direct selection on the QTL, while only about 30% of the loci reached fixation with trait-based selection. Even after 15 generations, only 60% of the loci reached fixation with trait-based selection.

As long as the residual and genetic correlations were similar, the direction of the correlation did not affect the RSE of MAS, as compared to trait-based selection. However, if the genetic and residual correlations were in opposite direction the RSE of MAS increased. Results are given in Table 15.6.

15.11 Summary

Again we must emphasize that a little bit of genetic gain can have a huge economic value. Thus, relatively large costs in genotyping can be justified to increase rates of genetic gain by only a few percent. It is not possible to consider within a single chapter all possible scenarios for MAS. As seen from the examples given, radically different results can be obtained depending on the breeding scheme and the assumptions employed. There does seem to be a consensus emerging that application of MAS could result in rather significant genetic gains, at least for several generations. Consideration of 10 or more generations does not seem very relevant, because profit horizons are at most 20 years, and breeding objectives tend to change over time anyway. Two other factors should also be considered within the context of long-term breeding programmes. First, some positive QTL alleles that are at very low frequency in the initial generations will be eventually become more common through trait-based selection. These alleles will only become candidates for MAS in later generations, after they reach a frequency high enough to be detected. Second, with normal rates of spontaneous mutation, it does not appear that the fixation of desirable alleles after a few generations of MAS is a serious problem.

Table 15.6 The effect of the environmental correlation on the efficiency of marker-assisted selection with all QTL known for a two-trait selection objective, relative to trait-based selection. The genetic correlation was –0.4 for all simulations. Heritabilities for the traits were 0.40 and 0.20. Results are the means of 15 replicates

	Environmental correlations		
Generation	–0.4	0	0.4
1	-	-	-
2	1.739	1.960	2.275
3	1.588	1.878	2.098
4	1.466	1.683	1.935
5	1.332	1.523	1.695
6	1.241	1.404	1.520
7	1.173	1.315	1.413
8	1.137	1.238	1.322
9	1.107	1.195	1.242
10	1.078	1.147	1.179

Chapter sixteen:

Marker-Assisted Introgression

16.1 Introduction

"Introgression" is the process whereby a trait, or a specific gene is transferred from one strain, denoted the "donor strain" to another strain, denoted the "recipient strain". It is generally assumed that, except for the desired gene in the donor strain, the recipient strain is economically superior. The prime example is disease resistance genes from wild relatives of domestic strains. Another example is a very advantageous gene that appears by mutation in a domestic population, such as the Booroola gene in sheep, which increases frequency of multiple births in females (Gootwine *et al.*, 1998). The traditional approach, illustrated in Figure 16.1, has been to first cross the donor and recipient strains to produce an F-1, which will be heterozygous for all loci that differ between the two strains. A series of BCes to the domestic strain is then performed, but only individuals carrying the donor allele for the gene being introgressed are selected as parents for the next BC generation. After the final BC generation the BC progeny are mated among themselves, and individuals homozygous for the donor allele of the introgressed gene are selected. The process of introgression generally requires between six and ten generations to obtain a population homozygous for the donor gene, but with more than 95% of the recipient genome.

Various studies, starting with Young and Tanksley (1989) and Hillel *et al.* (1990), have suggested that introgression can be accelerated by selecting backcross (BC) individuals based on a series of genetic markers with differing alleles in the donor and recipient strains. Hospital and Charcosset (1997) denoted this process "marker-assisted introgression" (MAI). Analytical equations to compute the expected fraction of the recipient genome retrieved with selection have been derived only for the first BC generation. Numerous simulation studies using different schemes have shown that, in general, MAI can decrease the time required for gene introgression by about two generations.

In the following section we will present general considerations of MAI. In Section 16.3 we will consider MAI of a major gene into an inbred line. Several recent studies have also considered MAI for QTL, which can be performed only using genetic markers. MAI for a single QTL will be considered in Section 16.4, and MAI for multiple QTL will be considered in Section 16.5.

MAI can also be applied to an outbred population under selection for quantitative traits. In this case, though, MAI will only be economically viable if the gain due to the introgressed gene is greater than the loss sustained by reduced selection on the remainder of the genome. MAI in an outbred population will also be considered in Section 16.4. If multiple QTL are introgressed, then a number of different breeding strategies can be applied, and these will be compared in Section 16.5, based on efficiency and costs.

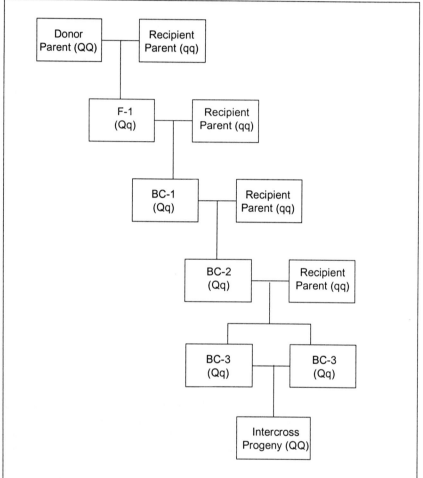

Figure 16.1 An introgression breeding scheme. The donor allele, Q, for the introgressed gene is transferred into the recipient strain. Although only three backcross generations are shown, in practice the number of BC generations will generally be greater

16.2 Marker-assisted introgression - general considerations

Under a classical BC breeding scheme, the expected fraction of the genome of the recipient parent in BC generation b, G(b) is computed as follows:

$$G(b) = 1 - (\tfrac{1}{2})^{b+1} \qquad \{16.1\}$$

Even without markers, G(b) can be increased by selection of BC progeny based on their similarity to the recipient phenotype, if the trait can be scored on the candidates for selection (Visscher *et al.*, 1996a). As noted in Chapter fourteen, this is not always possible. Furthermore, in an introgression breeding scheme, G(b) will be decreased slightly relative to Equation {16.1} due to "linkage drag", the persistence of donor genetic material linked to the introgressed gene (Brinkman and Frey, 1977). Linkage drag becomes more important in the later BC generations, in which the chromosomal segment containing the introgressed gene will be a major component of the donor genome remaining in the BC population.

Young and Tanksley (1989) suggested that linkage drag could be reduced by selection on genetic markers tightly linked to the introgressed gene. Assuming that the two strains have different alleles for the linked genetic markers, it should be possible to select for the donor allele of the introgressed gene and the recipient alleles for the flanking markers. If the introgressed gene is flanked by two genetic markers, individuals with the desired genotype would be produced only in the event of double recombination, which will be exceedingly rare, if all three loci are tightly linked. Therefore, Young and Tanksley (1989) suggested that individuals with the desired genotype for the introgressed gene and one of the two flanking markers could be selected in alternating generations.

Hillel *et al.* (1990) suggested that a large battery of genetic markers scattered throughout the genome could be used to select BC progeny containing a greater than expected fraction of the recipient genome. This can be denoted "background selection", as opposed to the "foreground selection" considered by Young and Tanksley (1989). Hillel *et al.* (1990) presented theoretical distributions and variances of the relative percentage of the donor genome in the selected BC progeny without considering information on the map location of the markers. Their analysis was based on using DNA fingerprint markers, and they assumed a random distribution of markers throughout the genome. Visscher *et al.* (1996a) noted that the formulas of Hillel *et al.* (1990) do not account for recombination around the marker loci.

Visscher *et al.* (1996a) also considered the situation in which the recipient strain is not an inbred line, but rather an outbred population in an ongoing selection program. In this case it is necessary to select the BC progeny for the donor gene and the desired selection index, rather than just maximum genetic content from the recipient strain. In addition, Visscher *et al.* (1996a) also considered the situation in which the introgressed gene is itself a QTL, rather than a major gene. This of course complicates the introgression breeding scheme. Markers flanking the QTL will be required in order to select BC progeny that received the donor QTL allele. Furthermore, as noted in Chapter ten, there will always be uncertainty with respect to the QTL location. Therefore the flanking markers must be sufficiently distant from the QTL so that it will be possible to determine with relative certainty that the QTL is in fact located between the flanking markers.

It should be noted that although MAI does decrease the number of generations required, it increases two key cost elements. First with traditional introgression, half of the progeny will carry the donor allele for the introgressed gene, and all of these can be used as parents in the next generation. However, if only a small fraction of the progeny is selected based on genetic markers, then many more individuals must be produced each generation. Second, genotyping costs for a large number of markers at each generation will also be significant.

16.3 Marker-assisted introgression of a major gene into an inbred line

MAI of a major gene to an inbred line was analyzed in detail by Hospital *et al.* (1992) using genetic markers for both foreground and background selection. They assumed that BC individuals to be used as parents in the next generation were selected by a linear selection index based on the progenies' marker genotypes. The general linear selection index formula for n traits is given in Equation {13.7}, and was modified as follows:

$$I_s = b_1 y_1 + b_2 y_2 + ... + b_n y_n = \mathbf{b_m' m_s} \qquad \{16.2\}$$

where $\mathbf{b_m}$ represents the index coefficient for $\mathbf{m_s}$, the marker scores. $\mathbf{m_s}$ is equal to zero or one for the donor or recipient allele respectively, and M is the total number of markers monitored. Hospital *et al.* (1992) assumed that only individuals carrying the donor allele for the introgressed gene are selected. In addition, differential weights are assigned to markers located on the chromosome containing the introgressed gene and to markers located on the other chromosomes. If the markers are equally spaced along all the other chromosomes, including markers at the chromosome ends, then the index weights are 0.5 for markers at the chromosome ends, and 1.0 for all other markers (Visscher, 1996).

Hospital *et al.* (1992) assumed that selection was based solely on marker genotypes, without considering phenotypes. Hillel *et al.* (1990) assumed a random distribution of genetic markers. Hospital *et al.* (1992) considered both a random distribution of markers, and a sample of markers selected to maximize the efficiency of MAI. The Haldane mapping function (Haldane 1919) i. e. zero interference, was assumed throughout.

For background selection on chromosomes that did not carry the gene being introgressed, two markers per chromosome of length 100 cM were nearly optimal. Increasing the number of markers had virtually no effect on the rate of recovery of the recipient genome. Optimal marker locations were at positions 20 and 80 cM. With a random distribution of markers, doubling the number of markers per chromosome resulted in nearly the same efficiency as optimally selected markers.

Hospital *et al.* (1992) provide formula to compute the optimum locations for markers on the chromosome containing the introgressed gene. As noted previously, the objective is to obtain the recipient genotype for the marker loci, and the donor allele for the introgressed gene. Since this requires a double crossing over, the probability for desired haplotype will be very low if the genes are tightly linked. However, if the markers are distant from the introgressed gene, then the selected individuals are likely to retain a significant segment from the donor genome. If 10% of the BC individuals are selected, nearly equal efficiency is obtained with spacing from 10 to 50 cM between each marker and the introgressed gene in the first BC generation. In later generations the optimal marker spacing decreases. By the third BC generation optimal marker spacing is 5 cM.

As noted previously, by employing MAI it is possible to decrease the number of generations by two, as compared to selection only on the introgressed gene, to obtain the same proportion of the recipient genome. For example, without markers six BC generations are required to obtain 99% of the recipient genome. The same fraction can be obtained after four BC generations of MAI.

16.4 Marker-assisted introgression of a QTL into a donor population under selection

Visscher *et al.* (1996a) assumed that the recipient population was under selection for a single quantitative trait with a known heritability. They considered both introgression on a major gene and a QTL. In the latter case they accounted for uncertainty with respect to the QTL location. They assumed two-stage selection among the BC progeny. In the first stage, BC progeny carrying the donor allele for the introgressed gene are selected. If the introgressed gene is a QTL, then selection will be for the donor marker haplotype for the two markers flanking the putative QTL location.

In the second stage, similar to the equation of Lande and Thompson (1990), given in Section 14.3, selection is for the composite index of the form:

$$I = b_y y + \mathbf{b_m}'\mathbf{m_s} \qquad \{16.3\}$$

where b_y represents the index coefficients for the quantitative trait records, y, and the other terms are as given in Equation {16.2}. In this case, unlike the model of Lande and Thompson (1990), b_y and y are scalars, because only a single trait is considered, while $\mathbf{b_m}$ and $\mathbf{m_s}$ are vectors.

In addition to selection in the second stage based on the index given in Equation {16.3}, Visscher *et al.* (1996a) also considered random selection, phenotypic selection, and selection based only on the genetic markers, similar to Hospital et al. (1992). Visscher et al. (1996a) assumed from one to 11 equally spaced markers per chromosome, and heritability of either 0.1 or 0.4 for the quantitative trait under selection. Selection proportions were 2.5% for males and 25% for females.

For background selection only with a heritability of 0.1 and selection on males, selection on a single marker was superior to phenotypic selection until the sixth BC generation. There was virtually no difference between selection on a single marker per chromosome up to 11 markers per chromosome, even to the sixth BC generation. There was virtually no gain from selection on the composite index including phenotypes, as compared to selection only on marker genotype.

If the introgressed gene is a QTL, selection of the donor QTL allele is based on flanking markers. In this case it will not be possible to determine with certainty which BC progeny received the donor QTL allele. Therefore, the frequency of the donor allele in the selected individuals will be less than 50% with either phenotypic selection, or selection based on additional markers. The reduction in allelic frequency is most severe if selection of the donor QTL allele is based on a single linked marker. The reduction in donor QTL allele frequency is even more severe if the QTL location is estimated from the data. A minimum marker bracket of four times the standard deviation of the estimated QTL position is required to obtain a 95% confidence interval that the QTL is in fact located within the marker bracket. For a 99% confidence interval the minimum bracket will be more than five times the standard deviation, but increases with increases in the standard deviation. If the standard deviation for the QTL location is 4 cM, it is not possible to obtain a 99% confidence interval for QTL location if the QTL is less than 25 cM from the end of the chromosome. Hospital and Charcosset (1997) found similar results.

Visscher et al. (1997) simulated introgression for a nucleus swine population under selection for a quantitative trait with a heritability of 0.25. They found that the reduction in genetic gain for the main objective of selection due to introgression without MAS was equivalent to between one and two generations. If MAS was employed, this loss could be slightly reduced if the number of generations of BCing was fewer than five. They did not consider the possibility of reducing the generation interval via MAS, by breeding prior to expression of the introgressed allele.

16.5 Marker-assisted introgression for multiple genes

Hospital and Charcosset (1997) and Koudande et al. (2000) considered MAI for up to three QTL. Hospital and Charcosset (1997) considered the following two schemes:

1. A "simultaneous design" in which a single BC population is monitored for all of the donor QTL alleles.
2. A "pyramidal design" in which each QTL is monitored in a separate BC

population. In the final generation these populations are mated to produce individuals carrying the donor alleles for all the introgressed QTL.

Many more individuals must be bred and genotyped if several QTL are monitored. For a traditional introgression breeding scheme for a single gene, one-half of the BC progeny at each generation will have the donor allele. However, if three unlinked genes are introgressed, only one-eighth of the progeny will have the desired genotype for all three loci. If 10% of the progeny are selected based on the index given in Equation {16.2} or {16.3} and only 10 individuals are required for mating, then 800 individuals must be genotyped in each generation. This of course assumes that it is possible to produce 160 progeny for each mating pair selected.

Koundande *et al.* (2000) noted that if multiple BC lines are maintained then several combinations are possible. For example, instead of three BC lines each maintaining a donor allele for one of the three QTL, it is possible to breed two BC lines one maintaining the donor alleles for one QTL, and the other BC line maintaining the donor alleles for the other two QTL. Alternatively, two of the donor QTL alleles can be maintained in each of the two BC populations with one locus in common between the two populations. The last alternative is apparently optimal. This option requires 76% fewer genotypes, 68% fewer animals to be genotyped, and costs 75% less than the simultaneous design.

16.6 Summary

In this final chapter we reviewed the literature on MAI. Analytical equations to compute the efficiency of MAI relative to traditional introgression can only be derived from the first BC generation. Therefore all of the studies that have considered MAI have been based on simulations. In general, MAI can decrease the number of generations required by about two, but requires producing many more individuals, which must also be genotyped. If the gene to be introgressed is a QTL, which cannot be scored phenotypically, then MAI is the only alternative. In order to transfer several genes from a donor to a recipient strain, pyramidal schemes, in which multiple BC lines are produced, are more efficient than selecting simultaneously for all loci within a single breeding population.

Glossary of Symbols

Matrices and vectors are listed in **bold** type. Matrices and vectors are listed before scalars with the same symbol. Capital letters are listed before the same lower case letters. The section in which the symbol is first mentioned is listed in parentheses after the definition. Latin symbols are listed first, then Greek, and then other symbols. Symbols that appear fewer than three times in the text are not listed.

Latin Symbols

A	Numerator relationship matrix (3.2)
a	Vector of additive genetic effects (3.9)
AI	Artificial insemination (13.6)
A_i	Effect of genotype i (8.3)
AIL	Advanced intercross lines (10.4)
a_i	Additive genetic effect for individual or trait i (3.9)
b	Vector of selection index coefficients (13.4)
b	Linear regression coefficient (2.5)
BC	Backcross, produced by mating F-1 individuals to one of the parental strains (4.3)
B_i	"Block" effect (4.4)
b_i	The index coefficient for trait i (13.4)
b_m	The index coefficient for the marker score (14.4)
bp	DNA base pairs (1.7)
$\mathbf{b}_y$	The vector of index coefficients for the quantitative trait records (14.4)
C	The genetic covariance matrix between the measured traits in **x** and the breeding values in **y** (13.4)

Glossary 251

C	The ratio of the cost of genotyping each individual to the cost of phenotyping each individual (9.3)
C_c	Annual costs of the breeding programme (13.5)
C_g	The cost of genotyping a single individual (9.3)
CI	Confidence interval (8.8)
C_{jk}	Effect of cow k, daughter of sire j (3.8)
cM	centi-Morgans = M/100 (1.7)
Cov(x,y)	Covariance between x and y (5.4)
C_p	The cost of phenotyping a single individual (9.3)
C_r	Coefficient of coincidence for genetic recombination (1.6).
C_T	The net present value of the total costs of the breeding programme (13.5)
CWER	"Comparison-wise" error rate (11.2)
d	The discount rate (13.5)
df	Degrees of freedom (2.9)
DH	Double hapliods (4.3)
D_k	Effect of dam k (3.11)
D_t	Difference between the mean of the tail samples for the quantitative trait (9.4)
DYD	Daughter yield deviations (6.11)
E(.)	Expectation of (.) (5.5)
EBV	Estimated breeding values (6.11)
ECM	Expectation/conditional maximization algorithm (6.7)
ELOD	Expectation of the log of the likelihood ratio (5.12)

e	Vector of residuals (2.4)
e	The base for natural logarithms and is approximately equal to 2.72 (2.7)
exp[.]	[.] to the power of e (3.14)
F	A matrix the relates the QTL additive effects of non-parents to parents (7.5)
F	The fraction of the genome under analysis for QTL (7.11)
F-1	Progeny of a mating between two inbred lines (4.3)
F-2	Progeny from self-breeding of F-1 individuals (4.3)
F-3	Progeny from self-breeding of F-2 individuals (4.8)
FDR	False discovery rate (11.4)
FS	Full-sibs (4.11)
FWER	"Family-wise" error rate (11.2)
f(.)	Statistical density function (3.12)
G	Additive genetic variance matrix (3.2)
GDD	Grand-daughter design (4.11)
GM	Gametic model (4.11)
GS_i	Effect of grandsire I (4.8)
$\mathbf{G_v}$	The variance matrix among the QTL gametic effects (4.10)
g_i	Genetic effect of individual i (4.7)
H	Herd effect (3.2)
H^2	The "heritability" of the QTL (12.4)
h^2	Heritability, the ratio of the additive genetic variance to the phenotypic variance (3.4)

HS	Half-sibs (4.11)
H_{xy}^2	The two-dimensional analog of H^2 (12.4)
I	Identity matrix (3.2)
i_A	The selection intensity for adults (14.6)
IAM	Individual animal model (3.9)
IBD	Identical by descent (4.7)
i_m	The selection intensity for immature individuals (14.6)
i_p	The selection intensity in standardized units when a fraction p of the sample is selected (9.4)
I_s	The linear index (13.4)
ISCS	Interval-specific congenic strains (10.7)
$i_{\male}$	The selection intensity in males (14.6)
$i_{\female}$	The selection intensity in females (14.6)
K	Number of hypotheses rejected (11.4)
k	Number of independent exponentially distributed variables, each with a parameter value of λ (10.2)
k_M	Effective number of alleles 911.6)
L	Likelihood function (2.7)
L_G	Generation length in years (13.2)
L_{ik}	Effect of "line" j nested within genotype I (8.3)
LOD	Log base 10 of the likelihoods ratio (6.18)
M	Matrix of phenotypic and marker data (7.12)
M	Morgans, expected number of events of recombination within a chromosomal segment (1.6)

m	Number of parameters, markers, or hypotheses tested (2.7)	
MAI	Marker-assisted introgression (16.1)	
MAS	Marker-assisted selection (13.5)	
M_G	Genome length in Morgans (11.2)	
M_i	Allele i of a marker locus (4.1)	
M_{ij}	The effect of the jth allele, nested within the ith parent (4.6)	
M_{ijkl}	Mendilian sampling effect of individual l with sire j and dam k (3.11)	
ML	Maximum likelihood (2.1)	
MLE	Maximum likelihood estimate (2.7)	
MOET	Multiple ovulation and embryo transplant (13.7)	
m_s	The net marker score (14.4)	
N	Sample size (2.3)	
n	Number of progeny per marker genotype class (8.2)	
Na	Number of marker alleles segregating in the population (4.5)	
N_c	Number of chromosomes (11.2)	
N_E	The effective number of loci (15.3)	
N_e	The effective population size (11.6)	
N_g	Number of inbred lines (8.3)	
N_k	Number of chromosomal intervals analysed (11.5)	
N_l	Number of individuals per line (8.3)	
N_o	The original effective population size (11.6)	
N_Q	The detectable number of QTL (7.11)	

Glossary 255

N_z	Number of individuals scored for the quantitative trait (9.4)
P	Matrix equal to: $\mathbf{V}^{-1} - \mathbf{V}^{-1}\mathbf{X}(\mathbf{X'V}^{-1}\mathbf{X})^{-1}\mathbf{XV}^{-1}$ (3.15)
p	Vector of permanent environmental effects (3.9)
p	Probability or allele frequency (2.7)
PCR	Polymerase chain reaction {1.5}
pev	Prediction error variance (3.5)
PFIM	Proportion of fully informative matings (4.5)
$P_{(i)}$	Probability for the result obtained if null hypothesis i is correct (11.4)
p_j	Permanent environmental effect of individual j (3.9)
PIC	Polymorphism information content (4.5)
p_m	The fraction of the additive genetic variance associated with the genetic markers (14.5)
PT	Progeny test (13.6)
P_v	Probability of sire QTL genotype v (6.12)
q	$mP_{(i)}/I$ where m is the number of hypotheses tested, and $P_{(i)}$ is the probability for the result obtained if null hypothesis i is correct (11.4)
q*	The level at which the FDR is controlled (11.4)
Q_i	Allele i of a quantitative trait locus (4.1)
Q^m_o	Maternal allele of individual o (7.3)
Q^p_o	Paternal allele of individual o (7.3)
QTL	Quantitative trait locus (loci) (1.1)
R	Residual variance matrix (3.2)
R	Recombination frequency between two markers (1.6)

256 *Quantitative Trait Loci Analysis in Animals*

R(.)	Reduction in sum of squares (3.13)
REML	Restricted maximum likelihood (3.1)
RFLP	Restriction fragment length polymorphism (1.5)
RIL	Recombinant inbred lines (4.3)
RSE	The relative selection efficiency of two different indices (14.5)
RSS	Residual sum of squares (5.3)
R_v	The cumulative discounted returns to year T (13.5)
r	Recombination frequency between a genetic marker and a quantitative trait locus (4.1)
r_1	Recombination frequencies between marker locus M and quantitative trait locus Q (5.3)
r_2	Recombination frequency between quantitative trait locus Q and marker locus N (5.3)
r_d	$1/(1+d)$ (13.5)
r_L	Recombination between a marker and a QTL in RIL (8.3)
r_t	Recombination frequency for AIL in generation t between two linked loci (10.4)
S	Sire effect (3.2)
SD	Standard deviation (8.4)
SE	Standard error (8.8)
SO_{ijk}	Effect of son k of grandsire i (4.8)
T	The profit horizon (13.5)
t	Generation number (10.4)
TC	Test cross, progeny of F-1 individuals and a third strain (4.3)

Glossary 257

T_C	Total costs (9.3)
T^m	The mth central moments of a sample (2.3)
Tr(.)	Trace of a matrix (3.13)
u	Vector of random effects (3.2)
u	Estimated genetic value of an individual (13.2)
V	Variance matrix for a random variable (2.6)
V	The nominal value of the annual rate of genetic gain (13.5)
v	Vector of economic values (13.4)
$\mathbf{v_g}$	Vector of gametic additive genetic effects (4.10)
v_i^m	Additive effect of the maternal allele of individual i (4.10)
v_i^p	Additive effect of the paternal allele of individual i (4.10)
$\mathbf{V_p}$	Phenotypic variance matrix (13.4)
V_Q	The variance due to a single detectable QTL (7.11)
V_π	The experimental error variance for π_f (9.6)
W	Incidence matrix for the gametic additive genetic effects (4.10)
X	Matrix of coefficients for the solutions in a linear model (2.4)
x	value of independent variable in an analysis model (2.5)
y	Vector of observations for the dependent variable (2.4)
y	Value of the dependent variable in an analysis model (2.3)
$\bar{y}$	Mean of sample of a dependent variable (2.3)
Z	Incidence matrix for random effects (3.2)
Z_p	The standard normal distribution value for probability p (8.2)

Greek Symbols

α	The type I error (8.1)
α_a	$2p(1-p)a$ where p is the allelic frequency and a is the additive effect (15.2)
α_c	The "comparison-wise" error rate (11.2)
α_f	The "family-wise error rate (11.2)
β	Vector of fixed effect solutions (3.2)
β	The type II error (8.1)
χ^2	The Chi-squared statistical distribution (2.9)
Δ	The mean map distance between markers in Morgans (11.2)
ΔG	Genetic gain per year (13.2)
Δp	The change in allele frequency due to selection (13.3)
δ	Distance to be minimized (2.15)
δ_g	Substitution effect in units of the residual standard deviation of the design (10.3)
δ_n	Expected contrast between marker groups (8.2)
δ_r	The maximum linkage distance at which linkage can be detected (7.11)
ε	Vector of residuals for the gametic model (7.4)
Φ	The cumulative normal distribution function (2.15)
ϕ	The response of the vector of individual traits, to one generation of selection on the selection index (13.4)
ϕ	The response due to one generation of selection on a single trait (13.2)

Glossary 259

ϕ_n	The deviation of the progeny polygenic value from the mean of the parental values (7.5)
γ	The ratio of the variances of residual and another random effect (3.8)
η	The mutation rate (11.6)
φ_p	The ordinate, or density, of the standard normal distribution at point of truncation p (9.4)
Λ	A matrix relating the QTL effects of parents to progeny (7.4)
λ	The parameter of the exponential distribution (7.11)
μ	Population mean (2.5)
μ_i	Mean of individuals with quantitative trait locus genotype i (5.3)
$\mu(Z)$	The expected number of regions with a standard normal distribution value greater than the critical value for α_c (11.2)
Π	Multiplicative sum (2.7)
π	The ratio of the circumference to the diameter of a circle, approximately 3.141 (2.7)
π_f	The mean of the genotype frequencies of Mm in the high tail and mm in the low tail (9.6)
π_j	Fraction of alleles identical by descent for sib-pair j (4.7)
θ	Vector of parameters (2.4)
θ	A parameter (2.2)
Σ	Arithmetic sum (2.3)
ρ	Residual correlation (3.7)
ρ_a	The accuracy of the genetic evaluation (13.2)
ρ_M	The expected rate of recombination per Morgan (11.2)

σ	Standard deviation of a population (2.7)
σ_A^2	The additive genetic variance (3.9)
σ_e^2	The residual variance (5.12)
σ_G^2	The genetic variance between lines (8.3)
σ_{Is}	The standard deviation of the selection index (13.4)
σ_m^2	The additive genetic variance explained by the genetic markers (14.5)
σ_m^{2*}	The variance of the marker score after selection on juveniles (14.7)
σ_s^2	The sire component of variance (3.22)
σ_t	Within marker genotype standard deviations for the tail samples (9.4)
σ_v^2	The variance due to the QTL (5.12)
σ_{xy}	Covariance between x and y (3.7)
σ_z^2	The phenotypic variance (14.5)
τ	The number of years from the beginning of a breeding programme until first returns are realized (13.5)
τ_j	The jth threshold on the scale of the continuous variable (6.17)

Other Symbols

∂	Partial derivative (2.9)
$\otimes$	The "Kronecker product" of two matrices or a matrix and a scalar (3.7)
$\lvert . \rvert$	Determinant of a matrix (3.14)

References

Andersson-Elkund, L., Danell, B. and Rendel, J. (1990) Associations between blood groups, blood protein polymorphisms and breeding values for production traits in Swedish Red & White dairy bulls. *Anim. Genet.* **21**: 361-376.

Bailey, N. T. (1961) *Introduction to the Mathematical Theory of Genetical Linkage.* Clarendon Press, Oxford.

Baret, P. V., Knott, S. A. and Vissher, P. M. (1998) Distribution of the maximum likelihood test statistic of QTL detection in a half-sib design. *Proc. 6th World Cong. Genet. Appl. Livest. Prod.* Armidale, NSW, Australia. **26**: 217-220.

Beavis, W. D. (1994) The power and deceit of QTL experiments: lessons for comparative QTL studies. *Ann. Corn Sorghum Research Conf.* Washington, D. C. **49**: 252-268.

Beckmann, J. S. and Soller, M. (1983) Restriction fragment length polymorphisms in genetic improvement: methodologies, mapping and costs. *Theor. Appl. Genet.* **67**: 35-43.

Benjamini, Y. and Hochberg, Y. (1995) Controlling the false discovery rate: a practical and powerful approach to multiple testing. *J. R. Statist. Soc. B.* **57**: 289-300.

Botstein, D., White, R. L., Skolnick, M. and Davis, R. W. (1980) Construction of a genetic linkage map in man using restriction fragment length polymorphisms. *Am. J. Human Genet.* **32**: 314-331.

Bovenhuis, H. and Weller, J. I. (1994) Mapping and analysis of dairy cattle quantitative trait loci by maximum likelihood methodology using milk protein genes as genetic markers. *Genetics* **137**: 267-280.

Bovenhuis, J., van Arendonk, J. A. M., Davis, G., Elsen, J.-M., Haley, C. S., Hill, W. G., Baret, P. V., Hetzel, D.J.S. and Nicholas, F. W. (1997) Detection and mapping of quantitative trait loci in farm animals. *Livest. Prod. Sci.* **52**: 134-144.

Brascamp, E. W. (1984) Selection indices with constraints. *Anim. Breed. Abs.* **52**: 645-654.

Brascamp, E. W., van Arendonk, J. A. M. and Groen, A. F. (1993) Economic appraisal of the utilization of genetic markers in dairy cattle breeding. *J. Dairy Sci.* **76**: 1204-1213.

Brinkman, M. A. and Frey, K. J. (1977) Yield component analysis of oat isolines that produce different grain yields. *Crop Sci.* **17**: 165-168.

Brookes, A. J. (1999) The essence of SNPs. *Gene* **234**: 177-186.

Cantet, R. J. C. and Smith, C. (1991) Reduced animal model for marker assisted selection using best linear unbiased prediction. *Genet. Sel. Evol.* **23**: 221-233

Churchill, G. A. and Doerge, R. W. (1994) Empirical threshold values for quantitative trait mapping. *Genetics* **138**: 963-971.

Coppieters, W. Kvasz, A., Farnir, F., Arranz, J. J., Grisart, B., Mackinnon, M. and Georges, M. (1998) A rank-based nonparametric method for mapping quantitative trait loci in outbred half-sib pedigrees: application to milk production in a granddaughter design. *Genetics* **149**: 1547-1555.

Cowan, C. M., Dentine, M. R. and Colye, T. (1992) Chromosome substitution effects associated with k-Casein and b-Lactoglobulin in Holstein cattle. *J. Dairy Sci.* **75**: 1097-1104.

Cunningham, E. P. (1969) The relative efficiencies of selection indexes. *Acta Agri. Scand.* **19**: 45-48.

Da, Y., VanRaden, P. M., Ron, M., Beever, J. M., Paszek, A. A., Song, J. Wiggans, G. R., Ma, R. Weller, J. I. and Lewin, H. A. (1999) Standardization and conversion of marker polymorphism measures. *Anim. Biotechnol.* **10**: 25-35.

Dahlquist, G. and Bjorck, A. (1974) *Numerical Methods.* Prentice Hall, Englewood Cliffs.

Darvasi, A. (1990) *Analysis of genes affecting quantitative traits with the aid of bracketed pairs of genetic markers and maximum likelihood methodology.* M. Sc. Thesis, The Hebrew University, Jerusalem, Israel.

Darvasi, A. (1998) Experimental strategies for the genetic dissection of complex traits in animal models. *Nat. Genet.* **18**: 19-24.

Darvasi, A. and Soller, M. (1992) Selective genotyping for determination of linkage between a marker locus and a quantitative trait locus. *Theor. Appl. Genet.* **85**: 353-359.

Darvasi, A. and Soller, M. (1994a) Optimum spacing of genetic markers for determining linkage between marker loci and quantitative trait loci. *Theor. Appl. Genet.* **89**: 351-357.

Darvasi, A. and Soller, M. (1994b) Selective DNA pooling for determination of linkage between a marker locus and a quantitative trait loci. *Genetics* **138**: 1365-1373.

Darvasi, A. and Soller, M. (1995) Advanced intercross lines, an experimental population for fine genetic mapping. *Genetics* **141**: 1199-1207.

Darvasi, A. and Soller, M. (1997) A simple method to calculate resolving power and confidence interval of QTL map location. *Behavior. Genet.* **27**: 125-132.

Darvasi, A., Vinreb, A., Minke, V., Weller, J. I. and Soller, M. (1993) Detecting marker-QTL linkage and estimating QTL gene effect and map location using a saturated genetic map. *Genetics* **134**: 943-951.

de Koning, G. J. and Weller, J. I. (1994) Efficiency of direct selection on quantitative trait loci for a two-trait breeding objective. *Theor. Appl. Genet.* **88**; 669-677.

Dekkers, J. C. M. and Shook, G. E. (1990) Economic evaluation of alternative breeding programs for commercial artificial insemination firms. *J. Dairy Sci.* **73**: 1902-1919.

Dentine, M. R. and Cowan, C. M. (1990) An analytical model for the estimation of chromosome substitution effects in the offspring of individuals heterozygous at a segregating marker locus. *Theor. Appl. Genet.* **79**: 775-780.

Ducrocq, V. and Quaas, R. L. (1988) Prediction of genetic response to truncation selection across generations. *J. Dairy Sci.* **71**: 2543-2553.

Edwards, M. D., Stuber, C. W. and Wendel, J. F. (1987) Molecular-marker-facilitated investigations of quantitative-trait loci in maize. I. Numbers, genomic distribution and types of gene action. *Genetics* **116**: 113-125.

Efron, B. and Tibshirani, R. J. (1993) *An Introduction to the Bootstrap.* Chapman and Hall, New York, NY.

Elkind, Y., Nir, B. and Weller, J. I. (1994) Maximum likelihood estimation of quantitative trait loci parameters with the aid of genetic markers using a standard statistical package. *CABIOS* **10**: 513-517.

Elsen, J. M., Khang, J. V. T. and Le Roy, P. (1988) A statistical model for genotype determination at a major locus in a progeny test design. *Genet. Sel. Evol.* **20**: 211-226.

Eshed, Y. and Zamir, D. (1996) Less-than-additive epistatic interactions of quantitative trait loci in tomato. *Genetics* **143**: 1807-1917.

Falconer, D. S. (1981) *Introduction to Quantitative Genetics*, 2nd Ed. Longman Inc., New York, NY.

Fernando, R. and Grossman, M. (1989) Marker assisted selection using best linear unbiased prediction. *Genet. Sel. Evol.* **21**: 467-477.

Fisher, R. A. (1918) The correlation between relatives on the supposition of Mendelian inheritance. *Trans. Royal Soc. Edinburgh* **52**: 399-433.

Fisher, R. A. (1930) *The Genetical Theory of Natural Selection.* Clarendon Press, Oxford.

Fulker, D. W. and Cardon, L. R. (1994) A sib-pair approach to interval mapping of quantitative trait loci. *Am. J. Hum. Genet.* **54**: 1092-1103.

Georges, M. and Massey, J. M. (1991) Velogenetics, or the synergistic use of marker assisted selection and germ-line manipulation. *Theriogenol.* **35**: 151-159.

Georges, M., Nielsen, D. Mackinnon, M., Mishra, A., Okimoto, R., Pasquino, A. T., Sargent, L. S., Sorensen, A., Steele, M. R., Zhao, X., Womack, J. E. and Hoeschele, I. (1995) Mapping quantitative trait loci controlling milk production in dairy cattle by exploiting progeny testing. *Genetics* **139**: 907-920.

Gianola, D. and Foulley, J. L. (1983) Sire evaluation for ordered categorical data with a threshold model. *Genet. Sel. Evol.* **15**: 201-223.

Gibson, J. P. (1994) Short-term gain at the expense of long-term response with selection on identified loci. *Proc. 5th World Cong. Genet. Appl. Livest. Prod.* Guelph, ON, Canada **21**: 201-204.

Goddard, M. E. (1992) A mixed model for analyses of data on multiple genetic markers. *Theor. Appl. Genet.* **83**: 878-886.

Gootwine, E., Yossefi, S., Zenou, A. and Bor, A. (1998) Marker assisted selection for FecB carriers in Booroola Awassi crosses. *Proc. 6th World Cong. Genet. Appl. Livest. Prod.* Armidale, NSW, Australia **24**: 161-164.

Gotz, K. U. and Ollivier, L. (1992) Theoretical aspects of applying sib-pair linkage tests to livestock species. *Genet. Sel. Evol.* **24**: 29-42.

Grignola, F. E., Hoeschele, I. and Tier, B. (1996a) Mapping quantitative trait loci in outcross populations via residual maximum likelihood. I. Methodology. *Genet. Sel. Evol.* **28**: 479-490.

Grignola, F. E., Hoeschele, I., Zhang, Q. and Thaller, G. (1996b) Mapping quantitative trait loci in outcross populations via residual maximum likelihood. II. A simulation study. *Genet. Sel. Evol.* **28**: 491-504.

Grodzicker, T., Williams, J., Sharp, P. and Sambrook, J. (1974) Physical mapping of temperature sensitive mutations of adenoviruses. *Cold Spring Harbor Symp. Quant. Biol.* **39**: 439-446.

Hackett, C. A. and Weller J. I. (1995) Genetic mapping of quantitative trait loci for traits with ordinal distributions. *Biometrics* **51**: 1252-1263.

Haley, C. S. and Knott, S. A. (1992) A simple regression method for mapping quantitative trait loci in line crosses using flanking markers. *Heredity* **69**: 315-324.

Haley, C. H., Knott, S. A. and Elsen, J.-M. (1994) Mapping quantitative trait loci in crosses between outbred lines using least squares. *Genetics* **136**: 1195-1207.

Hardy, G. H. (1908) Mendelian proportions in mixed population. *Science* **28**: 49.

Haldane, J. B. S. (1919) The combination of linkage values and the calculation of distances between the loci of linked factors. *J. Genet.* **8**: 299.

Haldane, J. B. S. (1932) *The Causes of Evolution.* Harper & Brothers, New York, NY.

Haseman, J. K. and Elston, R. C. (1972) The investigation of linkage between a quantitative trait and a marker locus. *Behav. Genet.* **2**: 3-19.

Hazel, L. N. (1943) The genetic basis for constructing selection indexes. *Genetics* **28:** 476-490.

Hazel, L. N. and Lush, J. L. (1942) The efficiency of three methods of selection. *J. Hered.* **33**: 393-399.

Henderson, C. R. (1973) Sire evaluation and genetic trends. In *Proc. Anim. Breed. Genet. Symp.* in Honor of Dr. D. L. Lush. ASAS and ADSA, Champaign, IL. pp 10-41.

Henderson, C. R. (1976) A simple method for the inverse of a numerator relationship matrix used in prediction of breeding values. *Biometrics* **32**: 69-83.

Henderson, C. R. (1984) *Applications of Linear Models in Animal Breeding.* University of Guelph, Guelph, ON, Canada.

Hill, W. G. (1971) Investment appraisal for national breeding programmes. *Anim. Prod.* **13**: 37-50.

Hillel, J., Schaap, T., Haberfeld, A., Jeffreys, A. J., Plotzky, Y., Cahaner, A. and Lavi, U. (1990) DNA fingerprints applied to gene introgression in breeding programs. *Genetics* **124**: 783-789.

Hoeschele, I. (1994) Bayesian QTL mapping via the Gibbs sampler. *Proc. 5th World Cong. Genet. Appl. Livest. Prod.* Guelph, ON, Canada **21**: 241-244.

Hoeschele, I. and VanRaden, P. M. (1993a) Bayesian analysis of linkage between genetic markers and quantitative trait loci. I. Prior knowledge. *Theor. Appl. Genet.* **85**: 953-960.

Hoeschele, I. and VanRaden, P. M. (1993b) Bayesian analysis of linkage between genetic markers and quantitative trait loci. II. Combining prior knowledge with experimental evidence. *Theor. Appl. Genet.* **85**: 946-952.

Hoeschele, I., Uimari, P., Gringnola, F. E., Zhang, Q. and Gage, K. M. (1997) Advances in statistical methods to map quantitative trait loci in outbred populations. *Genetics* **147**: 1445-1457.

Hospital, F. and Charcosset, A. (1997) Marker-assisted introgression of quantitative trait loci. *Genetics* **147**: 1469-1485.

Hospital, F., Chevalet, C. and Mulsant, P. (1992) Using markers in gene introgression breeding programs. *Genetics* **132**: 1199-1210.

Israel, C. and Weller, J. I. (1998) Estimation of candidate gene effects in dairy cattle populations. *J. Dairy Sci.* **81**: 1653-1662.

Jansen, R. C. (1992) A general mixture model for mapping quantitative trait loci by using molecular markers. *Theor. Appl. Genet.* **85**: 252-260.

Jansen, R. C. (1994) Controlling the type I and type II errors in mapping quantitative trait loci. *Genetics* **138**: 871-881.

Jansen, R. C. and Stam, P. (1994) High resolution of quantitative traits into multiple loci via interval mapping. *Genetics* **136**: 1447-1455.

Jayakar, S. D. (1970) On the detection and estimation of linkage between a locus influencing a quantitative character and a marker locus. *Biometrics* **26**: 451-464.

Jenson, J. (1989) Estimation of recombination parameters between a quantitative trait locus (QTL) and two marker gene loci. *Theor. Appl. Genet.* **78**: 613-618.

Jiang, C. and Zeng, Z.-B. (1995) Multiple trait analysis of genetic mapping for quantitative trait loci. *Genetics* **140**: 1111-1127.

Johanssen, W. (1903) *Uber Erblichkeit in Polulationen und in reinen Linien.* G. Fisher, Jena.

Kadarmideen, H. N. and Dekkers, J.C.M. (1999) Regression on markers with uncertain allele transmission for QTL mapping in half-sib designs. *Genet. Sel. Evol.* **31**: 437-455.

Kahler, A. L. and Wherhahn, C. F. (1986) Association between quantitative traits and enzyme loci in the F2 population of a maize hybrid. *Theor. Appl. Genet.* **72**: 15-26.

Kan, Y. S. and Dozy, A. M. (1978) Antenatal diagnosis of sickle-cell anemia by DNA analysis of amniotic fluid cells. *Lancet* **2**: 910-912.

Kashi, Y., Hallerman, E. and Soller, M. (1990) Marker-assisted selection of candidate bulls for progeny testing programmes. *Anim. Prod.* **51**: 63-74.

Kennedy, B. W., Quinton, M. and van Arendonk, J.A.M. (1992) Estimation of effects of single genes on quantitative traits. *J. Anim. Sci.* **70**: 2000-2012.

Khatib, H., Darvasi, A., Plotski, Y. and Soller, M. (1994). Determining relative microsatellite allele frequencies in pooled DNA samples. *PCR Methods Appl.* **4**: 13-19.

Knott, S. A. and Haley, C. S. (1992) Maximum likelihood mapping of quantitative trait loci using full-sib families. *Genetics* **132**: 1211-1222.

Knott, S. A., Elsen, J. M. and Haley, C. S. (1994) Multiple marker mapping of quantitative trait loci in half-sib populations. *Proc. 4th World Cong. Genet. Appl. Livest. Prod.* Guelph, ON, Canada. **21**: 33-36.

Knott, S. A., Elsen, J. M. and Haley, C. S. (1996) Methods for multiple-marker mapping of quantitative trait loci in half-sib populations. *Theor. Appl. Genet.* **93**: 71-80.

Knott, S. A., Marklund, L., Haley, C. S., Anderson, K., Davies, W., Ellegren, H., Fredholm, M., Hansson, I. Hoyheim, B. Lundstrom, K. Moller, M. and Anderson, L. (1998) Multiple marker mapping of quantitative trait loci in a cross between outbred wild boar and large white pigs. *Genetics* **149**: 1069-1080.

Korol, A. B., Preygel, I. A. and Bocharnikova, N. I. (1987) Linkage between loci of quantitative characters and marker loci. 5. Combined analysis of several markers and quantitative characters. *Genetika* **23**: 1421-1431.

Korol, A. B., Ronin, Y. I. and Kirzhner, V. M. (1995) Interval mapping of quantitative trait loci employing correlated trait complexes. *Genetics* **140**: 1137-1147.

Korol, A. B., Ronin, Y. I. and Nevo, E. (1998) Approximate analysis of QTL-environment interaction with no limits on the number of environments. *Genetics* **148**: 2015-2028.

Kosambi, D. D. (1944) The estimation of map distances from recombination values. *Ann. Eugen.* **12**: 172-175.

Koudande, O. D., Iraqi, F., Thomson, P. C., Teale, A. J., Van Arendonk, J.A.M. (2000) Strategies to optimize marker-assisted introgression of multiple unlinked QTL. *Mam. Genome* **11**: 145-150.

Kruglyak, L. and Lander, E. S. (1995a) A nonparametric approach for mapping quantitative trait loci. *Genetics* **139**: 1421-1428.

Kruglyak, L. and Lander, E. S. (1995b) Complete multipoint sib-pair analysis of qualitative and quantitative traits. *Am. J. Hum. Genet.* **57**: 439-454.

Kruglyak, L. and Lander, E. S. (1995c) High-resolution genetic mapping of complex traits. *Am. J. Hum. Genet.* **56**: 1212-1223.

Lande, R. and Thompson, R. (1990) Efficiency of marker-assisted selection in the improvement of quantitative traits. *Genetics* **124**: 743-756.

Lander, E. S. and Botstein, D. (1989) Mapping Mendelian factors underlying quantitative traits using RFLP linkage maps. *Genetics* **121**: 185-199.

Lander, E. S. and Kruglyak, L. (1995) Genetic dissection of complex traits: guidelines for interpreting and reporting linkage results. *Nature Genetics* **11**: 241-247.

Law, C. N. (1965) The location of genetic factors affecting a quantitative character in wheat. *Genetics* **53**: 487-498.

Lebowitz, R. J., Soller, M. and Beckmann, J S. (1987) Trait-based analyses for the detection of linkage between marker loci and quantitative trait loci in crosses between inbred lines. *Theor. Appl. Genet.* **73**: 556-562.

Lewontin, R. C. and Hubby, J. L. (1966) A molecular approach to the study of genic heterozygosity in natural populations. II. Amount of variation and degree of heterozygosity in natural populations of *Drosophila pseudoobscura*. *Genetics* **54**: 595-609.

Lipkin, E., Mosig, M. O., Darvasi, A., Ezra, E., Shalom, A., Friedman, A. and Soller, M. (1998) Quantitative trait locus mapping in dairy cattle by means of selective milk DNA pooling using dinucleotide microsatellite markers: analysis of milk protein percentage. *Genetics* **149**: 1557-1567.

Litt, M. and Luty, J. A. (1989) A hypervariable microsatellite revealed by in vitro amplification of a dinucleotide repeat within the cardiac muscle actin gene. *Am. J. Hum. Genet.* **44**: 397.

Lui, B. H. (1998) *Statistical Genomics: Linkage, Mapping and QTL Analysis*. CRC Press, Boca Raton, FL.

Lush, J. L. (1935) The inheritance of productivity in farm livestock. Part V. Discussion of preceding contributions. *Emp. J. Exp. Agri.* **3**: 25.

Lynch M. and Walsh, B. (1998) *Genetics and Analysis of Quantitative Traits*. Sinauer Associates, Inc. Sunderland, MA.

Mackinnon, M. J. and Weller, J. I. (1995) Methodology and accuracy of estimation of quantitative trait loci parameters in a half-sib design using maximum likelihood. *Genetics* **141**: 755-770.

Mackinnon, M. J. and Georges, M. A. J. (1998) Marker-assisted preselection of young diary sires prior to progeny-testing. *Livest. Prod. Sci.* **54**: 229-250.

Mangin, B., Goffinet, B. and Rebai, A. (1994) Constructing confidence intervals for QTL location. *Genetics* **138**: 1301-1308.

Mangin, B., Thoquet, P. and Grimsley, N. (1998) Pleiotropic QTL analysis. *Biometrics* **54**: 88-90.

Martinez, O. and Curnow, R. N. (1992) Estimating the locations and the sizes of the effects of quantitative trait loci using flanking markers. *Theor. Appl. Genet.* **85:** 480-488.

Martinez, O. and Curnow, R. N. (1994) Missing markers when estimating quantitative trait loci using regression mapping. *Heredity* **73**: 198-206.

Maruyama, F. and Fuerst, P. A. (1985) Population bottlenecks and equilibrium models in population genetics. II. Number of alleles in a small population that was formed by a recent bottleneck. *Genetics* **111**: 675-689.

Meng, X.-L. and Rubin, D. B. (1993) Maximum likelihood estimation via the ECM algorithm: a general framework. *Biometrika* **80**: 267-268.

Meuwissen, T. H. E. and Van Arendonk, J. A. M. (1992) Potential improvements in rate of genetic gain from marker assisted selection in dairy cattle breeding schemes. *J. Dairy Sci.* **75**: 1651-1659.

Meuwissen, T. H. E. and Goddard, M. E. (1996) the use of marker haplotypes in animal breeding. *Genet. Sel. Evol.* **28**: 161-172.

Meyer, K. (1989) Restricted maximum likelihood to estimate variance components for animal models with several random effects using a derivative-free algorithm. *Genet. Sel. Evol.* **21**: 317-340.

Michelmore, R. W., Paran, L. and Kesselli, R. (1991) Identification of markers linked to disease resistance genes by bulked segregant analysis: a rapid method to detect markers in specific genome regions using segreganting populations. *Proc Natl. Acad Sci. USA.* **88**: 9828-9832.

Moav, R. (1966) Specialized sire and dam lines. I. Economic evaluation of crossbreeds. *Anim. Prod.* **8**: 193-202.

Morgan, T. H. (1910) Chromosomes and heredity. *Amer. Nat.* **44**:194.

Morgan, T. H. (1928) *The Theory of Genes*. Yale University Press, New Haven, CN.

Motro, U. and Soller, M. (1993) Sequential sampling in determining linkage between marker loci and quantitative trait loci. *Theor. Appl. Genet.* **85**: 658-664.

Mullis, K., Faloona, F., Scharf, S., Saiki, R., Horn, G. and Erlich, H. (1986) Specific enzymatic amplification of DNA in vitro: the polymerase chain reaction. *Cold Spring Harbor Symp. Quant. Biol.* **51**: 263-273.

Neimann-Sprensen, A. and Robertson, A. (1961) The association between blood groups and several production characters in three Danish cattle breeds. *Acta. Agr. Scand.* **11**: 163-196.

Nicholas, F. W. and Smith, C. (1983) Increased rates of genetic change in dairy cattle by embryo transfer and splitting. *Anim Prod.* **36**: 341-353.

Ott, J. (1985) *Analysis of Human Genetic Linkage*. Johns Hopkins University Press, Baltimore, MD.

Paterson, A. H., Lander, E. S., Hewitt, J. D., Peterson, S., Lincoln, S. E. and Tanksley, S. D. (1988) Resolution of quantitative traits into Mendelian factors by using a complete linkage map of restriction fragment length polymorphisms. *Nature* **335**: 721-726.

Pauling, L., Itano, H. A., Singer, S. J. and Wells, I. C. (1949) Sickle cell anemia, a molecular disease. *Science* **110**: 543-548.

Payne, F. (1918) The effect of artificial selection on bristle number in *Drosophila ampelophila* and its interpretation. *Proc. Natl. Acad. Sci.* USA **4**: 55-58.

Perez-Enciso, M. and Toro, M. A. (1999) Robust QTL effect estimation using the Minimum Distance method. *Heredity* **83**: 347-353.

Plotsky, Y., Cahaner, A., Haberfeld, A., Lavi, U., Lamont, S. J. and Hillel, J. (1993) DNA fingerprint bands applied to linkage analysis with quantitative trait loci in chickens. *Anim. Genet.* **24**: 105-110.

Quaas, R. L. and Pollak, E. J. (1980) Mixed model methodology for farm and ranch beef cattle testing programs. *J. Anim. Sci.* **51**: 1277-1287.

Quaas, R. L. (1988) Additive genetic model with groups and relationships. *J. Dairy Sci.* **71**: 1338-1345.

Rendel, J. M. and Robertson, A. (1950) Estimation of genetic gain in milk yield by selection in a close herd of dairy cattle. *J. Genet.* **50**: 1-8.

Riquet, J., Coppieters, W., Cambisano, N., Arranz, J. J., Berzi, P., Davis, S. K., Grisart, B., Farnir, F., Karim, L., Mni, M., Simon, P., Taylor, J. F., Vanmanshoven, P., Wagenaar, D., Womack, J. E. and Georges, M. (1999) Fine-mapping of quantitative trait loci by identity by descent in outbred populations: Application to milk production in dairy cattle. *Proc. Natl. Acad. Sci. USA* **96**: 9252-9257.

Risch, N. (1990) Linkage strategies for genetically complex traits. II. The power of affected relative pairs. *Am. J. Hum. Genet.* **46**: 229-241.

Ron, M., Yoffe, O., Ezra, E., Medrano, J. F. and Weller, J. I. (1994) Determination of milk protein effects on production traits of Israeli Holsteins. *J. Dairy Sci.* **77**: 1106-1113.

Ronin, Y. I., Korol, A. B. and Weller, J. I. (1998) Selective genotyping to detect quantitative trait loci affecting multiple traits: interval mapping analysis. *Theor. Appl. Genet.* **97**: 1169-1178.

Sax, K. (1923) The association of size differences with seed-coat pattern and pigmentation in *Phaseeolus vulgaris*. *Genetics* **8**: 552-560.

Searle, S. R. (1982) *Matrix Algebra Useful for Statistics*. John Wiley & Sons, New York, NY.

Searle, S. R., Casella, G. and McCulloch, C. E. (1992) *Variance Components*. John Wiley & Sons, New York, NY.

Schulman, N. F., De Vires, M. J. and Dentine, M. R. (1999) Linkage disequilibrium in two-stage marker-assisted selection. *J. Anim Breed. Genet.* **116**: 99-110.

Simes, R. J. (1986) An improved Bonferroni procedure for multiple tests of significance. *Biometrika* **73**: 751-754.

Simpson, S. P. (1989) Detection of linkage between quantitative trait loci and restriction fragment length polymorphisms using inbred lines. *Theor. Appl. Genet.* **77**: 815-819.

Simpson, S. P. (1992) Correction: Detection of linkage between quantitative trait loci and restriction fragment length polymorphisms using inbred lines. *Theor. Appl. Genet.* **85**: 110-111.

Smith, C. (1967) Improvement of metric traits through specific genetic loci. *Anim. Prod.* **9**: 349-358.

Smith, C. and Simpson, S. P. (1986) The use of genetic polymorphisms in livestock improvement. *J. Anim. Breed. Genet.* **103**: 205-217.

Smith, C. and Smith, D. B. (1993) The need for close linkages in marker-assisted selection for economic merit in livestock. *Anim. Breed. Abs.* **61**: 197-204.

Soller, M. (1994) Marker assisted selection - an overview. *Anim. Biotechnol.* **5**: 193-207.
Soller, M. and Genizi, A. (1978) The efficiency of experimental designs for the detection of linkage between a marker locus and a locus affecting a quantitative trait in segregating populations. *Biometrics* **34**: 47-55.
Soller, M. and Beckmann, J. S. (1990) Marker-based mapping of quantitative trait loci using replicated progeny. *Theor. Appl. Genet.* **80**: 205-208.
Soller, M., Genizi, A. and Brody, T. (1976) On the power of experimental designs for the detection of linkage between marker loci and quantitative loci in crosses between inbred lines. *Theor. Appl. Genet.* **47**: 35-59.
Solomon, E. and Bodmer, W. F. (1979) Evolution of a sickle variant gene. *Lancet* **1**: 923.
Southern, E. M. (1975) Detection of specific sequences among DNA fragments separated by gel electrophoresis. *J. Mol. Biol.* **98**: 503-517.
Southey, B. R. and Fernando, R. L. (1998) Controlling the proportion of false positives among significant results in QTL detection. *Proc. 6th World Cong. Genet. Appl. Livest. Prod.* Armidale, NSW, Australia. **26**: 221-224.
Song, J. Z. and Weller, J. I. (1998) Maximum likelihood estimation of quantitative trait loci parameters with flanking markers in a half-sib population. *Proc. 6th World Cong. Genet. Appl. Livest. Prod.* Armidale, NSW, Australia. **26**: 341- 344.
Spelman, R. and Bovenhuis, H. (1998) Genetic response from marker assisted selection in an outbred population for differing marker bracket sizes and with two identified quantitative trait loci. *Genetics* **148**: 1389-1396.
Spelman, R. J., Garrick, D. J. and van Arendonk, J. A. M. (1999) Utilization of genetic variation by marker assisted selection in commercial diary cattle populations. *Livest. Prod. Sci.* **59**: 51-60.
Spiess, E. B. (1977) *Genes in Populations.* John Wiley and Sons, New York, NY.
Sribney, W. M. and Swift, M. (1992) Power of sib-pair and sib-trio linkage analysis with assortative mating and multiple disease loci. *Am. J. Hum. Genet.* **51**: 773-784.
Stam, P. (1986) The use of marker loci in selection for quantitative characters. In: Smith, C., King, J. W. B. and McKay, J. C. (eds.) *Exploiting New Technologies in Animal Breeding Genetic Developments.* Oxford University Press, Oxford, pp. 170-182.
Sutton, W. S. (1903) The chromosomes in heredity. *Biol. Bull.* **4**: 213-251.
Tautz, D. (1989) Hypervariability of simple sequences as a general source of polymorphic DNA markers. *Nucl. Acids Res.* **17**: 6463-6471.
Tanksley, S. D., Medina-Filho, H. and Rick, C. M. (1982) Use of naturally occurring enzyme variation to detect and map genes controlling quantitative trait in an interspecific backcross of tomato. *Heredity* **49**: 11-25.

Thaller, G. and Hoeschele, I. (1996a) A Monte Carlo method for Bayesian analysis of linkage between single markers and quantitative trait loci: I. Methodology. *Theor. Appl. Genet.* **93**: 1161-1166.

Thaller, G. and Hoeschele, I. (1996b) A Monte Carlo method for Bayesian analysis of linkage between single markers and quantitative trait loci: I. A simulation study. *Theor. Appl. Genet.* **93**: 1167-1174.

Thompson, R. (1979) Sire evaluations. *Biometrics* **35**:339-353.

Titterington, D. M., Smith, A. F. M. and Makov, U. E. (1985) *Statistical Analysis of Finite Mixture Distributions.* John Wiley & Sons, New York, NY.

Ufford, G. R., Henderson, C. R. and Van Vleck, L. D. (1979) Computing algorithms for sire evaluation with all lactations records and natural service sires. *J. Dairy Sci.* **62**: 511-513.

Uimari, P. and Hoeschele, I. (1997) Mapping two linked quantitative trait loci using Bayesian analysis and Markov chain Monte Carlo algorithms. *Genetics* **146**: 735-743.

van Arendonk, J. A. M., Bovehuis, H. van der Beek, S. and Groen, A. F. (1994a) Detection and exploitation of markers linked to quantitative traits in farm animals. *Proc. 5th World Cong. Genet. Appl. Livest. Prod.* Guelph, ON, Canada, **21**: 193-200.

van Arendonk, J. A. M., Tier, B. and Kinghorn, B. P. (1994b) Use of multiple genetic marker in prediction of breeding values. *Genetics* **137**: 319-329.

VanRaden, P. M. and Wiggans, G. R. (1991) Derivation, calculation and use of national animal model information. *J. Dairy Sci.* **74**: 2737-2746.

VanRaden, P. M. and Weller, J. I. (1994) A simple method to locate and estimate effects of individual genes with a saturated genetic marker map. *J. Dairy Sci.* **77**(Supl. 1): 249.

Villanueva, B., Pong-Wong, R., Grundy, B. and Woolliams, J. A. (1999) Potential benefit from using an identified major gene in BLUP evaluation with truncation and optimal selection. *Genet. Sel. Evol.* **31**: 115-133.

Visscher, P. M. (1996) Proportion of the variation in genetic composition in backcrossing programs explained by genetic markers. *J. Hered.* **87**: 136-138.

Visscher, P. M., Haley, C. S. and Thompson, R. (1996a) Marker-assisted introgression in backcross breeding programs. *Genetics* **144**: 1923-1932.

Visscher, P. M., Thompson, R. and Haley, C. S. (1996b) Confidence intervals in QTL mapping by bootstraping. *Genetics* **143**: 1013-1020.

Visscher, P. M., Mackinnon, M. and Haley, C. S. (1997) Efficiency of marker assisted selection. *Anim. Biotech.* **8**: 99-106.

Weber, J. L. and May, P. E. (1989) Abundant class of Human DNA polymorphisms which can be typed using the polymerase chain reaction. *Am. J. Hum. Genet.* **44**: 388.

Weller, J. I. (1986) Maximum likelihood techniques for the mapping and analysis of quantitative trait loci with the aid of genetic markers. *Biometrics* **42**: 627-640.

Weller, J. I. (1992) Statistical methodologies for mapping and analysis of quantitative trait loci. In: J. S. Beckmann and T. C. Osborn (Eds.) *Plant Genomes: Methods for Genetic and Physical Mapping.* pp. 181-207. Kluwer Academic Publishers Group, Dordrecht, The Netherlands.

Weller, J. I. (1994) *Economic Aspects of Animal Breeding.* Chapman & Hall. London.

Weller, J. I. and Fernando, R. L. (1991) Strategies for the improvement of animal production using marker assisted selection. In: L. B. Schook, H. A. Lewin and D. G. McLaren (Ed.) *Gene Mapping: Strategies, Techniques and Applications.* pp. 305-328. Marcel Dekker, Inc. New York, NY.

Weller, J. I. and Soller, M. (1981) Methods for production of multimarker strains. *Theor. Appl. Genet.* **59**: 73-78.

Weller, J. I. and Wyler, A. (1992) Power of different sampling strategies to detect quantitative trait loci variance effects. *Theor. Appl. Genet.* **83**: 582-588.

Weller, J. I., Soller, M. and Brody, T. (1988) Linkage analysis of quantitative traits in an interspecific cross of tomato (*L. esculentum* x *L. pimpinellifolium*) by means of genetic markers. *Genetics* **118**; 329-339.

Weller, J. I., Kashi, Y. and Soller, M. (1990) Power of "daughter" and "granddaughter" designs for genetic mapping of quantitative traits in dairy cattle using genetic markers. *J. Dairy Sci.* **73**: 2525-2537.

Weller, J. I., Wiggans, G. R., VanRaden, P. M. and Ron, M. (1996) Application of a canonical transformation to detection of quantitative trait loci with the aid of genetic markers in a multi-trait experiment. *Theor. Appl. Genet.* **92**: 998-1002.

Weller, J. I., Song, J. Z., Heyen, D. W., Lewin, H. A. and Ron, M. (1998) A new approach to the problem of multiple comparisons in the genetic dissection of complex traits. *Genetics* **150**: 1699-1706.

Westell, R. A., Quaas, R. L. and Van Vleck, L. D. (1988) Genetic groups in an animal model. *J. Dairy Sci.* **71**: 1310-1318.

Whittaker, J. C., Curnow, R. N., Haley, C. S. and Thompsom, R. (1995) Using marker-maps in marker-assisted selection. *Genet. Res. Camb.* **66**: 255-265.

Whittaker, J. C., Thompsom, R. and Visscher, P. M. (1996) On the mapping of QTL by regression of phenotype on marker-type. *Heredity* **77**: 23-32.

Xu, S. and Atchley, W. R. (1995) A random model approach to interval mapping of quantitative trait loci. *Genetics* **141**: 1189-1197.

Young, N. D. and Tanksley, S. D. (1989) RFLP analysis of the size of chromosomal segments retained around the *Tm*-2 locus of tomato during backcross breeding. *Theor. Appl. Genet.* **77**: 353-359.

Yule, G. U. (1906) On the theory of inheritance of quantitative compound characters on the basis of Mendel's laws - a preliminary note. *Rept. 3rd Intern. Confr. Genet.*, pp. 140-142.

Zeng, Z.-B. (1993) Theoretical basis for separation of multiple linked gene effects in mapping quantitative trait loci. *Proc. Natl. Acad. Sci. USA* **90**: 10972-10976.

Zeng, Z.-B. (1994) A composite interval mapping method of locating multiple QTLs. *Proc. 4th World Cong. Genet. Appl. Livest. Prod.* Guelph, ON, Canada, **21**: 37-40.

Zhang, W. and Smith, C. (1992) Computer simulation of marker-assisted selection utilizing linkage disequilibrium. *Theor. Appl. Genet.* **83**: 813-820.

Zhang, W. and Smith, C. (1993) Simulation of marker-assisted selection utilizing linkage disequilibrium: the effects of several additional factors. *Theor. Appl. Genet.* **86**: 492-496.

Zhang, Q., Boichard, D., Hoeschele, I., Ernst, C., Eggen, A., Murkve, B., Pfister-Genskow, M., Witte, L.A., Grignola, F.E., Uimari, P., Thaller, G. and Bishop M. D. (1998) Mapping quantitative trait loci for milk production and health of dairy cattle in a large outbred pedigree. *Genetics* **149**: 1959-1973.

Zhuchenko, A. A., Korol, A. B. and Andryushchenko, V. K. (1979a) Linkage between loci for quantitative characters and marker loci. I. Model. *Genetika* **14**: 6771-778.

Zhuchenko, A. A., Samovol, A. P., Korol, A. B. and Andryushchenko, V. K. (1979b) Linkage between loci of quantitative characters and marker loci. II. Influence of three tomato chromosomes on variability of five quantitative characters in backcross progenies. *Genetika* **15**: 672-683.

Author Index

(Only names of authors actually cited in the text are listed.)

Andersson-Elkund, L. 107
Atchley, W. R. 121, 122, 123, 133, 134, 151
Bailey, N. T. 26
Baret, P. V. 93
Beavis, 188
Beckmann, J. S. 8, 144, 145, 146
Benjamini, Y. 181,182
Bjorck, A. 26
Bodmer, 8
Botstein, D., 8, 59, 89, 90, 94, 123, 152, 155, 160, 179, 180, 191, 200
Bovenhuis, H. 50, 81, 111, 187
Boveri, 3
Brascamp, E. W. 209, 211, 234
Brinkman, M. A. 245
Brookes, A. J. 9
Cantet, R. J. C. 72, 126, 128, 133, 225
Cardon, L. R. 81, 82, 83, 122, 151
Charcosset, A. 243, 248
Churchill, G. A. 181, 200
Coppieters, W. 116
Cowan, C. M. 60, 107
Cunningham, E. P. 240
Curnow, R. N. 51, 77, 85, 92, 99, 100, 112, 153
Da, Y. 58
Dahlquist, G. 26

Darvasi, A. 51, 150, 154, 155, 157, 158, 160, 161, 162, 163, 164, 165, 166, 169, 171, 172, 173, 174, 175, 191, 200, 202
de Koning, G. J. 228, 236, 237, 238, 239, 241
Dekkers, J. C. M. 93, 113, 209
Dentine, M. R., 60
Doerge, R. W. 181, 200
Dozy, A. M. 8
Ducrocq, V. 207
Edwards, M. D. 8, 51
Efron, B. 155
Elkind, Y. 20
Elston, R. C. 7, 48, 50, 59, 63, 65, 66, 67, 81, 82, 83, 118, 120, 121, 151
Eshed, Y. 98, 188, 189
Falconer, D. S. 60, 65, 161, 207, 218
Fernando, R., 51, 71, 72, 73, 105, 120, 123, 125, 126, 128, 129, 132, 185, 186, 187, 210, 225
Fisher, R. A. 5, 6
Foulley, J. L. 117
Frey, K. J. 245
Fuerst P.A. 187, 188
Fulker, D. W. 81, 82, 83, 122, 151
Georges, M. 72, 108, 109, 178, 187, 188,

225, 228, 230, 232, 233, 234
Genizi, A. 7, 50, 63, 146
Gianola, D. 117
Gibson, J. P. 227, 237
Goddard M. E. 72, 128, 130, 131, 133, 187, 225, 236
Gootwine, E. 224, 243
Gotz, K. U. 59
Grignola, F. E. 72, 73, 133, 187
Grodzicker, T. 8
Grossman, M. 51, 71, 72, 73, 105, 120, 123, 125, 126, 128, 129, 132, 187, 225
Hackett, C. A. 50, 117
Haldane, J. B. S. 4, 5, 9, 10, 11, 79, 83, 84, 89, 136, 157, 170, 246
Haley, C. H. 77, 92, 114, 151
Hardy, G. H. 4, 63, 65, 110
Haseman, J. K. 7, 48, 50, 59, 63, 65, 66, 67, 81, 82, 83, 118, 120, 121, 151
Hazel, L. N. 5, 205
Henderson, C. M. 6, 30, 32, 33, 34, 38, 42, 46, 72, 106
Hill, W. G. 210
Hillel, J. 243, 245, 246
Hochberg, Y. 181, 182

Author Index

Hoeschele, I. 105, 107, 134, 135, 136, 137, 138, 140, 141, 186, 189, 228
Hospital, F. 243, 246, 247, 248
Hubby, J. L. 7
Israel, C., 108
Jansen, R. C. 88, 90, 91, 93, 94, 100, 101, 111, 117, 192, 196
Jayakar, S. D., 7
Jenson, J. 26
Jiang, C. 190, 196, 197
Johanssen, W. 5
Kadarmideen, H. N. 93, 113
Kahler, A. L. 8
Kan, Y. S. 8
Kashi, Y. 222, 230, 232, 233, 234
Kennedy, B. W. 51, 106, 237
Khatib, H. 163
Knott, S. A. 77, 87, 92, 109, 112, 116, 151, 187
Korol, A. B. 68, 99, 190, 194, 195, 196
Kosambi, D. D. 9, 11, 136
Koudande, O. D. 248, 249
Kruglyak, L. 85, 115, 119, 170, 171, 179, 180, 182, 186
Lande, R. 210, 219, 220, 222, 223, 224, 228, 229, 234, 236, 238, 239, 240, 247
Lander, E. S. 85, 89, 90, 94, 115, 119, 123, 152, 155, 160, 170, 171, 179, 180, 182, 186, 191, 200
Law, C. N. 7
Lebowitz, R. J. 160, 191, 200
Lewontin, R. C. 7
Lipkin E. 163
Litt, M. 8
Lui, B. H. 9
Luty, J. A. 8
Lush, J. L. 5, 205
Lynch, M. 15, 43, 46
Mackinnon, M. J. 109, 110, 111, 112, 113, 153, 154, 187, 228, 230, 232, 233, 234
Mangin, B. 92, 153, 155, 196, 199
Martinez, O. 51, 77, 85, 92, 99, 100, 112, 153
Maruyama, F. 187, 188
Massey, J. M. 225
May, P. E. 8
Meng, X.-L. 103
Meuwissen, T. H. E., 230, 231, 236
Meyer, K. 133
Michelmore, R. W. 163
Moav, R. 218
Morgan, T. H. 3, 9
Motro, U. 167
Mullis, K. 8
Neimann-Soressen, A. 6, 60, 116, 146
Nicholas, F. W. 215
Ollivier, L. 59
Ott, J. 11
Paterson, A. H. 8
Pauling, L. 7
Payne, F. 5
Perez-Enciso, M. 28
Plotsky, Y. 163
Pollak, E. J. 33, 40, 126, 127, 128
Quaas, R. L. 33, 40, 125, 126, 127, 128, 207
Rendel, J. M. 206
Riquet, J. 176, 177, 187
Risch, N. 118
Robertson, A. 6, 60, 116, 146, 206
Ron, M. 68, 107, 145
Ronin, Y. I. 162, 202, 203
Rubin, D. B. 103
Sax, K. 3, 5
Searle, S. R. 15, 41, 42, 43, 45, 197
Shook, G. E. 209
Simes, R. J. 179
Simpson, S. P. 72, 93, 120, 142, 150, 188, 217
Smith, C. 13, 72, 120, 126, 128, 131, 133, 169, 188, 189, 215, 217, 221, 225, 228, 236, 237
Smith, D. B. 13, 169
Soller, M. 6, 7, 8, 50, 63, 143, 144, 145, 146, 157, 160, 161, 162, 163, 164, 165, 166, 167, 171, 172, 191, 200, 202, 208, 225
Solomon, 8
Song, J. Z. 111, 187
Southern, E. M. 8
Southey, B. R. 185, 186
Spelman, R. 85, 86, 114, 230, 234, 235
Spiess, E. B. 187
Sribney, W. M. 151
Stam, P. 100, 101, 217

Sutton, W. S. 3
Swift, M. 151
Tanksley, S. D. 8, 243, 245
Tautz, D. 8
Thaller, G. 140
Thompson, R. 39, 210, 219, 220, 222, 223, 224, 228, 229, 234, 236, 238, 239, 240, 247
Tibshirani, R. J. 155
Titterington, D. M. 41, 114
Toro, M. A. 28
Ufford, G. R., 37
Uimari, P. 141
van Arendonk, J.A.M. 72, 132, 230, 231
VanRaden, P. M. 62, 69, 107, 108, 134, 135, 136, 137, 138, 170, 182, 186, 189, 200, 228
Villanueva, B. 227, 237
Visscher, P. M. 155, 245, 246, 247, 248
Walsh, B. 15, 43, 46
Weber, J. L. 8
Weller, J. I. 8, 15, 50, 51, 63, 68, 81, 88, 97, 98, 108, 109, 110, 111, 112, 113, 117, 132, 137, 144, 153, 154, 162, 170, 182, 187, 190, 197, 198, 199, 208, 210, 211, 220, 228, 233, 236, 237, 238, 239, 241
Westell, R. A. 40
Wherhahn, C. F. 8
Whittaker, J. C. 83, 85, 100, 104, 105, 236, 237
Wiggans, G. R. 62, 69, 107, 108, 182, 200
Wyler, A. 162
Xu, S. 121, 122, 123, 133, 134, 151
Young, N. D. 243, 245
Yule, G. U. 5
Zamir, D. 98, 188, 189
Zeng, Z.-B. 92, 100, 101, 102, 103, 190, 196, 197
Zhang, W. 131, 189, 228, 236, 237
Zhuchenko, A. A. 17, 50, 51, 76, 97

Subject Index

Figures in **bold** indicate major references. Figures in *italic* refer to diagrams, photographs and tables.

absorption 35
additional generations 67–70, 106–107
additive genetic effects 38, 40, 71, 86–87, 122, 229–230, *242*
adults, selection of 222–223
advanced intercross lines (AIL) 173–174
agricultural species, genetic maps 9
AI (artificial insemination) 69, 188–189
allele origin 58–59
allele substitution effect 60, 109
allele-sharing method 118–119
allelic frequencies 165–167, 229
    changes in 208–209, *209*
alternative hypothesis 24, 165, 197–198
ancestors, unknown 39–40
animal models
    genetic evaluations 226
    individual (IAM) 38–39
ANOVA (analysis of variance) 7, 50, 55, 62, 148, 151
assumptions, parameter estimation 48–51, 97

backcross design 115–116, 156
    contrast, evaluation of 144–145, *145*
    least squares estimation 77–81, *78, 80*
    linear model analysis 53–56, *54, 56*
    marker-assisted introgression 245–247, *245*, 248, 249–250
    maximum likelihood estimation 87–88
    moments method estimation 76–77, *77*
    QTL interaction effects 97–99, *98*
    sample pooling 165–166
    selective genotyping *161*
    statistical power 144–145, *145, 168*
    whole genome scans 180–181
backcross progeny (BC) 52, *54*
Bayesian estimation 27–28, 135–139
    significance tests, segregating QTL 139–140

Best Linear Unbiased Estimates (BLUE) 34
Best Linear Unbiased Predictors (BLUP) 34, 72
biased estimates 55, 92–93, 104, 106, 163, 189–190
binomial distribution 21
biochemical polymorphism 7
biometrical methodology 6
bivariate analysis 195–197
bivariate density plot *194, 195, 196*
bivariate normal distribution 193
block effect 54
blood groups 6–7,
Bonferroni adjustment 180
bootstrap 156–157
bovine genome 12–13, 181, 183–186, *184, 185*
breeding programs 206–212, *209, 215–216*
    dairy cattle 212–215, *213, 214, 215*
    marker-assisted introgression 245–247, *245*
    selection index *see* selection index
Bulk Segregant Analysis 164
bulls 234–235
    breeding values 30–31
burn-in cycles 141

canonical transformation 198–200
categorical traits 115–118
central F-distribution 55, 80, 82
central t-distribution 55, 82
chromosomal segments 60, 138
chromosomes 12–13
codominance 65, 148
coefficient matrix 32, 33
    additive genetic effects 38
    permanent environmental effect 38
companion-wise error rate (CWER) 179–186, *184, 185*, 187

277

complete genome scans 179
  analysis of multiple pedigrees 187–189
  biases with estimation 189–190
  false discovery rate 182–187, *184, 185*
  multiple markers 180–181
  permutation tests 182
complete model *see* alternative hypothesis
complex pedigrees
  linear regression estimation 113–114
  maximum likelihood estimation 111–112
  non-linear regression estimation 112–113
composite interval mapping
  hypothesis testing 103–104
  maximum likelihood parameter estimates 102–103
  principles 101
  properties 102
confidence intervals 23–24, 172–173
  estimation 153–154, 156–157
consistency 16–17
continuous distribution 4–5, 21, 23
contrast, evaluation of 144–145, *145*
  paternal alleles 148
convergence 25, 26
correlated traits 35–37, 192–193, 198–200, *202*
correlation coefficient 3
covariance matrix 82, 124–126
Cramer-von Mises distance 28
critical interval, determination of 170–172, *172*
crosses between inbred lines 51–53, 144–145
  estimation of power 144–145
  experiment design 52–53
  family analysis 108–109
  linear model analysis 53–57
  linear regression mapping of QTL 83–85
  maximum likelihood analysis 89–90
  QTL parameter estimation *see* QTL parameter estimation
  random gametic model 132
  replicate progeny 145–147, *147*

crossover interference *see* recombination interference
cytogenetics 3–5

dairy cattle 60, 68–69
  breeding programmes
    half-sib and progeny tests 212–215, *213, 214, 215*
    simulation studies, MAS 231
dam additive genetic component 62
dam effect 40–41
data distribution 28
data specification 26
daughter design
  biases with estimation 189
  breeding program *213, 233–234*
  canonical transformation 200
  estimation of power 147–151, *149*
  large families 60–63, *61, 62*
  marker information 112–113
  maximum likelihood analysis 109–111, 116
    fixed polygenic sire effect 111–112
    random effects 114–115
daughter-yield deviations (DYD) 69–70, 183, 107–108, *202*
dense maps 180, 181
density functions 89, 171–172, *172, 180, 192*
derivative-based methods 25, 26–27
derivative-free methods 25–26
discrete distribution 50
disease traits 118–119
DNA base pairs (bp) 12, 13, *13*
DNA-level polymorphisms 8
DNA-microsatellites 8–9, 158
dominance 51, 56, 86–87, *145*
double haploid lines (DHL) 145, 146
doubled haploid (DH) 52
Drosophilia 3, 5, 7

economic factors 15, 158–160
eigenvectors 198–199
electrophoresis 7–8
EM algorithm 112
environmental effects 5, 54, 99
enzyme polymorphisms 7–8

epistasis 51, 97, 104
error variances 155
errors 143, 179–187
estimate breeding values (EBV) 107–108
estimates within parameter space 16
expectation of the log of the likelihood ratio (ELOD) 94, 195
expectation/conditional maximization (ECM) algorithm 103, 117
expectation maximization (EM) 25, 26–27
    algorithm 90–92
experiments, design of 49
    additional generations 67–70
    assumptions and problems 48–51
    comparison of 70–71
    complete population analyses 71–73
    crosses between inbred lines 51–53, *52*
    linear model analysis 53–57
    optimization 158–169
    segregating populations 57–60
    large families 60–63
    small families 63–67
experiments, size of 6

F-2 design 86, 98
    confidence interval 173
    contrast, evaluation of 144–145, *145*
    equal power 147, *147*
    regression model 104–105
    sample pooling 165–166
    statistical power 144–145, *145*
    whole genome scans 180–181
F-2 generation 52
    linear model analysis 56–57, *57*
    replicate progeny 146, 147
F-3 generation 67, 145, 147, *147*
F-4 generation 145, *147*
false discovery rate 182–186, *184*, *185*
false positives 186–187
family analysis 60–67, 108–109, 112–114, 148, 223
family-wise error rate (FWER) 179–186, *184*, *185*, 187
Fernando and Grossman model 50, **71–73**, 133, 106, 124–126, 127, 129, 133
field data, analysis of 107–109

fine mapping
    advanced intercross lines 173–174
    confidence interval 172–173
    critical interval, determination of 170–172, *172*
    identity by descent 177–178
    interval specific congenic strains (ISCS) 175–176
    recombinant inbred segregation test 177
    recombinant progeny testing 175, *176*
    selective phenotyping 174
first derivative based methods (EM) 25, 26–27
fixed effects 30–31, 33, 35–47
    least squares solutions 32
    parental 128
    prediction error variances 34
    sires 111–112
flanking markers 77–79, *78*, 81–83, 85, 92
    linear regression mapping of QTL 83–85
    maximum likelihood estimation 89–90
F-test 80, 81

gametic effect models
    complete population analyses 71–74
    crosses between inbred lines 132
gametic effect variance matrix 130–131
Gamma distribution 171
Gauss–Seidel iteration 33, 39
general linear model 19–20
general product rule of probability 90–91
generalized least squares solutions 20
genes, number in genome 12–13
genetic gain
    breeding schemes 214, 215–216, *215*, 231–233, *232*, 235–236, *236*
    computation of 207–208
    value of 210–212
genetic map units 12, 13, 137
genetic mapping 3–4
    functions 9–12, *13*, 137
    scale 12–13, 13
genetic maps 180–181
    Internet sites 9

genetic markers 50–51
    saturated map 170–73
    selection of sires 233–236, *236*
genetic penetrance 49, 118
genetic standard deviations 138
genetic variance 33, 67, 146–147, 238
Genetics and Analysis of Quantitative Traits 15
genome
    bovine 181,183–186, *184, 185*
    information content 85
genome scans 179–190, *184, 185*
genotype distribution 62
genotype effect 55
genotypes
    missing marker 85–87
    probabilities 55–57, *56, 58, 62*
genotyping
    cost of 160, 162
    selective 161–164, *161, 163, 201–204, 203, 204*
germ-line manipulation 226
ghost QTL 51
Gibbs sampling 141–142
granddaughter design 68, 107–108, 116, 134–135, 233
    Bayesian estimation 138, 139–141
    complex pedigrees 112–114
    estimation of power 148–151, *150*
    false discovery rate 183–186, *184, 185*
Gv 72, 124–126, 133
    inverse of 126–127

haemoglobin gene, human 8
Haldane mapping function 10–11, 79, 84, 89, 137, 159, 171, 174
half-sib design *see* daughter design
half-sib tests 212–214, *214, 215*
haploid lines 52
Hardy–Weinberg distribution 62, 65, 110
Haseman-Elston sib-pair model 50, 122–124, 152
Henderson's Method III 42
herd effect 31
heritability 33, 47, 134, 138, 149, 160, *160*, 237, *242*
    genetic variance 147
    low 69

heterogenous variance 88
heterozygote mean contrast 57
heterozygotes 56, 87
higher order QTL effects 97
Holsteins 183, 188, 200, *202*
homogenous variance 88
homozygote mean contrast 56
homozygotes 56, 87
human populations 9, 63

identity by descent (IBD) 63, 65, 118, 145, 177–178
    marker alleles 81, 122–123
inbred lines 48
    crosses between *see* crosses between inbred lines
    major genes 247–248
    mean squares 146
individual animal model (IAM) 38–39
infinitesimal model 6
information content, genome 85
informative markers 58
informativity 11–12
interaction effects 97–99, 98
interval mapping 85–87, 123–124, 152, 153
    biases in 92–93
    likelihood ratio test 93–94
    multitrait analyses 200–201
interval specific congenic strains (ISCS) 175–176
intuitive estimate value 21
isozymes 8
iterative methods 25, 33, 43

jackknife methods 156–157
joint density function 43
juveniles, selection of 222–223

Kosambi mapping function 11, 137
Kronecker product 36
kurtosis 50, 51

large families 60–63
least squares analysis 77–81, 81–83, 86
least squares solutions
    general linear models 19–20
    single parameter 18–20

Index 281

likelihood function 102, 104, 154, 192–193
  maximizing 25, 123–124
likelihood ratio test statistic (LR) 93, 197
likelihood ratio tests 24, 88, 93–94, 124, 151, 153
linear loss function 27
linear models
  crosses between inbred lines 51–57
  daughter design 60–61
  general 19–20, 100–101
  mixed 30–31
  paternal effect 126
  power 152
linear regression estimation 112–114
  mapping of QTL with flanking markers 83–85
linear regression models 18–19
linkage 88, 100, 197–198
  complete 65, 94, 144
  distance 137
  drag 246
  effect of recombination 146
  incomplete 66
  probability 137, 140
  significance 181
  single marker 109–111
linkage disequilibrium 48–73
linkage groups 4
linkage studies 7
linked QTL 105
loci interactions 51
loci, effective number 230
LOD (log of likelihood) values 157, 172, 195
logistic distribution 117
loss functions 27
loss, economic value 27, 28
Lycopersicon esculentum 98, 189–190
Lycopersicon pennellii 98, 190

Mackinnon and Weller model 110–111
map distances 9–11, *12, 137*
mapping functions 9–11
marker alleles 81
marker brackets 91, 103, 129–130, 134–135
  detection power 145, 151–152
  length of 83, 155
  multiple 99–101, 129–130
marker genotype heterozygote 55
marker genotype homozygote 55
marker genotypes 104–105
  density functions 89
  missing marker 85–87
  trait expectation 55–56, *56, 62*
marker information 58, 85–87, 112–113, 114
marker intervals 113, 155
marker-assisted introgression 244–247, *245*
  major gene, inbred line 247–248
  multiple genes 249–250
  QTL into a donor population 248–249
marker-assisted selection (MAS)
  'animal model' genetic evaluations 226
  breeding schemes 231–233, *232, 239–242*
    sire selection 233–236, *236*
  effective number of QTL 230
  germ-line manipulation 226
  maximum selection efficiency 224–225
  and phenotypic information
    adults 222–223
    individuals 220–221
    relatives 223–224
  phenotypic selection vs. MAS 220–221
  polygenic variance 228–230
  segregating populations 225
  selection within a breed 219–220
  sex-limited traits 221–222
  simulation studies *see* simulation studies
  two-stage selection 222–223
  vs. selection index 218–219, 236–239, *239*
markers
  information content 85–87
  multiple 11–12, 100, 180–181, 129
    QTL analysis 104–105
  single 87–88, 138

Index

markers *Continued*
   spacing 153, 157, 158–159
     economic optimization 158–159
   two flanking 89–90, 192
Markov Chain Monte Carlo (MCMC)
   algorithms 141
maternal effect 126–127, 128
matrix algebra 15–16
Matrix Algebra Useful for Statistics 15
maximum likelihood analysis 7
   categorical traits 115–117
   confidence intervals 23–24
   daughter design 109–111
   hypothesis testing 23–24
   methods to maximize likelihood
     functions 25
   mixed models 41
   multi-parameter 22–23
   power 152
   QTL parameters, single marker
     109–111
   random effects 114–115
   single parameter 20–22
   variance components 43–46
maximum likelihood estimation 87–88,
   114–115
   complex pedigrees 111–112
   composite interval mapping 102–103
   confidence intervals 23–24
   crosses between inbred lines 87–88,
     89–90
   Haseman–Elston sib-pair model
     122–124
   hypothesis testing 23–24
   map distances 11
   mixed models 41
   multi-parameter 22–23
   significance for segregating QTL
     88–89
   single marker 87–88
   single parameter 20–22
   two flanking markers 89–90
   variance components 43–46
maximum selection efficiency 224–225
mean squares 146
mean within-parent differences 62–63
meiosis 49, 171–172, *171*
Mendelian genetics 3–4, 5, 7, 49

Mendelian sampling 40–41, 128
microsatellites *see* DNA-microsatellites
milk production 30–31, 35, 39, 200
minimum difference estimation 28–29
minimum estimation error variance 16
missing marker genotypes 85–87
mixed model methodology 6
mixed models
   equations 32
     absorption 35
     solutions 33–34
   linear 30–31
   maximum likelihood estimation 41,
     43–46
   multivariate analysis 35–37
   parental effects 128–129
   segregating populations 107–109
MOET nucleus breeding schemes
   231–233
moments method 17, 50, 76–77
Morgan mapping function 82
Morgans 4, 9, 10, 171–172
morphological markers 7
multiple pedigrees, analysis of 187–189
multiple QTL
   biases with estimation 189–190
multiple records 37, 38
multiple regression models 83–85,
   100–101
multitrait analyses 191–192, 200–201
   correlated traits 192–193
     canonical transformation 198–200
     determination of statistical
       significance 200–201
   pleiotropy vs. linkage 197–198
   power 194–197, *194*, *195*, *196*
   selective genotyping 201–204, *202*,
     203, *204*
multitrait breeding
   multiple identified QTL 241–242, 242
   single identified QTL 239–241, *240*
multitrait models 46
multitrait selection 209–210
multivariate analysis 35–37, 192–193
multivariate normal distribution 43

nested alleles 61
nested hypotheses 24

Newton–Raphson method **26**, 29
non-linear least squares estimation 86
non-linear regression 80–82, 112–114
non-linear regression interval mapping *80*
non-parametric bootstrap 156
normal distribution 50
normal equations 20, 34
nucleus breeding schemes 215–216, 231–233
nuisance parameters 27, 53, 91
null hypothesis **24**, 55, 62, 197–198
    BC design 88
    likelihood ratio 93, 104, 134–135
    mixed model 106
    genotype frequencies 165

optimization of experimental designs
    economic optimization
        marker spacing 158–159
        replicate progeny 159–160, 160
    sample pooling
        estimation of power 165–167
        general considerations 164
    sample sizes 26, 167–168
    selective genotyping 161–164, 161, 163, 167–168, 168
    sequential sampling 168–169
outbred populations
    identity by descent 177–178
    linkage disequilibrium 48–50
    QTL parameter estimation 105–107

parameter estimation 15–16, 103
    Bayesian estimation 27–28
    derivative free methods 25–26
    estimator properties 16–17
    first derivative based methods (EM) 26–27
    least squares 18–20
    maximum likelihood estimation
        confidence intervals 23–24
        hypothesis testing 23–24
        mixed models 41
        multi-parameter 22–23
        single parameter 20–22
        variance components 43–46
    methods to maximize likelihood functions 25

minimum difference estimation 28–29
moments method 17
outbred populations 105–107
second derivative based methods 25, **26**
parameter space 16
parametric bootstrap 156
parental information 66–67
partial derivatives 22–23
partial dominance 65
paternal alleles 113
    contrasts 148
paternal effect 126–127, 128, 130–131
permanent environmental effect 37, 38
permutation tests 182
phenotype, regression of 104–105
phenotypic selection 174, 220–221
    adults 222–223
    cost of 159–160, 162–163, *163*
    individuals 220–221
    relatives 223–224
    sample size 167–168, *168*
phenotypic standard deviation (SDU) 144, 149, 150–151
physical mapping 12–13, *13*
pleiotropy 55, 197–198
Poisson distribution 10
poly(TG) sites 8–9
polygenic breeding value 128
polygenic effects 71, 106–107, 108
    additive 122
    sire 111–112, 114
polygenic variance 133, 134, 228–230
polymerase chain reaction (PCR) 8
polymorphism information content (PIC) 59
population analyses 71–74
populations, size of 188, 213
posterior probability 27, 139–140
prediction error variance 23–24, 34, 72–73, 88
prior distribution 27, 135–139
probabilities, progeny QTL 110–111, *111*
progeny
    genotypes 63, 110–111, *111*
    number 144–145, *145*
    test schemes 231–235, *232*
    types 52, *147*

progeny tests 214–215, *214, 215*
proportion of fully informative matings (PFIM) 59–60
p-values 182–183, *184*
pyramidal design 249

QTL analysis
   multiple trait *see* multiple trait QTL analysis
   random effects *see* random effects
   regression of phenotype 104–105
QTL detection
   experimental designs 48–51, 52, *73*
      additional generations 67–70
      comparison of 70–71
      crosses between inbred lines 51–57, *54, 56, 57*
      gametic effect models 71–74
      segregating populations 57–67
   false discovery rate 182–186, *184, 185*
      a priori determination 186–187
   milestones in 3–5
   permutation tests 182
   power of *see* statistical power
   statistical methods *see* statistical methods
QTL effects 51, 70–71
   degrees of freedom 81, 93, 98
QTL genotype probability 55
QTL parameter estimation
   correlated traits 192–193
      canonical transformation 198–200
   crosses between inbred lines 75
      expectation-maximization algorithm 90–92
      interval mapping 85–87, 92–94
      least squares 77–83
      linear regression mapping 83–85
      maximum likelihood estimation 87–90
      moments method 76–77
   outbred populations 105–107
   statistical methods *see* statistical methods
QTL properties 16–17
QTL substitution effect 109, 112, 144, 148, 155

QTL variance 70–71, *70, 133–134*
QTL, mapping of 83–85, 155
quadratic loss function 27
quantitative genetics (1920–1980) 5–6

random effects 30–33, 35–47, 121–122
   Bayesian estimation 135–139
      significance tests, segregating QTL 139–140
   Gibbs sampling 141–142
   granddaughter design 139–141
   Markov Chain Monte Carlo (MCMC) algorithms 141
   maximum likelihood estimation 114–115
      Haseman–Elston sib-pair model 122–124
   prediction error variances 34
   random gametic model
      computing Gv 124–126
      computing inverse of Gv 126–127
      crosses between inbred lines 132
      multiple QTL and marker brackets 129–130
      reduced animal model (RAM) 127–129
      variance matrix 130–131
   reduced maximum likelihood estimation (REML), Fernando and Grossman model 133–135
random effects 30–47, 71, 106
random QTL models 152–153
random residuals 19, 31
random selection 106
recombinant inbred lines (RIL) 67, 99, 145, 159
recombinant inbred lines (RILB) 52
recombinant inbred lines (RILF) 52
recombinant inbred segregation test 177
recombinant progeny testing 175, *176*
recombination frequencies 9–11, *12, 79, 115–116, 130*
   AIL 173–174
   estimation of power 145
recombination interference 10
recombination parameters 133

records 127, 129
reduced animal model (RAM) 40–41, 72, 127–129
reduced maximum likelihood estimation (REML) 122
  Fernando and Grossman model 133
  marker brackets 134–135
reduced model *see* null hypothesis
regression model 65, 152
  F-2 design 104–105
  linear *see* linear regression
  non-linear *see* non-linear regression
regression of phenotype 104–105
relative selection efficiency (RSE) 221, 222–224, 241, *242*
  reduction in 224–22
repeatability model 37–38
repetitive DNA 8
replicate progeny 146, 159–160, *160*
residual sum of squares 79–80, 84
residual variances 32, 67, 69, 147–146
residuals 55
restricted maximum likelihood estimation (REML) 43, 45–46, 133–135
restriction fragment length polymorphisms (RFLP) 8
robustness 17, 51

sample pooling 164
  estimation of power 165–167
  sample sizes 167–168, *168*
sample size 7, 23–24, 50, 70, 167–168, *168*
  estimates of CI 154–155, 156
  estimation of power 144–145, *145*
  selective genotyping 162–163, *163*
sampling variance 224–225
SAS (statistical package) 29, 80
saturated genetic marker map
  confidence interval 172–173
  critical interval 170–172, *172*
saturated genetic marker map 170–173
Sax, K. 5
scale, mapping 12–13, *13*
second derivative based methods 26
segregating marker-alleles 61
segregating marker-linked QTL 69, 107
segregating populations *52*, 57–60
  analysis of field data 107–109
  estimation of power 147–151, *149*, 150
  large families 60–63
  marker information 225
  small families 63–67
segregating QTL 82
  detection of 148–151, *149*, *150*
  significance of 56, 124
selection efficiency 224–225
selection index 5–6, 223–224, 236–239, 240
  inefficiencies 218–219
  traditional breeding programmes
    changes in allelic frequencies 208–209, *209*
    dairy cattle 212–215, *213*, *214*, *215*
    multitrait selection 209–210
    nucleus breeding schemes 215–216
    single trait selection 206–208
    value of genetic gain 210–212
selective genotyping 161–164, *161*, *163*, 167–168, *168*
  multiple traits 201–204, *202*, *203*, *204*
selective phenotyping 174
self-fertilizing plants 67
selfing 145–146
sequential sampling 168–169
sex-limited traits 221–222
sib-pair analysis 152
  flanking markers 81–83
  Haseman–Elston model 50, 122–124, 152
  small families 63–67, *64*, *66*
sickle cell anaemia 7
significance tests, segregating QTL 139–140
simple sequence repeats (SSR) *see* DNA-microsatellites
simulation studies, MAS
  dairy cattle breeding schemes 231
  effective number of QTL 230
  MAS vs. selection index 236, *239*
  modelling polygenic variance 228–230
  MOET nucleus breeding schemes 231–233

286 Index

simulation studies, MAS *Continued*
   multitrait breeding
      single identified QTL 239–241, *240*
      multiple identified QTL 241–242, 242
      progeny test schemes 231–235, *232*
      selection of sires 233–236, *236*
simultaneous design 249
single identified QTL 239–241, *240*
single markers 87–88
   QTL parameter analysis 109–111
single nucleotide polymorphisms (SNPs) 9
single parameter
   least squares solutions 18–19
   maximum likelihood estimation 20–22
single trait
   analysis 194–197, *194*, *195*, *196*
   selection index 206–208, 237
   selective genotyping *203*, *204*
sire effect 31, 37, 40, 111–112, 114
sires 60, 69, 214
   detection of segregating QTL 148–151, *149*, *150*
   genotypes 110–111, *111*, *130–131*
   models of 32, 33, 39
      mulitrait 35–37, 47
   selection 233–236, 236
skewness 50, 51
small families 63–67
software 20, 29
sparse maps 180
standard deviation 22
statistical density 21, 41
statistical methods 96
   allele-sharing method 118–119
   composite interval mapping *see* composite interval mapping
   field data from segregating populations 107–109
   higher order QTL effects 97
   maximum likelihood analysis *see* maximum likelihood analysis
   outbred populations, QTL parameter estimation 105–107
   QTL interaction effects 97–99, 98
   regression of phenotype 104–105

simultaneous analysis, multiple marker brackets 99–101
threshold model 117–118
statistical power 73, 94, 143–144, 167–168, *168*, 194–197
   confidence intervals, estimation
      analytical methods 153–154
      jackknife methods 156–157
      parametric and non-parametric bootstrap 156–157
      simulation studies 154–155
   crosses between inbred lines 7, 144–145
   replicate progeny 145–147, 147
   effect of methodology 151–152
   likelihood ratio tests 24, 151
   marker spacing 159
   random QTL models 152–153
   replicate progeny 159–160
   sample pooling 165–167, *168*
   segregating populations 147–151, 149, 150
statistical significance, multitrait analyses 200–201
sufficient statistic 27, 90
support intervals 153–154, 157
swine 249

technical error 164, 167
testcross (TC) progeny 52
threshold model 117–118
tomatoes 8, 76, 98, 189–190
trait distribution 50
trait space 194
trait value 55–56, *56, 77*
trait-based selection 224–225
traits
   correlated 35–37, 192–193, 198–200
   multitrait analysis *see* multitrait analysis
   sex-limited 221–222
   single *see* single traits
t-test 55, 56, 144, 151
two flanking markers 89–90, 92
two-stage selection 222–223
type I error 143, 153, 179
type II error 143

unbiased estimates 6, 163
unbiasedness 16
uninformative marker genotypes 85–87
units, genome measurement 12

variables 15
variance components 43–46
    estimation of 41–46, 122–124
    outside parameter space 46–47
    progeny group 147
variance matrix 20, 31, 46–47
    additive effects 86–87

dominance effects 86–87
fixed effects 32
QTL gametic effects 124–126, 130–131
vegetative clones 145, 146
velogenetics 226–227

wheat 7
Wilcox rank-sum test 115–117

zero interference 10, 89–90
Zw statistic 115–116

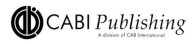